# Data Sanity

a Quantum Leap to Unprecedented Results

## Sanity
### 2nd edition

by Davis Balestracci, MS

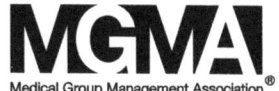

Medical Group Management Association® (MGMA®) publications are intended to provide current and accurate information and are designed to assist readers in becoming more familiar with the subject matter covered. Such publications are distributed with the understanding that MGMA does not render any legal, accounting, or other professional advice that may be construed as specifically applicable to an individual situation. No representations or warranties are made concerning the application of legal or other principles discussed by the authors to any specific factual situation, nor is any prediction made concerning how any particular judge, government official, or other person will interpret or apply such principles. Specific factual situations should be discussed with professional advisors.

**Library of Congress Cataloging-in-Publication Data**
Balestracci, Davis, Jr., author.
 Data sanity : a quantum leap to unprecedented results / Davis Balestracci. -- Second edition.
    p. ; cm.
Includes bibliographical references and index.
ISBN 978-1-56829-438-4
I. Medical Group Management Association, issuing body. II. Title.
 [DNLM: 1. Group Practice--standards. 2. Efficiency, Organizational. 3. Health Care Evaluation Mechanisms. 4. Organizational Culture. W 92]
R729.5.G6
610.6'5--dc23
                          2015002658

Item: 8803

ISBN: 978-1-56829-438-4

Copyright © 2015 Medical Group Management Association

All rights reserved. No part of this publication may be reproduced, stored in a retrieval system or transmitted, in any form or by any means, electronic, mechanical, photocopying, recording or otherwise, without the prior written permission of the copyright owner.

*The Paradoxical Commandments* © 1968, renewed 2001, by Kent M. Keith.
*Quality Digest* articles © *Quality Digest*. Reprinted with permission. www.qualitydigest.com.
All material © Donald M. Berwick, MD, MPP, FRCP, used with permission.
Material from all editions of *The TEAM Handbook* © Joiner Associates Inc. used with permission.
All material © Jim Clemmer, leadership and organization development author, speaker, and workshop/retreat leader (www.ClemmerGroup.com) used with permission.

Medical Group Management Association
104 Inverness Terrace East
Englewood, CO 80112-5306

Printed in the United States of America

10 9 8 7 6 5 4 3 2 1

# Dedication

I dedicate this book to two very special people — the two finest, most decent men who have ever been part of my life.

My dad, **Davis Balestracci** — a simple, loving, working-class man and policeman who died on August 18, 2007, right after I started writing the first edition of this book. He was a man who never failed to support me, even when he did not quite understand me (and, given the child I was, that was often). One of my fondest memories has to do, coincidentally, with the first edition of my previous book, *Quality Improvement: Practical Applications for Medical Group Practice* (Englewood, CO: Center for Research in Ambulatory Health Care Administration of Medical Group Management Association, 1994). He and my mother attended a half-day seminar I gave at the 1994 Medical Group Management Association national conference in Boston. He came up to me at the break with that teasing, loving twinkle in his eyes and said, with mock seriousness, "Hey, you certainly sound like you know what you're talking about (pause) *Where did you come from?*" Well, Dad, I proudly came from you. One other memory during his last days was when he looked at a picture of his father with tears in his eyes and said, "You know, they don't come any better than that guy." I disagree: Sorry, Dad, you're at least a tie — I would not be the man I am without your influence. His family was always first and foremost.

He was a rather direct communicator — you always knew where he stood — so as you will see, I come by my style honestly. It was only late in his life that Dad shared with me an incident that may give you an idea of his character. Early in his police career, he refused to lie under oath when told to by his boss. He told the truth, implicating his boss in a graft case. It ultimately cost him dearly, and he never regretted it. Lying would have been anathema to him, tantamount to disgracing the badge and his own integrity. Every time a frontline person says to me, "Davis, your walk matches your talk," I smile. It has occasionally cost me dearly, too. I remember describing these incidents to my dad, and he would smile, proudly.

**Dr. Rodney Dueck** — one of the finest human beings I have ever met. He was my boss in my first healthcare job, but he never acted like it. He always treated me as a colleague with utmost respect and mentored me in a way that is still blossoming to make me a better consultant. He could see through the transparency of my anger and frustration, without judgment, and coach me on how to convey the passion that he *knew* was underlying it all without alienating people. As a result, I grew in effectiveness. He would deliver the most blistering feedback with genuine love and concern in his eyes that conveyed the message, "Davis, no judgment, I just want you (and us) to be successful. Can you help me understand what's *really* going on?" His friendship, collegiality, and deep respect have helped me attain more personal inner peace and growth than I have ever thought possible (and I appreciated his feedback on Chapter 3).

# Contents

Foreword .................................................................................. ix
Preface ................................................................................... xiii
Acknowledgments ........................................................................ xvii
Introduction ............................................................................. xix

**CHAPTER 1: Quality in Healthcare: The Importance of Process** .................. 1
    Quality Assurance vs. Quality Improvement ........................................ 2
    Overarching Framework of Quality Improvement .................................... 3
    The Increasing Problem of Medical Tragedies ..................................... 10
    Improvement Models and the Role of Statistics ................................... 12
    A Change in Managerial Perspective and Behavior ................................. 15
    Some Thoughts on Benchmarking ................................................... 17
    Summary ......................................................................... 19

**CHAPTER 2: Data Sanity: Statistical Thinking as a Conduit to Transformation** ..... 21
    The Need for Statistical Thinking in Everyday Work .............................. 22
    The Role of Data: A New Perspective on Statistics ............................... 22
    Data "Insanity": Management by Graphics ......................................... 23
    The Lens of Statistical Thinking ................................................ 26
    Data Sanity: 10 Lessons to Simple, Enlightening, and Productive
        Alternatives to Routine Data Presentation .................................. 29
    Summary ......................................................................... 64
    Appendix 2A: Calculating Common Cause Limits for a Time-Ordered
        Sequence ................................................................... 66

**CHAPTER 3: A Leadership Belief System: Basic Skills for Transforming Culture** ..... 69
    Feeling Stuck? ................................................................... 69
    A Deeper Cultural Context for Understanding Resistance to Change ................ 79
    Deconstructing the Culture ...................................................... 86
    Summary ......................................................................... 98

**CHAPTER 4: A Leadership Handbook: Creating the Culture to Deliver Desired New Results** ..... 101
    Eight Errors to Avoid ........................................................... 102
    A Message From My Seminar Participants ......................................... 104
    The Need to Shift Cultural $B_1$ Beliefs ....................................... 104
    The Role of the Leadership Team ................................................ 118
    They're Watching You ........................................................... 122

Create Educational Moments ..................................................... 122
Summary............................................................................ 124

**CHAPTER 5: Deeper Implications of Process-Oriented Thinking:
Data and Improvement Processes**................................................... 129
Introduction ....................................................................... 130
Variation and Process Analysis: Improvement Process Cornerstones............. 132
Information Gathering as a Process ............................................. 148
A New Perspective for Statistics.................................................. 158
Summary............................................................................ 163

**CHAPTER 6: Process-Oriented Statistics: Studying a Process in
Time Sequence**..................................................................... 169
Old Habits Die Hard ............................................................... 169
Statistics and Reality: The Inference Gap ....................................... 176
Deeper Issues of Collecting Data over Time ..................................... 177
Run Chart Analysis ................................................................ 190
Converting a Run Chart into an I-Chart.......................................... 195
Beyond Mechanics ................................................................. 207
Sentinel Event, Root Cause Analysis, and Near-Miss Investigations ............. 232
Summary............................................................................ 240

**CHAPTER 7: Statistical Stratification: Analysis of Means**....................... 245
Revisiting Quality Assurance vs. Quality Improvement.......................... 245
Analysis of Means vs. Research.................................................... 246
A Handy Technique to Have in Your Back Pocket ............................... 258
Analysis of Means for Continuous Data ......................................... 265
Case Study: Using Analysis of Means as a Diagnostic Tool ..................... 268
Summary............................................................................ 281
Appendix 7A: Deeper Issues and Advanced Statistical Concepts................. 282

**CHAPTER 8: Beyond Methodology: New Perspectives on Teams,
Tools, Data Skills, and Standardization** .......................................... 297
Teams as Part of Larger Systems .................................................. 297
Some Wisdom from Juran ......................................................... 299
A Process for Improvement ....................................................... 302
What about the Tools?............................................................. 311
No More Tools — It's Time for the Remedial Journey.......................... 319
Summary............................................................................ 324
Appendix 8A: Simple Data Issues and Studying the Current Process ............ 326

**CHAPTER 9: Cultural Education and Learning as a Process**...................... 341
A Friendly Warning................................................................ 341
Implications for Organizational Education ...................................... 342
Keep the Projects High Level ..................................................... 345
An Innovative Approach to Organizational Education.......................... 347
What About the Physicians? ...................................................... 351

Summary ............................................................. 353
    Appendix 9A: Key Quality Improvement Concepts Needed by the
        Entire Culture ............................................................ 353

**CHAPTER 10: The Ins and Outs of Surveys: Understanding the Customer**..... 363
    More than One Method for Customer Feedback ............................... 363
    Twelve Basic Steps of Survey Design ........................................... 367
    More on Sample Size ........................................................ 374
    Stoplight Metrics Revisited .................................................. 374
    Summary ................................................................... 377

**Afterword: Just Between Us Change Agents** ...................................... 381
    A Belief System for Change Agents ........................................... 382
    10 Commandments .......................................................... 382
    The Paradoxical Commandments .............................................. 383

**Appendix: The Physician's World** ................................................ 385
    Quality Assurance vs. Quality Improvement .................................... 385
    Deming and Juran .......................................................... 388
    Clinical Trials vs. Quality Improvement ....................................... 389
    Enumerative Statistics vs. Analytic Statistics ................................... 390

**About the Author** ............................................................. 393
**Index** ....................................................................... 395

# Foreword

When I first encountered modern quality theory, I thought it was simple: a pinch of new statistical devices, a dash of participative management, a teaspoon of processes-mindedness, and voilà: breakthrough. I was wrong, but good fortune gave me mentors with the patience to let me learn step by step. Otherwise, I might have run away, daunted, from what has since become a lifelong learning task.

There were clues that I underestimated the field. The 4th edition of Joseph Juran and Frank Gryna's magisterial *Juran's Quality Handbook* (New York: McGraw-Hill, 1988) numbered more than 1,800 dense pages; Blanton Godfrey and colleagues' award-winning *Modern Methods of Quality Control and Improvement* (New York: Wiley, 1986) — the first text I ever read on the subject — contained exercises too tough for me in every chapter; the American Society for Quality Control's technical *Journal of Quality Technology*, to which I subscribed, blew past my limited training in statistics on every page; and W. Edwards Deming's *Out of the Crisis* (Cambridge, MA: MIT Center for Advanced Engineering Studies, 1982) seemed inscrutable. It took me a year to begin to feel any comfort with statistical process control theory, and when I read Walter Shewhart's disastrously named but pathfinding book, *Economic Control of Quality of Manufactured Product* (Milwaukee, WI: ASQ Quality Press, 1980), I felt the thrill of doors opening to insights I had never even imagined.

Newcomers to the sciences of quality, especially if, like me, they were already experts in related topics, easily become dismissive in the first stage of encountering challenging new theories of such grand reach. Indeed, I thought myself way beyond what Deming was teaching in the first day of the four-day seminar I attended in Washington, D.C., in 1986 at the urging of my pioneering colleague, Dr. Paul Batalden. At midstream on the second day, fed up with the obscurity and incanted slogans in his course — What, for pity's sake, was this "constancy of purpose" stuff? — I flew home to Massachusetts to sleep that night in my own bed. At 3:00 a.m., I awoke, literally sweating. I was on the first plane that morning back to Washington to finish the course. My wife, frankly, thought I had gone insane, but what actually had happened was that I had mustered just enough insight to recognize that my allergic reaction to Deming's teaching was not because he was wrong, but because I was wrong. His framing was the first I had ever encountered in my life that could explain the performance of healthcare systems scientifically and offer approaches to their improvement. The corollary, almost too hard to see, was that my own activities in quality assessment and assurance — a big part of my career — had no theory of similar power underpinning it. It was an apotheosis of the very "reliance on inspection for improvement" that Shewhart had begun to unlearn more than a half-century before.

In the mid-1980s, unexpectedly and not without discomfort, my intellectual development took a sharp turn as I gradually began to see the science of improvement to be not a small toolbox but a mountain range. I have been climbing there ever since.

Jim Bakken was a founding member of the board of the Institute for Healthcare Improvement, the nonprofit organization that a group of similarly entranced friends formed in 1991 to help accelerate progress toward better care. Bakken was a protégé of Deming's and a former vice president of Ford Motor Company, which was one of the first American homes to serious quality management. It was he who first told me about Deming's late formulation of categories of knowledge that a thorough student of continual improvement might want to master. Deming called the framework "profound knowledge," to distinguish it from the also-necessary "subject-matter knowledge" or "disciplinary knowledge." It is the combination that holds the keys to rapid and significant improvement. The elements of profound knowledge, Deming asserted, are four:

1. Knowledge of systems, rooted in general systems theory and mindful of such characteristics as system dynamics, interdependency, flow, queuing theory, and more;
2. Knowledge of variation, beginning in part with Shewhart's insights about statistical process control, but extending widely into branches of theoretical and applied statistics;
3. Knowledge of psychology, a grab bag of theory and practice applied in human systems, including theories of motivation, adult learning, cognitive science, cooperation, communication, and group process, for example; and
4. Knowledge of how knowledge grows, perhaps the most central of the four domains, linking epistemology to the real-world processes of learning and prediction. Its hallmark is the deceptively simple plan-do-study-act cycle.

Even a cursory inspection of these four large categories suggests the breadth of Deming's view of what forms of scholarship and study the practice and leadership of system improvement must engage. Omit even one, and trouble lies ahead: Omit statistical knowledge, and inference goes astray. Omit system knowledge, and imagination goes blind. Omit the elements of knowledge of psychology, and misunderstanding, conflict, and suboptimization gain control. Omit the epistemology that links knowledge to action, and learning over time slows and stalls.

To master it all is nearly impossible for a single person. That is, perhaps, why system improvement efforts with traction almost always comprise teams whose members each bring intellectual and emotional assets that others lack. The sharp-minded statistician gains guidance and balance from the intuitions of the psychologist, and both take instruction from the engineer.

In organizational contexts, the needed skill mix is even broader, reaching into management and executive leadership competence and deeds. Indeed, it becomes impossible for improvement in organizations to last long or thrive without proper leadership; that is what teachers of system improvement largely mean by the word *transformation* — continual improvement demands different leadership systems from the currently normal ones. Thus, the four "technical" components of profound knowledge always need a fifth — proper context, especially leadership — to yield their benefits.

Deming produced his "14 Points for the Leadership of Improvement" as a strong, almost formulaic description of what that proper context should look like. The 14 Points were his translation of the technical requirements of improvement into the behavioral requirements of organizational leaders. They sound soft, but each has roots deep in the sciences that profound knowledge categorizes. Deming's recommendations to top leaders are not philosophical; they are derived almost as directly from his knowledge of systems as Euclid's theorems are derived from the axioms.

To guide us properly through this immense landscape — the vast technical terrain of each of the elements of profound knowledge, the adaptation of technique to the world of executive behavior and organizational leadership, the linkages among all of that, and the translation of theory into recommendations one can act on — requires either a large faculty or a rare polymath. Davis Balestracci is the latter.

I have known Davis for almost two decades and have seen time and again the reach of his intellect and imagination. One manifestation is his almost unparalleled mastery of the writings and literature of quality improvement. He can cite more authors with more authority and inclusiveness in the fields of improvement than perhaps any other writer of the last few decades except Juran himself. By no means does Davis stops at the usual boundaries. He explores ideas in Eastern philosophy, poetry, and history and brings back to us lessons, insights, and pregnant quotation over and over again. My e-mail inbox has a folder called "Davis," in which I have learned over the years to store his messages with clever, unexpected references and stories that later on, often years later, will become relevant to my own learning or projects.

In this book, as in the earlier editions of *Quality Improvement: Practical Applications for Medical Group Practice* (Englewood, CO: Center for Research in Ambulatory Health Care Administration of Medical Group Management Association, 1994, 1996), Davis packs together his decades of study and experience in a form accessible to readers at almost any level of maturation. So wide is his reach and so clear are his interpretations that, in offering this resource, he can save learners a great deal of the time and energy they would need to devote on their own to knitting together the lessons from dozens of scholars on dozens of topics. For the novice, no single book on improvement offers a more complete and accessible summary. For the intermediate, no other source is more likely to resolve areas of chronic confusion, such as in statistics or the psychology of motivation. For the master, no overview will have a longer shelf life in offering great examples, pithy vignettes, or linkages among topics to draw upon for both personal learning and resources for teaching others.

And, for anyone interested in the wide, wide field of improvement and its related sciences, no other book offers more discipline and wit wrapped into a single, enjoyable package.

Donald M. Berwick, MD, MPP, FRCP
President Emeritus and Senior Fellow, Institute for Healthcare Improvement

# Preface

This book remains an ongoing labor of love that began in 1994. It summarizes the wisdom I have obtained by relentlessly applying quality improvement philosophy.

As so many of us have painfully discovered, true progress can seem virtually glacial (see the introduction). If there is to be the "quantum leap to unprecedented results" in the book title, the time has come for people in improvement roles to be far more proactive in working cooperatively in true partnership with boards, executive management, and physician leadership in addition to staff. I hope this book will provide you with both a catalyst and conduit to do this. It demonstrates a new way of *thinking* via a *common organizational language* based in *process* and understanding *variation* to motivate *more productive daily conversations* for *everyone*. This shift in thinking will take nothing less than a shift to a vision of "the transformed organization" with improvement actually built into organizational DNA. I'm providing an innovative road map that most of you will find quite challenging, but the rewards awaiting you are many.

## DATA INSANITY CONTINUES UNABATED

The rampant waste caused by poor *everyday* organizational use of data continues. Many high-level executives have no idea of the vast potential that exists to have their organizations take "a quantum leap to unprecedented results" through the common language alluded to in the preceding paragraph. I call it "data sanity," which is a new, more productive conversation in reaction to the everyday use of data and the resulting meetings and actions.

In executives' defense, given their experiences with business school statistics courses and the statistics taught by the consulting groups many hire, I must say this lack of awareness truly isn't their fault. It's time for people working in improvement to own this fact, stop the excuses, stop training that is nothing short of legalized torture, stop tolerating the executive attitude of "give me the 10-minute overview," and *do* something about changing their perceptions of improvement and, especially, statistics. To be fair, many people in improvement have had the exact same experiences with statistics in required courses, on-line belt training, and project facilitation training and are naively passing on the only experience they know. All of this is the wrong focus – *and the wrong material*. Implicit in these is an approach that is "bolt-on" to the current ways of doing work.

I hope to show you an intriguing alternative that can be hardwired or built into your current culture. All it requires of participants are the abilities to (1) count to eight; (2) subtract two numbers (this advanced technique could involve some borrowing); (3) sort a list of numbers; (4) use simple multiplication and addition; and (4) think critically, which is missing in most training.

The time is far overdue to stop the everyday madness of meetings where data are involved, much of which I like to call "management by little circles" (MBLC), poring over data tables drawing little circles and demanding explanations for why a number is different from either its predecessor or an arbitrary goal. Unfortunately, in these meetings, there are as many different sets of circles as there are people in the room. And then there are other meetings where pages and pages of data displays such as bar graphs, trend lines, and traffic light and variance reports are handed out (shown in Chapter 2 to be virtually useless), which make a person wish, "When I die, let it be in a meeting. The difference between life and death will be barely perceptible."

*All this activity, in addition to the activity that actually produces these reports and analyses, is waste*, pure and simple. In fact, it is far worse than that. Well-meaning but incorrect conclusions and actions resulting from these meetings unwittingly inflict damage on good, hard-working frontline people, demoralize culture, and actually make things worse. I challenge Lean enterprise practitioners to recognize this as a source of waste and calculate its cost.

Chapter 2, which has been improved for this edition, is targeted to boards, executives, and middle management to show the unknown and untapped power of some *basic* tools that will cause a *profound* change in conversations and results. It is also targeted to improvement professionals. This is your chance to learn how to stop boring these powerful people to death and, instead, become willing allies in getting them desired results beyond their wildest dreams.

The 10 Lessons in Chapter 2 are designed to show how routine meetings with everyday data can be transformed and create the awareness that you are swimming in more daily opportunity than you (and your leadership) ever could have imagined. It will create far more impact than many current "bolt-on" projects that fall into the trap of using vague teams generating vague data on vague problems resulting in vague solutions and getting vague results. I am talking here about built-in transformation, which will make such projects more focused on key strategic areas (Chapter 9). Your job will become far more interesting – and effective.

## PLOT THE DOTS AND WATCH THE CONVERSATIONS CHANGE

Please stop delivering or studying statistical training that continues to perpetuate the perception of statistics as "sadistics" and makes participants wish they were in a dental chair instead. The wrong things are being taught, perpetuated and misused. Some of the biggest myths perpetuated relate to the concept of *normal distribution*, which will rarely be mentioned in this book. Statistical training needs major surgery. It should no longer teach people statistics, but instead *teach them how to solve their problems* and make *lasting* improvements by thinking critically. Organizational education is another major revision in this edition and is discussed in Chapter 9.

As the case study in Chapter 2 will show, leaders can no longer continue to abdicate their responsibility for learning basic methods for understanding and dealing with variation. It's time that promotions reflected a person's willingness to use them routinely, be successful with them, and teach them to their direct reports.

I will provide in-depth discussion on the use and interpretation of the statistical techniques of *run charts* and *control charts* of process data. I continue to be amazed at the awesome power of simply plotting the dots, as are the audiences I address. Trust me: An increased emphasis on process in the context of understanding variation will develop your intuition as to proper tool use, and you won't need as many (traditional tools are covered in Chapter 8). One other purpose of this book is to show the importance of *critical thinking* in conjunction with the use of simple tools and respect for the process.

## LOGIC + HUMANS = CHANGE?

Chapters 3 and 4 cover essential leadership skills and present a context that will create an atmosphere where improvement can flourish. However, as shown in Exhibit 1.2 and described further in Chapter 9, a crucial step to transformation is to create a critical mass of 25 to 30 percent of leadership employing both data sanity principles and the leadership skills of Chapters 3 and 4.

Ongoing change continues to be relentless in people's everyday lives with the perceived need being "even bigger, even better, even faster, even more, right now!" Given this and the economic woes of the past five years, people's anxiety levels still guarantee that "you name it and *somebody's* angry."

I hope this book gives you the skills to see your job through a newer (and saner) lens and to anticipate and manage the inevitable "disgustingly predictable" resistance you *will* encounter without getting an ulcer (my leadership mantras in Chapter 3 should help). My wish is for you to use its principles to gain the support and respect of your organizational culture.

## NO MAGIC BULLET

Be careful: Books and consultants continue to try their best to seduce you with easy answers, templates, and fancy Japanese words — this book isn't one of them. I do, however, promise you realistic, practical answers that may not initially seem easy, but will address *deep* causes, get your desired results and hold these gains, if you do your homework.

At this moment, a technique called "rapid cycle PDSA" (plan-do-study-act) is ubiquitously being touted as the cure-all; but it requires a certain discipline, which is inherent in the principles within this book. If any of you have tried it and are frustrated, *you have good reason*. Read my article series in the Resources of Chapter 8. If you read this book and learn its lessons about human variation, I promise you success in dealing with the lurking realities of rapid-cycle PDSA.

## CHANGES IN THIS EDITION

The book has been tightened up, eliminating Chapter 3 from the previous edition and radically revising Chapters 2 and what is now Chapter 9.

Projects are still necessary for organizational improvement, but they must be seen in the context of cultural transformation. *Data Sanity* will catalyze this process and the use of everyday data to create the time to make effective, more strategic projects.

Chapters 1 through 4 present a needed executive overview and leadership development plan of what it takes to commit to using "improvement" to transform an organization. The plan is meant to be read by boards, executives, physician leadership, middle management, and people having formal improvement responsibility. I hope this book will help you begin to create a common language among these groups and motivate their need to become allies in leading improvement, mentoring the front line in this language, and dealing with the predictable resistance that *will* be released.

These chapters are also designed as an education for people with formal improvement responsibilities to motivate their responsibility and gain organizational credibility to relentlessly educate the executives, board, and middle management by showing them how to get results.

Chapters 3 and 4 address the continued woeful lack of understanding of the cultural and leadership issues involved in transforming to a culture of improvement and creating the culture where improvement can thrive. It is a synthesis of an approach based in results-orientated cognitive psychology. In my consulting practice, it has proven itself over and over again to be simple, practical, and robust both in terms of understanding and dealing with organizational and individual workers' behaviors. It also provides a catalyst for one's leadership development.

Chapters 5 through 10 contain the deeper knowledge of data concepts (including keeping data collections simple and efficient). They show how to plot data statistically, and most importantly, how to apply critical thinking to a situation. This is the in-depth knowledge required for people who have more formal responsibility for improvement.

Chapter 8 focuses on built-in projects aligned with key strategic issues as a context for improvement. It also takes a realistic view of teams and their inevitable problems that we've all experienced, both as members and facilitators. Taking a key concept from Lean enterprise, there is an extensive discussion of the wisdom and need for process standardization and how it actually leads to more effective innovation. Additional improvement tools are in there. Appendix 8A shows examples of their application to everyday situations but is more advanced than the lessons presented in Chapter 2. This is the work that a leader in improvement would do behind the scenes.

Chapter 9 considers organizational education in a much deeper context than its corresponding Chapter 10 in the previous edition. It uses Exhibit 1.2 for its road map. Chapter 9 emphasizes "teachable moments" *to solve everyday problems*. There is one caveat; the important problems aren't necessarily the ones that walk into managers' offices. The most important problems *are the ones of which no one is aware.*

Chapter 10 discusses the correct use of surveys and their proper design. Surveys are yet another huge source of waste, especially with the current emphasis on measuring and getting a good score in customer satisfaction rather than improving it. A robust context is given as well as a process for integrating customer involvement into everyday decision making.

## WELCOME

My hope is that I can motivate you to keep learning and imbibe passion for wanting to make a difference and have the wherewithal to keep a tenacious attitude going beyond learning the tools to truly make a difference. It is a most interesting journey.

Using my language of Chapter 3, I hope this book will be an "**a**ctivating event" to change your current "**b**eliefs" about improvement, resulting in "**c**onsequential behaviors" that will lead to your desired "results." I wish I could say that it was as easy as ABC, but it isn't.

To my newfound companion and colleague, welcome to a transformational journey. I hope you will respond to and learn from the many challenges that await!

# Acknowledgments

The following people have directly influenced the material in this book in some way, shape, or form through our formal and informal interactions. Their support and generosity have helped me write a book whose quality is several quantum leaps above what it would have been otherwise.

I offer a big thank-you to the following people:

- *Everyone* involved with the previous edition, all of whom helped to make it a success, especially Stu Janis.
- Donald Berwick, MD, for inspiring me to pursue a career change to healthcare improvement; offering me an ongoing laboratory for my ideas through inviting me to present at the Institute for Healthcare Improvement's annual forum every year since 1994, where I have addressed literally thousands of people hungry to improve healthcare; and graciously agreeing to write the foreword.
- Mike Richman, publisher of *Quality Digest*, for giving me a forum since 2005 to share and develop the "method to Balestracci's madness," being a pleasure to work with, and graciously allowing me to use material from many of these columns and articles for this edition.
- To the thousands of people who have attended my seminars over the past 22 years, through whom I tested many versions of this book's material, for your e-mails and feedback: I smile as I think of the hundreds of people who have said to me at the end of my statistical thinking seminars, "You know, I'm probably the biggest mathphobe in this room. But, now I get it!" One person even called me a healer!
- To Betsy Holt and Mary Mourar, who respected my material, rationale, and passionate style during their editing for this edition.
- A very special acknowledgement to Paige Hector, who is a social worker with a national reputation in the long-term care industry. I met her in 2012 when I gave a plenary speech to the national conference of the American Medical Directors Association for long-term care. She told me that the last edition of *Data Sanity* changed her life. I have since mentored her, and no one has ever made a mentor feel so proud. She was a true partner in this new edition as she helped me see things through a new reader's eyes. Not only that, she "edits me perfectly" to get things back to earth, for which I know a lot of people will silently thank her. This is a *much* better book than it would have been without her collaboration.

In reflecting on the past 30 years, I thought about a number of other people I would also like to acknowledge with gratitude. They influenced my thinking and the material of this book in a more indirect way. So another big thank-you to Prof. Stanley Wasserman, W. Edwards Deming (for his personal correspondence and encouragement), Ginny Agresti, Heero Hacquebord, Faith Ralston, Tom Nolan, Connie Koran, Joseph Mitlyng, Robert Mitchell, and John Miller.

And one final thank-you to Debbie, my best friend and spouse, who changed my life in 2010 and whose unwavering love and support have enriched my life beyond what I ever thought could be possible.

# Introduction

## TIME TO MOVE FROM QUALITY AS BOLT-ON TO IMPROVEMENT AS BUILT-IN

I remember back in the early 1990s when I was writing my first book, total quality management (TQM) was on its last legs and continuous quality improvement (CQI) was the new fad. Reengineering crept in for a little while, but then it became all about Six Sigma (and its ensuing subindustry of statistical belt training). The presence of Lean enterprise caused some guru vs. guru wars. An uneasy alliance called Lean Six Sigma seems to currently predominate with some nontrivial smatterings of Toyota Production System.

### Lessons Still Not Learned

My respected colleague Ron Snee talks about six common mistakes that continue to be made despite what has been learned in the last 30 years:

1. Failing to design improvement approaches that require the active involvement of top management;
2. Focusing on training rather than improvement;
3. Failing to use top talent to conduct improvement initiatives;
4. Failing to build the supporting infrastructure, including personnel skilled in improvement and management systems to guide improvement;
5. Failing to work on the right projects, which are those that deliver significant bottom-line results; and
6. Failing to plan for sustaining the improvements at the beginning of the initiative.

I remain more convinced than ever that any solid improvement theory comes from the late W. Edwards Deming's teachings. (Henry Neave's *The Deming Dimension* [see Resources] is probably the absolute best resource for understanding Deming's work. It reads like a novel.) Deming died in 1993 and each new fad du jour seems to incorporate more principles of his teachings, albeit piecemeal.

For all intents and purposes, the basic tools and statistical theory underlying Deming's teachings have barely changed. In this new edition, I have made their applications even simpler. Through development of his "system of profound knowledge" as a context for improvement, Deming considered his approach to be a *theory of management* that needed to be built into an organization's DNA.

I agree with Snee's observations and just haven't seen much progress on the six listed mistakes. I hope this book can make a modest contribution to remedying this. My goal remains to create organizational cultures where the words *quality* and *statistical* are dropped as adjectives from programs because they are givens. And by the way, *you* are the "top talent" to which Snee alludes.

## BEYOND BOLT-ON PROJECTS: A BUILT-IN STRATEGY TO ATTAIN ORGANIZATIONAL GOALS

In one of Dr. Donald Berwick's most underrated annual plenary talks at the Institute for Healthcare Improvement (IHI) forum ("Why the *Vasa* Sank"), he said:

> I want to see healthcare become world class. I want us to promise our patients and their families things that we have never before been able to promise them. …I am not satisfied with what we give them today. …And as much respect as I have for the stresses and demoralizing erosion of trust in our industry, I am getting tired of excuses…
>
> To get there we must become bold. We are never going to get there if timidity guides our aims. …Marginal aims can be achieved with marginal change, but bold aims require bold changes. The managerial systems and culture that support progress at the world-class level…don't look like business as usual.
>
> (1) Bold aims, with tight deadlines; (2) "improvement" as the strategy; (3) signals and monitors — providing evidence of commitment to aim, giving visible evidence of strategy via management of monitors; (4) idealized designs; (5) insatiable curiosity and incessant search; (6) total relationships with customers; (7) redefining productivity and throughput; (8) understanding waste; (9) cooperation; (10) extreme levels of trust.
>
> The lesson about the *Vasa* is not about the risk of ambition. It is about the risk of ambition without change, ambition without method.[1]

What is the *Vasa*? It was a Swedish war ship built in 1628. It was supposed to be the grandest, largest, and most powerful warship of its time. King Gustavus Adolphus himself took a keen personal interest and insisted on an entire extra deck above the waterline to add to the majesty and comfort of the ship and to make room for the 64 guns he wanted it to carry. This innovation went beyond the shipbuilder knowledge of the time and made the ship unstable. No one dared tell the king. On its maiden voyage, the ship sailed less than a mile and sank to the bottom of Stockholm harbor.

Berwick's speech was given in 1997. Look once again at his 10 challenges and ask, "What has changed?"

I know my answer and I wonder: Has improvement become an industry getting better at building quality improvement *Vasas*? Especially because of Six Sigma, is this industry justifying its existence by creating a culture of "qualicrats?" (a term coined by Jim Clemmer): "The quality movement [has given] rise to a new breed of techno-manager — the qualicrat. These support professionals see the world strictly through data and analysis and their quality improvement tools and techniques. While they work hard to quantify the 'voice of the customer,' the face of current customers (and especially potential new customers) is often lost."[2]

What is the quality profession doing to change that perception? I see it adding more tools and creating more fads du jour, promising instant results to attention-deficit executives who continue to spout what Clemmer calls "passionate lip service" about improvement.

Do improvement leaders even recognize that they have to change that perception? I think it's time to connect the dots for executives regarding the integration of improvement into organizational culture. The process of doing this will have serious implications (1) for the management and leadership of people (the organizational hiring, development, and promotion processes) and (2) for needed changes to the bolt-on culture of many improvement leaders and how they currently interact (or not) with executives. And when improvement leaders do get such an opportunity, they must *stop boring them to death* and instead *solve their biggest problems*.

Improvement methods may come and go, but the need to improve performance and the bottom line never goes out of style. And for those of you who are willing to take a much broader view of your role, this book is for you and it's designed to help keep you employable.

## GIVEN TWO DIFFERENT NUMBERS, ONE WILL BE LARGER

Does one need a huge salary to make that distinction, then either reflexively say, "Good job!" or throw some semblance of a tantrum saying "I don't like it! This is unacceptable! Do something about it!" in response?

What if it were possible to create a culture where people know that the deeper and more important questions to ask are:

- "Is the process that produced the second number the same as the process that produced the first number? May I please see a chart of the data in its time order?"
- And if a number is different from a desired goal, "Is this variation from the goal due to common cause or special cause? May I please see a chart of the data in its time order?"

According to Mark Graham Brown,[3] proper organizational use of data has the potential to reduce senior management meeting time by 50 percent and eliminate one hour of a middle manager's time every day poring over useless data. This is time that can then be spent on organizational transformation using the principles in this book and generating more time for your front line to do what it likes best — patient care.

## CONDONING "VAGUE" AS A STRATEGY

Although controversial in some academic circles, IHI's December 2004–June 2006 "100K Lives Campaign" was a huge boost to healthcare improvement awareness. The trouble is, if you put focused attention on anything, it will improve. The following situation made me suspicious.

The day the results of the campaign were announced, I was giving a seminar for the Michigan Hospital Association, and I asked if any hospitals represented were part of the campaign. Quite a few hands went up. I then asked how they felt about their results and their level of executive commitment and was met with dead silence. One brave person raised her hand and said, "Our executives were nowhere to be seen during it, except to cajole us for results, but they all seem to have the time to go to Atlanta and sip champagne," to which I saw nodding heads and heard snickers. *What is wrong with this picture?*

Campaigns such as this remind me of my respected colleague Brian Joiner's warning: "Vague solutions to vague problems yield vague results."[4] I am not faulting IHI's efforts, but what were the deeper motivations of the organizations that joined: a true passion for improvement or peer pressure to look good supported by the aforementioned "passionate lip service"? In my opinion, executive lack of visible passion for excellence remains the major barrier to healthcare transformation. If only it was as easy as Captain Jean-Luc Picard of *Star Trek: The Next Generation* saying, "Make it so." It's not. And yes, I know the current way of running the business is perceived as occupying more than 100 percent of executives' time. There's a way to fix that and it's called *data sanity*.

## TIME FOR CULTURAL HARDWIRING

### The Front Line Wants Answers Not More Models

Understanding work as "processes" or "systems" is a revelation to most people, as well as an initial counterintuitive leap in thinking. Frontline workers tend to see their jobs as a bunch of isolated activities uniquely tailored to each customer interaction. And they are very proud of how *hard* they work. To them, *that's* quality: "And-it-already-takes-up-100-percent-of-my-time-to-the-point-where-I-can-barely-keep-up-with-it-thank-you-very-much!"

Deming would set a trap right at the beginning of every one of his four-day seminars. He would glare at the audience and ask, "What's it going to take to take an organization to unprecedented levels of quality?" He could always count on one person to stand up and say, "By everyone doing their best," after which Deming would give the person his famous scowl and growl, "They already are, and that's the problem."

### Improvement Activity Translating into Lasting Impact

Berwick gave a heartfelt speech at the 1999 IHI annual forum, "Escape Fire," about a horrific experience he had with the healthcare system because his wife, Ann, had contracted a mysterious illness (contained in his book *Escape Fire*[1]). In one of our occasional chats, I asked Berwick, given the success of the 100K Lives Campaign, if his wife were in the hospital now (it was seven years later), would the same thing happen? His answer was "I have absolutely no doubt, yes."

In Berwick's 1993 plenary speech ("Buckling Down to Change"[1]), he outlined 11 things that needed to be done in healthcare within two years:

(1) Reduce the use of inappropriate surgery, hospital admissions, and diagnostic tests; (2) improve health status through reduction in underlying root causes of illness; (3) reduce cesarean-section rates to below 10 percent without compromise in maternal or fetal outcomes; (4) reduce the use of unwanted and ineffective medical procedures at the end of life; (5) adopt simplified formularies and streamline pharmaceutical use; (6) increase the frequency with which patients participate in decision making about medical interventions; (7) decrease uninformative waiting of all types; (8) reduce inventory levels; (9) record only useful information only once; (10) reduce the total supply of high-technology medical and surgical care and consolidate high-technology services into regional and community-wide centers; (11) reduce the racial gap in health status, beginning with infant mortality and low birth weight.

Awareness has probably increased, but would you agree with me that these fundamental issues remain? There has been some token progress on issue 6, less so issue 8, and, with recent emphasis on an electronic medical record, issue 9 is making some, but glacial, progress. Are any of these less important today? I don't think so. As I've emphasized, we need to talk about transformation, especially transformation of healthcare leadership.

## TRUE ROOT CAUSES

With the increased focus on horrific hospital events and insurance companies refusing to pay for what they deem "never events" that "shouldn't" happen, the past five years have seen a growing subindustry of root cause analyses sprout up in most organizations, led by improvement personnel. In an article from 2003 by John Dew[5] that is no less relevant today, he says to be very careful about so-called root cause analyses. The *true* root causes usually go even deeper into cultural issues (see Chapter 1). I ask you to consider them seriously because they are also probably unintentional — good people doing their best:

- Placing budgetary considerations ahead of quality;
- Placing schedule considerations ahead of quality;
- Placing political considerations ahead of quality;
- Being arrogant;
- Lacking fundamental knowledge, research or education;
- Pervasively believing in entitlement; and
- Exhibiting autocratic leadership behaviors, resulting in "endullment" rather than empowerment.

Improvement leaders have been forced to, and made huge strides in, speaking the language of senior management. Dew believes that in many organizations, senior management still doesn't understand the fundamental lessons of quality and isn't interested in learning them. Could it be that few improvement leaders make it into senior management positions because senior management doesn't really believe in quality concepts?

No doubt, these are very difficult for you as leaders to read. But, let me give you a lesson about feedback discussed much more thoroughly in Chapters 3 and 4: Feedback is *a perception being shared, not a truth being declared*. If these perceptions are being created by you and your leadership team in the culture, you have to ask yourself three questions:

1. Is this a perception I want them to have?
2. If this perception continues, will we be able to achieve the organizational results to which we aspire?
3. *How do I have to change* to create the perceptions I want them to have?

Creating healthier perceptions in the culture will motivate the right actions to produce desired results. But be aware, *this process will involve some deeper understanding and visible behavior changes on your part as well* (see Chapters 3 and 4).

I urge you to read the article, "Quality Turf Wars"[6]; it is nearly 20 years old and could have been written yesterday. Most of my clients agree, and it has also been my experience in many organizations, these battles *will* go on right under your noses during a transition to a culture of improvement. It is only when a critical mass of 25 to 30 percent of leaders deals with these issues head on that transformation will begin to take hold.

Exhibit 1.2 is a robust road map for this journey. Getting through its first two steps is discussed in Chapter 9, but the material in Chapters 1 to 4 is the catalyst to make it happen faster and more smoothly.

## IT'S ALL ABOUT PEOPLE

A lot of executives ask in frustration, "How do we motivate our people?" It makes me think of a Dilbert cartoon where, to improve morale, the management put everyone on antidepressants. One woman was so depressed, she took all of the pills. Everyone was frantic, "We need to get her to vomit. What should we do?" And someone said, "I've got it! Let's go get the mission statement from the boardroom and read it to her" and they *all* vomited.

Let me offer some friendly and frank advice: If executives and management don't "walk the talk," any quality improvement effort is dead in the water and just creates better cynics for the next grand announcement after the annual retreat. As I once said to an executive whose cultural reputation was famous for this, "I'm sorry, your behavior is speaking so loudly that I can't hear what you're saying."

You can use Heero Hacquebord's article[7] as a barometer for your efforts. In the early 1990s, a respected colleague of mine who is considered one of the best Deming proponents in the world wrote a brilliant article about his back surgery experience entirely through the lens of Deming's improvement theory. I suggest that you and your team read it occasionally and ask yourselves, "Could this have happened yesterday in our facility?"

## ARE YOU READY TO SAY "ENOUGH!"?

I attended a conference in the late 1980s that gave me a pearl of wisdom every bit as applicable today. A successful improvement effort requires: (1) the personal *will* to want to change; (2) the *belief* that the organization is capable of change; (3) the *wherewithal* to undo old habits by a tenacious commitment to learning *all* aspects of quality; (4) *creating the change*; and to which I am now adding (5) saying "Enough!" and then getting your leadership to say "Enough!"

> Enough of attending meetings that lead to building a bridge to nowhere, enough of asking what I'm supposed to ask rather than what needs to be asked, enough of praising people who are undeserving of praise, enough of valuing form over substance, enough of accepting good when what is needed is outstanding, enough of enabling people to act as victims when they need to take personal responsibility.
>
> Inevitably, this kind of shift doesn't happen unless a substantial number of leaders put their collective foot down and say enough in unison.[8]

The time is *now* to manifest more effective executive engagement (and development), use everyday "data sanity" as a philosophy and conduit for organizational transformation, use data more deliberately and efficiently in improvement, and create an everyday culture of improvement through leadership where key results can be hardwired and built into cultural DNA.

I leave you with one last nugget from Berwick from what might be his best speech of all time, "Run to Space":

> Plotting measurements over time turns out, in my view, to be one of the most powerful devices we have for systemic learning. …Several important things happen when you plot data over time. First, you have to ask what data to plot. In the exploration of the answer you begin to clarify aims, and also to see the system from a wider viewpoint. Where are the data? What do they mean? To whom? Who should see them? Why? These are questions that integrate and clarify aims and systems all at once. Second, you get a leg up on improvement. When important indicators are continuously monitored, it becomes easier and easier to study the effects of innovation in real time, without deadening delays for setting up measurement systems or obsessive collections during baseline periods of inaction. Tests of change get simpler to interpret when we use time as a teacher. …So convinced am I of the power of this principle

of tracking over time that I would suggest this: If you follow only one piece of advice from this lecture when you get home, pick a measurement you care about and begin to plot it regularly over time. You won't be sorry.[1]

As you will shortly discover, if you follow only that "one piece of advice" from Berwick's talk, you will indeed take "a quantum leap to unprecedented results."

As you begin (or even retrace) your quality journey, let me share some wonderful advice from the absolute best mentor I ever had, who is one of the dedicatees of this book, Dr. Rodney Dueck, who smiled and said to me one time when he saw my frustration: "Davis, just think of it all as entertainment."

## REFERENCES

1. Berwick, Donald M. 2004. *Escape Fire: Designs for the Future of Health Care*, 11–42, 61–94, 127–154. San Francisco, CA: Jossey-Bass.
2. Clemmer, Jim. n.d. "Technomanagement: A Deadly Mix of Bureaucracy and Technology." The Clemmer Group. www.clemmergroup.com/technomanagement-a-deadly-mix-of-bureaucracy-and-technology.php.
3. Brown, Mark Graham. 1996. *Keeping Score: Using the Right Metrics to Drive World-Class Performance*. New York: American Management Association.
4. Joiner, Brian L. 1994. *Fourth Generation Management*. New York: McGraw-Hill.
5. Dew, John. 2003. "Root Cause Analysis: The Seven Deadly Sins of Quality Management," *Quality Progress* (September).
6. Simmons, Annette, and J. Michael Crouch. 1997. "Quality Turf Wars." *Quality Digest* (October). www.qualitydigest.com/oct97/html/cover.html.
7. Hacquebord, Heero. 1994. "Health Care from the Perspective of a Patient: Theories for Improvement." *Quality Management in Health Care* 2 (2): 68–75. www.qualitydigest.com/IQedit/Images/Articles_and_Columns/December_2011/Special_Health/Heero_back_surgery.pdf.
8. Dabbah, Mariela. 2011. "Protests: When Enough Is Enough." *The Huffington Post: The Blog*. www.huffingtonpost.com/mariela-dabbah/protests-when-enough-is-e_b_1035047.html.

## RESOURCE

Neave, Henry R. 1990. *The Deming Dimension*. Knoxville, TN: SPC Press.

CHAPTER 1

# Quality in Healthcare: The Importance of Process

*If I had to reduce my message for management to just a few words, I'd say that it all had to do with reducing variation.* — W. Edwards Deming

## KEY IDEAS

- The concept of quality improvement has a much different, more robust mind-set than that of traditional quality assurance.
- Process-oriented thinking is the anchoring concept of any good improvement framework: *All* work is a process.
- Process-oriented thinking creates a common organizational language that will reduce defensiveness.
- At least 85 percent of an organization's problems are caused by bad processes, not the workers. Routinely blaming processes and not people will cause a quantum leap in morale.
- Concentrate on the four C's besides costs: Strive to reduce confusion, conflict, complexity, and chaos instead and this *will* reduce costs.
- It is not the problems that march into your office that are important — the important ones are those *no one is aware of.*
- A broader understanding is needed of the concept of variation, with an ultimate goal of reducing *inappropriate and unintended* variation while pushing for *deep-level fixes.*
- There is no such thing as "improvement in general." The 80/20 rule (or the Pareto principle, which is the startling realization that 80 percent of job "heartburn" is due to only 20 percent of work processes) needs to be applied to the overall improvement process via specific initiatives related to high-level organizational strategy.
- Most current quality fads come out of sound theory that is more than 30 years old. Deeper understanding of the theory is what is needed, not blindly applying its most recent straightjacketed manifestation.
- Quality, when integrated into a business strategy, is present in virtually *every* aspect of *every* employee's *everyday* work.
- A road map is provided for implementing a culture of improvement. It has five distinct steps and represents a 5- to 10-year journey.

## QUALITY ASSURANCE VS. QUALITY IMPROVEMENT

Quality can be an elusive goal. The traditional approach to healthcare service quality, quality assurance (QA), has perhaps focused more on activities required to satisfy regulators and identify outliers than quality improvement (QI), which focuses on continuous efforts to meet customer needs. (See the appendix at the end of this book for an explanation of their fundamental differences.) Now, faced with increasingly sophisticated consumers making renewed demands for quality, medical groups and other providers are seeking effective ways to serve and retain patients within the realities of resource constraints.

Much has been written about defining, measuring, and evaluating quality in healthcare delivery. A variety of philosophies and approaches greets the manager who asks, "How can our practice improve quality?" Further complicating the issue are questions such as, "Can we afford a QI program?" and "Will the physicians and other clinical staff accept further demands on their time and decision-making power?"

Leaders from all parts of the healthcare spectrum have come to believe that an efficient system resulting in demonstrable quality constitutes the key to continued provider survival. Private and publicly funded projects are providing productive responses to these questions. Entities such as the Institute for Healthcare Improvement (IHI) have further developed the QI approach in healthcare. Most of its projects have focused on hospital settings. More recently, the organization has begun various access and idealized design projects for group practices and is studying "flow" concepts over the entire continuum of care. However, much still remains to be learned about translating earlier QI principles to medical group practice.

A growing number of medical group practice providers are adopting more QI tools and techniques to attain significant administrative and clinical improvements. Numerous Medical Group Management Association® member groups continue to implement their own programs focusing on a wide variety of practice management concerns. QI seems to have definitively evolved as a more robust preference to the QA approach by moving beyond:

- Quality control (quality by inspection);
- Quality assurance (quality by attempting to prevent recurrence of outliers found by inspection);
- Quality circles (quality by forming teams closest to the work); and
- Motivation and awareness (zero defects; quality is free).

In moving to a sounder context, QI has integrated the following three key concepts:

1. Customer needs must be met;
2. Most inefficiencies are the result of measurable variations in a process; and
3. An interdepartmental, cross-functional team approach is often the most effective means of identifying process problems and improving the process to meet customer needs.

QI combines quantitative quality measurements and team efforts in an ongoing, systematically monitored process. As interdisciplinary practice staff seeks to coordinate the complex clinical and administrative processes involved in patient service, QI becomes a logical model for improving medical group practice.

In addition to organizing improvement and ensuring that it lasts beyond initial implementation, QI involves people from all disciplines relevant to a process. Processes

**EXHIBIT 1.1** ▪ The "Universal" Process Flowchart

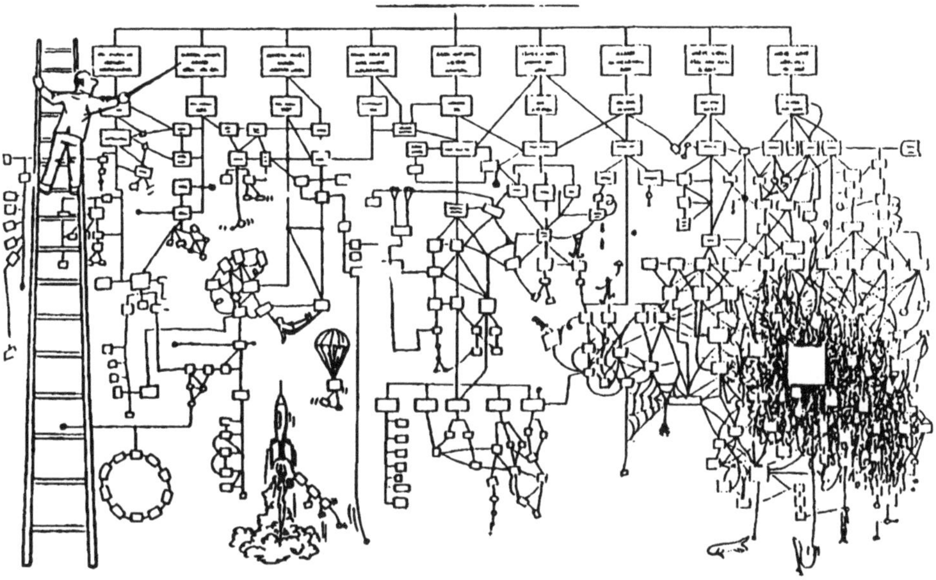

extend across departmental and traditional lines, and the people needed to improve them will cross departmental lines as well. Key to this cross-functional effort is the support of both upper management and clinical leaders. Although QI can improve specific areas without a guiding vision and proactive leaders, a reworked and transformed organization cannot occur without them.

## OVERARCHING FRAMEWORK OF QUALITY IMPROVEMENT

Donald Berwick, MD, president and chief executive officer of IHI, is fond of the following quote: "Each system is perfectly designed to get the results it is already getting." Indeed, and most systems look like Exhibit 1.1, the "universal" process flowchart, which is generally undocumented in terms of what *really* happens.

Despite the intentional humor of the figure, wouldn't you say that it characterizes *every* process needing improvement? Or it would not need improvement. And not only is such a process perfectly designed to get the results it is already getting — and will continue to get — but the results actually fall into three categories:

1. Organizational results;
2. Tolerated organizational management behaviors; and
3. Tolerated individual behaviors.

Working under such unintended chaos can escalate the workforce's emotions — and customers' incivility.

As the late Scottish academic David Kerridge says, "All organizations suffer from the five C's: confusion, conflict, complexity, chaos, and cost. ...The order in which we have listed the five C's is a guide to strategy for *whole system* improvement. If we reduce confusion and conflict, the benefits are not easy to see in advance, but they are long term, widespread, and increasing. They reduce complexity and chaos, and make improvements of other kinds possible. Direct cost-cutting appears to give good short-term results, but even if it does no harm, there is no long-term bonus."[1]

Consider Berwick's questions from his seminal 1989 editorial on QI, "Continuous Improvement as an Ideal in Health Care":[2]

- Do you ever waste time waiting, when you should not have to?
- Do you ever redo your work because something failed the first time?
- Do the procedures you use waste steps, duplicate efforts, or frustrate you through their unpredictability?
- Is information that you need ever lost?
- Does communication ever fail?

These are all process breakdowns that cause waste — in time, money, and efficiency. And I hope it has created a realization in you that QI is not about the problems that march into your offices; the important problems are the ones *no one is aware of*. In addition, healthcare systems have the ongoing presence of three relentless sources of stress: patient flow, clinical stress, and provider differences.

To name a few obvious daily problems, patient flow issues (delays, lost opportunities, increased length of stay), laboratory defect issues (label, ID band, order entry defects; unsuccessful draws, recollects), information or matching issues (patient ID error, lack of precertification, nurses calling physician offices, lost use of funds in accounts receivables), and various instances of noncompliance to established Joint Commission standards are quite common. Such challenges are generally symptomatic of much deeper poor process design and human frustration in reaction to these processes: patient or customer dissatisfaction, rework, inconsistent handoffs, unreliable information, duplicate information (that is inconsistent), liability and risk, physician and clinical staff dissatisfaction, lost business, customized work-arounds, clinical decision or treatment delays, wrong treatment, instrument downtime, and so forth. As another quality giant of the 20th century, the late Joseph Juran observed, these latter issues have become so entrenched in the current culture that people have "disconnected their alarm signals"[3] to them as opportunities for improvement.

W. Edwards Deming used to ask audiences, "What is it going to take to attain unprecedented levels of quality and productivity?" He could always count on a person to answer, "By everyone doing his or her best!" And he would glare at them and growl, "They already are, and that's the problem!"

As I am emphasizing, it is all about process. The chaos shown in Exhibit 1.1 is undesirable variation. And what people do not realize is that traditional statistics courses actually *deny* its existence, making application of the usual techniques (called *enumerative statistics*) incorrect. What QI needs is statistical techniques that allow for this variation, *expose* the variation (called *analytic* or *process-oriented statistics*), and measure the effects of interventions to reduce this inappropriate and unintended variation. The ultimate goal is more consistent prediction. (The contrast between enumerative and analytic statistics is summarized more thoroughly in Chapter 6 and the appendix because the enumerative approach is so entrenched in academic culture and in the clinical trial mind-set of physician culture.)

So, to summarize QI in a process-oriented context:
- Principle 1: Your current processes are perfectly designed to get the results they are already getting, and will continue to get. *Insanity is doing things the way you have always done them while expecting different results.*
- Principle 2: The current processes are also perfectly designed to take up more than 100 percent of the people's time working in them. *It is amazing how much waste can be disguised as useful work.*
- Principle 3: Improving quality improves processes. *There is no such thing as "improvement in general."*

Because of Principle 2, the perception exists that no time can be found for improvement. This would be analogous to driving a car with four flat tires while going 65 miles per hour on the freeway and claiming not to have time to stop and change the tires because you are in too much of a hurry. In other words, the current way of doing business takes the entire digestive capacity of the organization, and although everyone knows it could be improved, it somehow works in spite of itself.

At a conference I attended 20 years ago, this excellent advice was given: The Pareto principle (or the 80/20 rule, which is covered in Chapter 5 and discussed shortly) is taught as an improvement tool, but most organizations' QI efforts fail because they neglect to apply it to their QI effort in a global sense. So in the language of the Pareto principle, what are the 20 percent of the organizational processes causing 80 percent of your problems and which of these problems are vital to your organization's future? Of course, everything needs improvement, but great solutions to small problems remain insignificant solutions in the greater scheme of things and they take just as much time to correct as making a significant improvement.

## All Work Is a Process

All clinicians and their patients are involved in processes, from the relatively simple ones used in local, private offices to the mammoth processes of national healthcare. Many of us have been victims of a lost test result, misinterpreted order, cumbersome paperwork, or an unreliable on-call system. However, some clinicians do not recognize the key role they can play in improving the processes (in the areas of patient scheduling, patient instruction, or claims management, for example) that lie behind these errors.

Think of how Berwick's questions affect a patient's perception of quality. What are the payers' perceptions when such events are related to them? Can financial losses caused by these events ever truly be quantified? Consider employee turnover and loss of morale.

Why do these problems happen and keep happening? They represent breakdowns in current work processes, or they occur because of the lack of a *consistent* work process. These breakdowns are generally not the fault of the people doing their jobs, but of the processes themselves. Assigning blame and responsibility to the individual perceived to be at fault will not fix the problems. The work-environmental odds are against them 85 to 15, as established empirically by Deming and Juran.

The 85/15 rule (not related to the Pareto principle) states that individuals have direct control over only approximately 15 percent of their work problems. The other 85 percent are controlled by the processes in their working environment. In fact, by the end of his life, Deming had come to the conclusion that the workers themselves can directly control only 3 to 6 percent of their work environment, so the odds against the workers could be as high as 97 to 3. Thus the problems alluded to by Berwick will not go away unless the processes in which the people operate are improved.

To quote Jim Clemmer from *Firing on All Cylinders*:

> Only about 15 percent of the [problems] can be traced to someone who didn't care or wasn't conscientious enough. But the last person to touch the process, pass the product, or deliver the service may have been burned out by ceaseless [problem solving]; overwhelmed with the volume of work or problems; turned off by a "snoopervising" manager; out of touch with who his or her team's customers are and what they value; unrewarded and unrecognized for efforts to improve things; poorly trained; given shoddy materials, tools, or information to work with; not given feedback on when and how products or services went wrong; measured (and rewarded or punished) by management for results conflicting with his or her immediate customer's needs; unsure of how to resolve issues and jointly fix a process with other functions; trying to protect himself or herself or the team from searches for the guilty; unaware of where to go for help. All this lies within the system, processes, structure, or practices of the organization.[4]

I have been using this insightful paragraph and never found any better explanation as to why it is the processes and not the people. It should be laminated and handed out to everyone in every work culture. If you are still not convinced, see the sidebar, "Faulty Systems, Not Faulty People," which is a brilliant editorial by Lucian Leape, MD, a professor at the Harvard School of Public Health. You may be familiar with the error in question — a massive chemotherapy overdose at the Dana–Farber Cancer Institute (DFCI) that resulted in the death of *Boston Globe* health reporter Betsy Lehman. James Conway, chief operating officer at DFCI, expressed strong support for Leape's opinion and his organization offered support for the 18 nurses involved.

Consider two quality principles that will begin to create the culture for improvement:

1. Have *zero* tolerance for blame; and
2. Blame *processes*, not people.

If in your behavior and what you facilitate in your meetings, you could entrench these two principles, it would cause a quantum leap in cultural morale. A lot of the processes ultimately involved will take some type of executive or managerial action to change.

A process can sabotage one's thinking, leading to the tendency to blame people in many subtle ways. People are visible; the processes, systems, and organizational culture that shape their behavior are not as easily seen. Yes, people do make mistakes (the 15 percent controllable by the individual in the 85/15 rule), but who hires, trains, coaches, measures, and rewards them? Do the processes allow the people to perform to expectations? (See the discussion in Chapter 4 of the elements that need to be in place for true employee empowerment.)

When something goes wrong, it is easy to find the last person who touched it and lay the blame there (or use the quality platitude, "Ask 'Why?' five times" until you find the "Who"). But many service breakdowns are caused by process issues: systems, procedures, policies, rules, and regulations. Process-oriented questions to ask when something fails are:

- Was this a unique event or an event waiting to happen?
- Could this just as easily have happened to another person (or group of people)?
- If we fired and replaced everyone, not just this person, could this happen again?

## Faulty Systems, Not Faulty People

The decision by the Massachusetts Board of Registration in Nursing to begin disciplinary hearings for 18 nurses involved in the tragic death of Betsy Lehman due to an overdose of chemotherapy is misguided, inappropriate, and harmful. It should be rescinded.

The decision is misguided because it focuses on the individuals when it has been shown that the errors were caused by major failures in the design of the medication system. It is inappropriate because it assumes that the errors resulted from carelessness or negligence which deserve punishment. It is harmful because it needlessly and publicly humiliated people by providing their names to the press. It is also harmful because the threat of such punishment is a powerful deterrent for other nurses to identify, report, and analyze errors in order to develop methods to prevent them.

The Board action is based on the traditional, now discredited, assumption that all errors are misconduct or negligence. In fact, errors are rarely misconduct, and in this case specifically they clearly were not. Rather, they resulted from a complicated system in which the doses of drugs received by patients varied widely according to which of 100 or more protocols were being used at the time in this research hospital. The doses in question were no higher than those nurses had seen used in other patients, so they were not questioned. This happened not once, but repeatedly over several days. Does the Board of Registration really believe that all 18 nurses involved in this case were careless?

The ostensible purposes of revocation or suspension of a license are to teach the individual to be more careful, to deter others from similar misconduct, and to protect the public by removing a dangerous person from practice. In the absence of misconduct or willful intent, punishment accomplishes none of these objectives. Specifically, there is no evidence whatever that punishment for unintentional errors makes the recipient less likely to make future mistakes, nor that it deters others.

This is not to say there is no role for punishment. Punishment is indicated for willful misconduct, reckless behavior, and unjustified deliberate violation of rules. But not for errors.

The delay in the Board's action raises important questions as to its intent. If the Board really believes that these 18 nurses are threats to patient safety, it is unconscionable that they waited four years to take action. That they did so suggests that neither reform of individuals nor protection of the public was their aim, but rather retribution stemming from the belief that error equals sin, and therefore it must be punished.

This concept of error as sin and the use of punishment for its control was abandoned long ago by industries outside of health care. There is an immense body of scientific knowledge that demonstrates both that errors are common — everyone makes errors every day — and that errors have causes. Many of the causes are familiar: hurry, interruption, anxiety, stress, fatigue, overwork, etc.

More importantly, error prevention specialists have learned how to design tasks and conditions of work to minimize the effects of these factors, to make errors more difficult to make. Simple things like standardization of processes, use of checklists to prevent forgetting, appropriate work loads, and adequate sleep all reduce the likelihood of an individual making an error. This focus on the design of systems rather than on the individual has been highly successful in reducing errors in a number of hazardous enterprises. The airlines are a familiar example.

Following Betsy Lehman's death, the Dana Farber Cancer Institute examined their systems and found them wanting. They overhauled the entire organization. In addition to extensive administrative reorganization, including changing leadership and assigning specific responsibility

(Continues)

(Continued)

for patient safety, they re-designed their entire medication system. Specific changes included a nurse, physician and pharmacist pre-approval system for all high dose chemotherapy, computerized maximum dose checking and potential error identification, multidisciplinary review of all medication errors, and nurse and pharmacist participation in protocol review and approval.

The institution did what the public would want a hospital to do after a tragic accident. It held itself accountable for the error and made extensive efforts to correct its faulty systems so it and other errors would not recur. In this process, it found the nurses involved were not at fault and therefore carried out no disciplinary actions against them. Subsequent review by both the Department of Public Health of the Commonwealth and the Joint Commission on the Accreditation of Healthcare Organizations led to approval, even commendation, for this aggressive response. To help others improve, over the last three years Dana Farber staff have openly shared their learning and improvements with other institutions nationwide.

It is important to emphasize that attention to systems design to prevent errors does not in any way diminish personal accountability. It does, however, redefine it somewhat. Since only the institution can modify its systems, it is the institution that must be held accountable for safe systems. In turn, the institution must hold individual nurses, doctors, and other health care workers accountable for maintaining high standards of performance, following rules, and working within their levels of competence. Hospitals can, should, and do, refer nurses and doctors to their respective Boards for disciplinary action when there is reckless, negligent, or irresponsible behavior.

Betsy Lehman's tragic death was a "wake-up call" for health care. Since then a sea-change has occurred in the willingness of hospitals, doctors, and nurses to face their mistakes and to make systems changes to prevent errors. Many hospitals, like the Dana Farber, are redesigning their medication systems. The AMA [American Medical Association] has formed a National Patient Safety Foundation to bring together all interested parties — health care professionals, regulators, industry, patient representatives, and even lawyers — to develop more effective means of preventing errors, disseminate information, and educate health professionals and the public about non-punitive systems approaches to error prevention.

The Veterans Health Administration has made patient safety a priority and initiated a number of programs, including computerized medication ordering, rewards for safety ideas, and a non-punitive reporting system. In Massachusetts, regulators, professional societies, consumer representatives, hospitals and safety experts have formed a Coalition for the Prevention of Medical Error to work together to develop more effective methods of error prevention. The Massachusetts Hospital Association has launched a medication safety improvement program with its member hospitals.

We have learned a great deal in the past few years about how to make health care safer. While we must still hold individuals responsible for high standards of performance, we now recognize that most errors result from faulty systems, not faulty people. To identify systems failures, we need to know about the errors they cause. We need to make it safe for all health care workers to report errors. It is time for the Board of Registration in Nursing to help that process by stopping punishment of nurses for their mistakes.

— Lucian L. Leape, MD, Harvard School of Public Health

Source: Lucian Leape, MD. "Faulty Systems Not Faulty People." Boston Globe, Op-Ed. January 12, 1999.
© Lucian L. Leape, MD, Harvard School of Public Health. Used with permission.

In another classic story of a nurse who, instead of injecting the correct drug, injected potassium chloride — a potentially fatal mistake — it would be so simple to dismiss the nurse or revoke her license because of incompetence. But in considering the process diagram, might that process be perfectly designed to result in people being tired and stressed, leading to an incident such as that described? In fact, an investigation of that incident showed the correct drug next to the potassium chloride in identical bottles, with identical labels, with the same (small) print except for the correct drug's name and the wrong drug. *This was an accident waiting to happen*, and it could easily have happened to someone else subsequently, even if the nurse had been dismissed.

In fact, a process has six sources of input: people, work methods, machines, materials, measurements (data), and environment. In this case, it had nothing to do with methods (that is, competence); it was the design of the work environment. It also should trigger the question: "Where else in our organization is a similar scenario (a dangerous drug next to a routine drug) waiting to happen?"

This discussion brings up another key concept in QI: All variation is caused and is one of two types, either *special cause* (specific) or *common cause* (systemic). It is vital to know the difference for any incident (any incident is an occurrence of undesirable variation) because *treating one as the other will generally make things worse* (certainly not better). The human tendency is to treat *all* variation as special cause: The nurse in the medication error example was seen as the problem (special cause), when in fact the process was unintentionally designed to have the incident occur (common cause) because of the high stress inherent in the current process, especially if it resembles Exhibit 1.1.

Because the important problems are the ones no one is aware of, you need to expand your concept of variation and, whenever possible, push for deeper-level fixes. The following three approaches can be taken to fix undesirable variation, from least to greatest impact (reactive to proactive) on long-term resolution of a problem:

- Level 1 fix (*incident*): Reacting immediately to the undesirable output to "make it right." Unfortunately, this fix is often followed by assigning blame to an individual for its occurrence because of "lack of accountability" (in this case, disciplining the nurse).
- Level 2 fix (*process*): Looking at the process that produced the specific incident and fixing it so that it does not happen again (e.g., separating these specific two drugs).
- Level 3 fix (*system*): Asking whether this incident is symptomatic of a deeper system issue where processes like these are unintentionally designed (e.g., where else does the organization have dangerous drugs next to commonly used drugs?). Do data exist on other similar occurrences that might shed insight?

The Level 1 fix is by far the most common and usually necessary reaction to problems because the situation is undesirable and needs immediate rectification. However, once the output and cause have been fixed, the assumption is implicit that the incident will not happen again (e.g., making sure the patient is out of danger, then finding out who injected the wrong drug and taking some type of action). In essence, a Level 1 fix is damage control and cleaning up the aftermath.

If all one did was solve organizational problems using Level 1 fixes, one would create high potential for treating common cause as special cause. For example, most healthcare systems have someone in charge of dealing with patient and family complaints, and each complaint is dutifully considered and dealt with (special cause strategy). But what if your system is perfectly designed to have complaints? Despite good customer service (recovery), the number of complaints would not necessarily decrease.

Another example is putting frontline people through customer service training in how to deal with angry customers. Of course, those skills are valuable and necessary, but an organization should also work on the processes that cause angry customers, which are not necessarily the frontline employee's fault. You would want staff to use these skills as seldom as possible, or they will burn out.

A more serious issue when such training is used as a Level 1 fix arises because, superficially, customers have complained on surveys that "Employees don't smile at us or look at us." The deeper question should be, "Why don't employees want to smile at customers or take time with them?" Employees will treat the customer no better than the way they are treated and "Smile or else!" will not fix anything.

Often people claim to just "know" that a specific person is the problem. In this case an interesting question is, "What kind of process (hiring, promotion, etc.) allowed a 'person like that' to get into that position?" The surprising revelation to most people is, yet once again, your current processes are perfectly designed to get the results you already observe.

Part of the change to QI is a change in focus from the 15 percent to the 85 percent. To cover the broader scope of the latter problems, projects will be fewer but executed at a higher level in the organization. Upper management should be brought directly into the improvement process and should integrate this focus into business strategy. Future significant opportunities for improvement will then be aligned to and based on customer needs.

## THE INCREASING PROBLEM OF MEDICAL TRAGEDIES

> If we are unhappy with the behavior of people on our team or in our organization, we need to take a closer look at the system and structure they're working in. If they behave like bureaucrats, they're likely working in a bureaucracy. If they're not customer focused, they're probably using systems and working in structure that wasn't designed to serve the servers and/or customers. If they're not innovative, they're likely working in a controlled and inflexible organization. If they resist change, they're probably not working in a learning organization that values growth and development. If they're not good team players, they're likely working in an organization designed for individual performance. Good performers, in a poorly designed structure, will take on the shape of the structure.[5]

There has been an increasing wave of publicity reporting tragic medical errors — true horror stories of events that shouldn't happen, which cause major public outrage. When a medical error occurs, executives jump on others to investigate and stop future errors.

I have introduced you to the concepts of two types of variation: common (systemic) and special (unique or specific) cause. The human tendency is to treat *all* variation as special. And because "never events" aren't supposed to happen, the well-meaning approach is to do a root cause analysis on every incident, that is, treat each as a special cause.

Have you wondered whether organizations are perfectly designed to have "never events"? It means they could be waiting to happen, *which is* common cause.

Root cause analyses have the luxury of hindsight and often result in actions based on biases and a lack of critical thinking. With a known outcome, it is so easy to oversimplify the inherent situational complexity and ignore the uncertainties of the circumstances the potentially "blamable" person or people faced. Unrealistic perfection becomes the standard, and human performance and error factors are overlooked or treated superficially. During class exercises in which a tragic case is presented, I often hear the contempt as people smugly ask: "How could he not have seen that was going to happen?" or "How could they have been so irresponsible and unprofessional?"

There is the illusion that what is common sense to the individuals doing the analysis is the only way to see the world. But the deeper questions become: "Why did these particular actions make perfect sense to the people at the time? *Would it also have made perfect sense to someone else in the same set of circumstances?*" If so, this points to the culture as the root cause. Without asking these questions, lengthy, overly judgmental discussions about the abilities and characters of the people closest in time and space to the mishap can result. This can overshadow more productive efforts and make it more difficult to uncover important underlying (i.e., cultural) and actionable causes of the event (as happened in the page 7 sidebar scenario).

It is all too obvious that another course of action was available; but why jump so quickly to condemn the "guilty" for what they failed to do to prevent the mishap? It's so easy to provide alternative scenarios after an undesired outcome is already known.

> To be of value, root cause analysis should focus primarily on identifying solutions to system design flaws, thereby preventing accidents and failures.... When it comes to causal analysis, organizations tend to be satisfied with a simplified, linear and proximal set of causes.
>
> However, studies of accidents in complex socio-technical systems show that they are begging to be looked at more broadly and deeply for causes.
>
> The human tendency is an expectation of quickly getting to the bottom of things, get the forms filled out, fix the problem identified and get back to work. Invariably, this leads to solutions aimed at the people involved on the front line — retrain them, supervise them better or just fire them — rather than at the conditions that led to the event.[6]

Could many possible Level 3 fixes relate to lack of empowerment, communication disconnect, and/or lack of information? Revisit Clemmer's words at the beginning of this section and ask the probing question, "Why did it make sense at the time for people to do what they did?"

These are deeper system issues that could mean you have other potential "never events" (seemingly unrelated) lurking in other parts of your organization — virtual ticking time bombs.

## IMPROVEMENT MODELS AND THE ROLE OF STATISTICS

I believe Deming's philosophy of quality has ultimately proven to be the most robust. As a friend of mine characterized almost 25 years ago, "Deming is true religion, Juran is a very good church historian, and Crosby is a TV evangelist." (The late Philip Crosby was considered by many to be the third quality giant of the 20th century, Deming and Juran being the other two. Crosby relied heavily on motivation and promoting what came to be known as the "Do it right the first time" philosophy.)

After recently hearing a world expert on Lean enterprise, it dawned on me that there was nothing new here. Many of the concepts were originally discussed in the first edition of the valuable reference *The TEAM Handbook*,[7] which was first published in 1988. What people do not realize is that all of these movements evolve out of the same sound, vigorous theory based in process-oriented thinking. It is when this theory manifests in a straight-jacketed fad du jour that people lose sight of the original intent and begin arguing over and drowning in minutiae.

As referenced in the introduction, Brian Joiner's book, *Fourth Generation Management*, may be the best overall quality book available. Everyone going through the legalized torture of Six Sigma belt training should read it to understand the role of statistics as it applies to QI. Clemmer's previously mentioned *Firing on All Cylinders*, which integrates improvement theory and its cultural aspects into a robust structure, runs a close second.

Every item of alleged monumental savings brought about by Six Sigma makes me think of a quote allegedly attributed to Deming: "All you've done is get your processes to where the hell they should have been in the first place. That is *not* improvement." Getting rid of underlying waste is indeed a most consequential accomplishment, but once that is accomplished, nothing is left to improve and that *rate* of savings will not sustain itself.

How deeply has the concept of "process" permeated the very fabric of your organization? In any organization, there is no lack of raw material needed for improvement: enthusiasm, focused attention on key issues, and hard-working people with good ideas. They may be necessary, but they are not sufficient. They need the catalyst of critical thinking inherent in process-oriented thinking. Process-oriented thinking is the anchoring concept of any sound improvement framework. It creates a common organizational language that looks at any undesirable variation objectively to reduce blame and defensiveness.

*The TEAM Handbook* also contains what I consider the best high-level summary of improvement (which serves as a project road map in Chapter 8). To repeat yet again: It is all about process. Problems that occur with a process have seven sources:[7]

- Source 1. There is inadequate knowledge of customer needs.
- Source 2. There is inadequate knowledge of how a process currently works.
  - There is variation in people's perceptions of how things currently work (variation in training or its comprehension, individual preferences caused by undocumented reactions to unforeseen inputs or situations).
- Source 3. There is inadequate knowledge of how a process should work.
  - There is variation in people's perceptions of how things should work, given the current process state (or objective) or poor process design (naive or obsolete design, poor training, expansion beyond initial needs and capacity).

These first three sources address the key issue of what is actually happening vs. what should be happening. Let's consider this gap as variation: what we know vs. what we don't know, much of it caused by nonquantifiable human variation. (But even with this variation reduced, as the project moves forward, the additional problems of human variation still remain in both the improvement process itself and any subsequent data collection.)

- Source 4. There are errors and mistakes in executing procedures. There are underlying process issues that cause *everyone* working in the process to make the same mistake, in which case the process is perfectly designed to tolerate the mistake, and it is a system issue. Telling people to "be more careful (or else)" will not work.

  With the increasing publicity of tragic medical errors, I'd like to propose a special subclass of errors and mistakes, that is, a series of errors and mistakes occurring *simultaneously* within a sequential series of key procedures for a single patient or customer — similar to "getting all the red lights" on one's way to work — which is a common cause. This results in unforeseen incidents and tragedies, often causing major outrage and unwanted publicity.
  - There is variation in how individuals are trained to do the work and in how people actually do the work.
  - Beneficial strategies to work around process design limitations are developed, which should then be implemented processwide.
- Source 5. Current practices fail to recognize the need for preventive measures.
  - Environmental factors make the process perfectly designed to have undesirable variation; incidents occur.
  - Human fatigue and attention deficit (sensory overload) cause poor short-term memory, confirmation bias, fixation, reversion under stress, and overgeneralization.
- Source 6. The process has unnecessary steps, inventory buffers, wasteful measures and data, including:
  - Complexity added in the past due to inappropriate reactions to experienced variation, resulting in non-value-added work;
  - Implementing untested solutions;
  - Using poorly collected data to make decisions; and
  - Routine data collections that are rarely or never used.
- Source 7. There is variation in inputs and outputs and challenges with "everyday" variation.

To explain *basic* differences:

- Six Sigma is obsessed with creating a process that is consistently, virtually defect free (or free of undesirable incidents) through studying the variation of the preceding Source 6 and intuiting issues inherent in Sources 1 through 5 as "theories to be tested" using planned data.
- Key elements of Lean production reflect obsessions with formally documenting the true current process up front (reducing human variation in perception), appropriate error proofing (Sources 2 and 5), and exposing waste (Source 6), generally in terms of complexity.

  The goal is to look at an entire process and have only the work occurring that benefits the customer (called *value-added* work vs. the *non-value-added* work many times designed for organizational convenience or to formally rework process errors that should not even be occurring).

Lean production cites eight examples of waste in healthcare: (1) defects (resticks, medication errors, label errors); (2) overproduction (blood draws done early to accommodate laboratory and extra diagnostic tests); (3) inventories (patients waiting for bed assignments, laboratory samples batched, dictation waiting for transcription); (4) movement (looking for patients, missing medications, missing charts or equipment); (5) excessive processing (multiple bed moves, retesting); (6) transportation (moving patients to tests); (7) waiting (inpatients waiting in the emergency department, patients waiting for discharge, physicians waiting for test results); and (8) underutilization (physicians transporting patients, equipment not being used because of upstream bottlenecks).

- The Toyota Production System takes the concept of "inventory buffers" one step further to an obsession with all aspects of *wasted time* that keep a process from "flowing." Think about the quality indicator "number of sleepless nights" while a patient waits for a potentially life-threatening test, its result, or his or her first scheduled chemotherapy. What if a patient could come to a clinic any time he or she wished, get a screening test, get the result, get further required diagnostics if needed, get those results, and get a doctor's visit leading to needed treatment in one visit? In other words, how does one avoid the various aspects of "batching" so ingrained in the current medical culture, in this case, one appointment vis-à-vis five potential appointments, usually set for the convenience of the medical personnel? Toyota focuses on "developing brilliant processes in which average employees may excel." The uncomfortable healthcare analog might be that healthcare systems have discontinuous processes in which brilliant staff struggle to produce average results.

The important role of statistical techniques in the six sources of problems with a process applies to Sources 2, 3, 4, and 7.

- Source 2 is the inadequate knowledge of how a process currently works. One of the two main reasons most projects fail is lack of a good baseline estimate of the extent of a problem (the other is too much detailed flowcharting). Do in-house data exist, or can a collection be designed to plot a simple chart for assessment, which then allows one to judge the effects of interventions?
- Resolving Source 3 will involve using statistical techniques to test theories, assess interventions, and hold gains to determine how the process truly "should work" if competing theories are available.
- To eliminate Source 4, patterns of errors and mistakes can be studied statistically to find hidden opportunity in a process.
  - If some people or departments are making the mistake and others are not, then knowledge exists in the system to prevent the mistake or expose inconsistency in trainers' results.
  - If *everyone* and *all* departments are making the mistake, then the process is perfectly designed to have the mistake occur: Removing the source of error will take a systemic intervention.
- Improving quality means improving processes to make them as consistently predictable as possible (reduced variation) and having staff react appropriately to everyday variation (Source 7).

## A CHANGE IN MANAGERIAL PERSPECTIVE AND BEHAVIOR

Successful change and QI require a customer orientation, modeling of QI skills and behavior at all staff levels, and reduction of inappropriate variation. Such modeling is a potentially powerful strategic weapon that calls for strong executive response and involvement.

In line with the preceding discussion, a surprisingly cohesive set of principles has evolved:[8]

- Customer-first orientation;
- Top management leadership of the QI process;
- Continuous improvement as a way of everyone's work life;
- Respect for employees and their knowledge, resulting in their active involvement in the improvement process;
- Reduction of product (e.g., clinical outcomes) and process variation;
- Provision of ongoing education and training of employees;
- Familiarity with a statistical way of thinking and the use of basic statistical methods throughout the organization;
- Emphasis on prevention rather than detection;
- View of vendors as long-term partners (to ensure consistent incoming quality of materials and services);
- Performance measures that are consistent with the goals of the organization;
- Standardization, or the development of and adherence to the best known ways to perform a given task;
- Emphasis on product and service quality in design;
- Cooperation and involvement of all functions within an organization;
- Awareness of the needs of internal customers; and
- Substantial culture change.

The concept of QI inherently makes common sense, but if it were only common sense, people would already be doing it and there would be no need for this book. Deming was in fact fond of saying, "Common sense has been our ruination." The concept at work here is actually counterintuitive common sense.

It is the implementation of QI and the associated transformation that require going beyond obvious common sense. Five major steps are involved in this long-term transition toward QI implementation (Exhibit 1.2). Because of the deliberate, majestic pace of change to be discussed in Chapters 3 and 10, keep Deming's warning in mind: "A good company will take five years to turn around. Most will take ten."

Why does this process take so long? Everyone knows that things need to change or improve. Why can't we set some goals, give everybody training, and start benefiting now? Everyone needs to change and, in their hearts, most want to change. However, an organization must remain in business, and although current methods may not be perfect, the organization knows only one way to stay in business: the current way. Change requires a lot of resources, but if all of its resources — time, staff, capital — are consumed by operating with the current methods, where do people find time to improve?

**EXHIBIT 1.2** ■ A Road Map: Major Steps to Transformation

1. Establish top management awareness and education.
   - See quality improvement as a balanced scorecard that will help the organization execute its strategy.
   - Establish focus, context, and clear results:
     – Mission, vision, and values;
     – Three to five strategic initiatives that cascade; and
     – Follow-up, follow-up, follow-up.
   - Learn and apply:
     – Process thinking;
     – Problem-solving tools;
     – Statistical thinking; and
     – The "accountable question" in responding to cultural victim behavior (Chapter 3).
2. Build a critical mass.
   - 25–30% of management demonstrating their commitment to quality (promotions reflect commitment to quality);
   - 20–30% of organization educated in quality philosophy;
   - 10–20% of organization trained in basic tools for quality improvement;
   - 1–2% of organization trained in advanced tools;
   - Zero tolerance for:
     – Blame, and
     – "Victim" behavior.
3. Achieve a quality culture.
   - All employees are educated in basic quality improvement tools and philosophy;
   - Use of data is integrated and statistically based;
   - Feedback is an integral part of organizational culture, is nonjudgmental, and is based entirely on:
     – Being sincerely commitment to people's success; and
     – Addressing behaviors seen as inconsistent with:
       - Organizational success; and
       - Individual success;
   - Suppliers are heavily involved; and
   - Improvement initiatives are given top priority at executive meetings.
4. Adopt the following ways of life:
   - Customer orientation;
   - Continuous improvement;
   - Elimination of waste;
   - Prevention, not detection;
   - Reduction of variation;
   - Statistical thinking and use of data;
   - Adherence to best-known methods;
   - Use of best available tools;
   - Respect for people and their knowledge; and
   - *Results-based* feedback: emotionally intelligent culture.
5. Provide world-class quality (quality permeates design efforts).
   - Reorganization is performed around key products/services and markets;
   - Quality improvement process is institutionalized and self-sustaining;
   - Totally consistent management practices are instituted; and
   - 50% of all staff members are trained in advanced tools.

Source: Adapted from E.C. Huge. 1990. "Measuring and Rewarding Performance" in *Total Quality: An Executive's Guide for the 1990s*, 19–20. Ernst & Young Quality Improvement Consulting Group (eds.). Homewood, IL: Richard D. Irwin.

The first edition of *The TEAM Handbook* once again shows its wisdom by defining the following laws of organizational change:[7]

1. Things are the way they are because they got that way.
2. Unless things change, they will likely remain the same.
3. Change would be easy if it weren't for all the people.
4. People don't resist change; they just resist being changed themselves.

Does this mean little value exists in the 5- to 10-year transition required for complete QI transformation? Not at all. It is an investment in the future. Think of it as an investment in reducing Kerridge's four C's: confusion, conflict, complexity, and chaos. Although, as he would say, the ultimate documented cost savings are "unknown and unknowable," can you intuit that there is untold value to your organization if this could take place? And consider the fact that many well-meaning ad hoc cost-cutting programs actually *increase* organizational confusion, conflict, complexity, and chaos.

Again, efforts to overcome the inertia of operating the business at the current level cannot be overestimated. Change is very difficult, with its own majestic, deliberate pace that cannot be hurried (see Chapter 3). However, just because the journey is long does not mean it should not begin; quoting the ancient wisdom of the Chinese philosopher Lao-Tzu, "A journey of a thousand miles begins with a single step."

Developing organizational enthusiasm for statistical thinking and the team process approach is an important step on the learning curve to full transformation. Creating a common organizational language based in process through awareness of the data-driven QI approach will provide increasing value. As people gain experience with statistical thinking and tools (and an atmosphere of zero tolerance for blame), organizational defensiveness will dramatically decrease as they develop, analyze, revise, implement, and evaluate various improvements through an objective approach using data.

## SOME THOUGHTS ON BENCHMARKING

Deming was at his most vehement when he said, "Examples without theory teach nothing!"

Benchmarking is *the art of asking process-oriented questions* about the gap (variation) between your performance and the (alleged) benchmark: What works, for whom, and under what circumstances? What you ultimately get is dependent on how you ask the questions.

Whole systems transformation is complex change against a shifting baseline. Many times, findings reveal factors that enable or constrain the fortunes of a change effort; however, when applied to your organization, *the presence of enabling factors does not necessarily ensure success* but rather, its absence makes failure more likely.

Beware of pat formulas such as Six Sigma, DMAIC (which refers to define, measure, analyze, improve, and control), and Lean enterprise; off-the-shelf improvement packages; or examples. They're often sold as a one-size-fits-all, step-by-step process that one can drop right into an organization. When that doesn't work, some managers or consultants try to alter the organization to fit the program rather than the other way around.

### Effective Benchmarking

Benchmarking requires several steps, done correctly, in order to be an effective tool. You must first do your homework by asking questions to find out how your operation works down to the smallest detail:

- What are you doing?
- How are you doing it?
- What is your measure of how well you are doing it?
- Why are you looking for improvement?
- Have you made recent improvements?
- What are you planning to do during the next year?

These must be tailored to your specific situation or you won't be able to see all the pieces of the puzzle. Only then can you ask the right questions in order to compare it with the operation of the true top performers.

Do not fall into the lurking trap of asking questions of your benchmarking peers to defend your own status quo. No two departments are 100 percent alike, and if you examine an organization or department with which to benchmark, looking for only the differences, that is exactly what you will find. It's much harder to ask questions to determine exactly what improvement they made to achieve their performance.

Besides conference examples, another common practice has become paying (big bucks) for the privilege of becoming part of a benchmarking database. The theory is to (allegedly) improve by gauging your performance among peer groups, usually created without much thought. I describe databases such as these with the acronym resulting from "continuous recording of administrative procedures."

As I've seen happen all too often, people average the top 10 percent performances and say, "I want us to be there. Make it so." Deming had another saying, "A goal without a method is nonsense!"

There are two questions that must always be asked, even in response to presented examples: (1) Are you statistically different from the benchmark and is the difference common or special cause? "Given a set of numbers, 10 percent will be the top 10 percent." (For a more in-depth discussion, see Lesson 10 in Chapter 2.) But, more importantly, (2) How did the organizations in the database actually define this measure?

Trust me, this second question is always an issue, especially in defining and counting occurrences of "events." Many exposed differences result from slightly different processes used to determine the measure. Yes, a different process may be exposed, but the observed variation is often caused by the "measurement" input to the benchmarking process, not necessarily the "methods" input, which is assumed. Then, even when people agree on the definition, you would be amazed at how much human variation (unintentional or even sometimes intentional cultural bias) manifests when the measures are actually made.

And, even if you do all of this well, *effective learning and capability development doesn't happen just because you want it to.*

If an organization's systems don't work well, if cultural skill levels aren't strong, if processes are out of control, if measurements are giving incomplete or false feedback, if communication channels are crossed, or if reward and recognition practices are unaligned, the clearest focus, strongest context, and best of intentions will result in wasted time and wasted money.

When Deming's preceding two statements start to make sense, then you are on your way to transforming your role and yourself.

## SUMMARY

Here is a summary of that most crucial concept of process-oriented thinking:

- All work is a process.
- A process is any sequence of tasks having inputs that undergo some type of conversion action to produce outputs.
- The six sources of inputs are people, work methods, machines, materials, environment, and measurements (data).
- All processes exhibit output variation, and any input can be a source of variation.
- Any time a process does not "go right," variation has occurred.
- All processes are potentially measurable: Processes speak to us through data.
- There is benefit to understanding variation and reducing *inappropriate and unintended* variation while pushing for deeper-level fixes.
- As will be discussed in subsequent chapters, the use of data involves four processes: definition, collection, analysis, and interpretation.
- Any variation can be one of two types (special cause or common cause). Treating one as the other makes things worse.

Meanwhile, as leaders:

- Develop a passion for delighting customers;
- Develop a passion for eliminating waste;
- Routinely use data to speed up learning and improvement;
- Develop process and system thinking;
- Optimize the system as a whole (seek deep fixes);
- Learn to hear the signal through the noise — it is all about understanding variation;
- Treat everyone as if we are all in the same boat together trying to row in the same direction;
- Practice win-win whenever possible;
- Believe in people; and
- Focus on releasing people's intrinsic motivation.

*The intent in QI is not to create a series of stiflingly formal special projects.* Rather, the intent is to align the entire organization toward key goals, focus more intensely on customers, and simultaneously create a workplace of joy and excellence.

Quality, when integrated into a business strategy, is present in virtually *every* aspect of *every* employee's *everyday* work. The following skills will be needed by everyone in the organization:

- Thinking in terms of processes and automatically blame processes, not people, when things go wrong;
- Identifying the unnecessary complexity and waste in current work processes that result in costs, but no added value, to customers;
- Using the Pareto principle to better focus job improvement activity;

- Designing and using simple, efficient data collection methods to improve the effectiveness of processes;
- Communicating with a common language to depersonalize problems, break down current barriers among departments, and unify organizational quality efforts; and
- Facilitating work teams to develop simple actions to study and prevent problems in everyday work that staff consistently finds frustrating.

As I cannot emphasize enough, you will know you have succeeded when the words *statistical* and *quality* are ultimately dropped as adjectives because they will be "givens."

## REFERENCES

1. Kerridge, David. 1996. "Dr. Deming's Cure for a Sick System." *Journal for Quality and Participation* 19 (7): 24.
2. Berwick, Donald M. 1989. "Sounding Board: Continuous Improvement as an Ideal in Health Care." *New England Journal of Medicine* 320 (1): 56.
3. Juran, Joseph M. 1970–1980. *Juran on Quality Improvement* video series. Boston: Juran Institute.
4. Clemmer, Jim. 1992. *Firing on All Cylinders: The Service/Quality System for High-Powered Corporate Performance*, 67–68. Homewood, IL: Business One Irwin.
5. Clemmer, Jim. 2014. "Organization Structure Limits or Liberates High Performance." The Clemmer Group. www.clemmergroup.com/organization-structure-limits-or-liberates-high-performance.php.
6. Brown, Meredith. 2010. "Letters." *Quality Progress* (December).
7. Scholtes, Peter R., and others. 1988. *The TEAM Handbook*, 5–20. Madison, WI: Joiner Associates.
8. Huge, Ernest C. 1990. *Total Quality: An Executive's Guide for the 1990s*. Homewood, IL: Richard D. Irwin.

CHAPTER 2

# Data Sanity: Statistical Thinking as a Conduit to Transformation

**KEY IDEAS**

- Traditional report formats do not accurately represent true variation.
- Data are usually heavily aggregated, and comparisons are based almost exclusively in "this month/last month/12 months ago" thinking with variances to goals.
- The routinely used managerial summary technique of rolling average actually renders statistical analysis invalid.
- Half of executive meeting time and almost one hour a day of middle management time is spent poring over data. It is a waste of time and results in subsequent organizational waste in futile activity.
- "Is the process that produced this observation the same as the process that produced other observations?" is a deeper, more profound question when discussing and comparing two different numbers.
- Run charts and control charts must become routine analysis tools.
- A true statistically defined trend is a relatively rare occurrence.
- It is easy to intuit patterns in data that are not really there. It is amazing how nonrandom randomness can look.
- Preconceived notions of special causes, especially seasonality, can result in biased, inappropriate displays of data.
- Tampering, which is reacting to common cause variation as though it is special cause variation, results in incalculable losses for the organization.
- The capability of any process being improved must be assessed, that is, its actual inherent performance vs. its desired performance. Any goals must be evaluated in the context of this capability, and an appropriate strategy must be developed to deal with gaps.
- Quality assurance thinking and analyses that use rankings must be reevaluated in a common cause context.
- Whether they realize it or not, people are already using variations of the ideas presented in this chapter.
- Understanding and reacting appropriately to variation is the key concept here.

## THE NEED FOR STATISTICAL THINKING IN EVERYDAY WORK

People generally do not perceive that they need statistics, they only see the need to solve their problems. Given the current rapid pace of change in the economic environment and frustration at rising medical costs, a clamoring has been seen for "accountability" and "paying for performance." This outcry has resulted in a well-meaning tendency for performance goals to be imposed from external sources and for outcome data to be made public with increasing specificity. It has also unintentionally created a defensive atmosphere, making improvement efforts flounder when:

- Results are mass produced in aggregated row-and-column formats, complete with rankings and variances to numerical goals;
- Perceived trends are acted on to reward and punish via "this month to last month" and "this month to the same month last year" comparisons;
- Labels, such as *above average* and *below average,* are attached to individuals and institutions; and
- Executives or politicians are "outraged" by certain results and impose even "tougher" standards.

These well-meaning strategies are simple, obvious, and wrong. They also exhibit several usual statistical traps that mislead analysis and interpretation and insidiously cloud decisions every day in virtually every work environment.

In addition to dealing with the need to generate and respond to this type of data, leaders also face the everyday necessity to generate the data to manage the business, and there is no difference between the approach to analyzing and improving a clinical process and that to an administrative process.

Despite what we have all been taught, statistics is not an arcane set of techniques used to "massage" data. These are the realities:

- Taking action to improve a situation is tantamount to using statistics.
- Traditionally taught academic statistics have severely limited value in real-world processes.
- Understanding of variation is more important than using techniques.
- Statistical thinking gives a knowledge base from which to ask the right questions.
- Unforeseen problems are caused by the exclusive use of arbitrary numerical goals, "stretch" goals, and "tougher" standards for driving improvement.
- Using heavily aggregated tables of numbers, variances to goals, traffic light or bar graph formats, or linear trend analysis as vehicles for making meaningful management decisions results in actions that are many times futile and inappropriate.
- Meetings during which data presentations, such as the graphics just mentioned, are discussed are usually wasteful, pure and simple.
- Interpreting percentages can be deceptive.
- There is poor awareness of the true meaning of the terms *trend, above average*, and *below average.*

## THE ROLE OF DATA: A NEW PERSPECTIVE ON STATISTICS

Because everything is a process, true understanding of any situation requires data, which provide an objective view of a situation. As you will see from the examples in this chapter, there is an elegant simplicity to this approach — initially seen as counterintuitive — and unlimited opportunity to apply it. However, management must make this transformation from a crisis-driven to a data-driven organization, or unwitting, inappropriate, and unintentionally destructive first-instinct reactions to everyday variation will continue to be the norm.

Statistical thinking involves simple skills that can be applied immediately by anyone to create an atmosphere of continuous improvement. This approach allows people, via a common language, to:

- View variation from a different, expanded perspective;
- Use a process-oriented approach to define and analyze improvement opportunities;
- Routinely use a variety of simple charts to display and analyze data;
- Recognize poor and useless data displays and analysis;
- Observe and interpret variation to take a productive, appropriate action; and
- Ask better questions to get to deeper improvements.

*Whether or not people understand statistics, they are already using statistics.* People make decisions in their jobs every day by reacting to observed variations in data. Whether the data are numerical, perceptual, or anecdotal, these decisions based on them are in essence predictions that the resulting actions will cause things to somehow get better as a result. These actions have consequences and carry two risks:

1. Acting on a perceived difference when none really exists; or
2. Failing to detect a real change and consequently taking no action.

## DATA "INSANITY": MANAGEMENT BY GRAPHICS

### How Many Meetings?

Do the data presentations in Exhibit 2.1 look familiar? These are real examples I have encountered that are typical of routine operational "how we are doing" meetings during which some data are handed out summarizing current performance. They may or may not also include "this month/last month/same month last year" comparisons (e.g., percentage change) and variances to goals. Everyone gets busy drawing little circles around numbers, and no one's circles match. Believe it or not, however, they are using statistics.

Why is this statistics? Because people look at a pattern on a graph or a number on a page and mentally compare it with what they *think* it should be in their heads. If that gap (variation) is unacceptable, they draw a circle because they want to take an action to close that gap. The trouble is, *there is variation in how people perceive variation.* So the meeting unravels to the point where everyone is arguing the merits of his or her individual circles to organize subsequent action (organizational time and resources). This exercise exposes the group to the two risks listed in the previous section, usually the first, acting on a perceived difference when none really exists, which W. Edwards Deming called "tampering."

Statistical knowledge and skills are needed to minimize these errors. However, traditional teaching of statistics still predominates, and the wrong concepts continue to be taught. Many people joke about their "Statistics from Hell 101" requirement, how it was one of the worst courses they took, and how they remember none of it, which is probably a good thing. But the routine calculation, presentation, and misapplication of "summary stats" is a hidden organizational plague.

Most people have minimal statistical skills and experience a lack of comfort with numbers. The success of quality improvement (QI) will depend on the appropriate organization-wide development of a basic set of statistical skills. Integration of these data skills into *all* aspects of an organization's culture will accelerate and enhance the improvement process. By far, the most frequent error is reacting to variation that is just random noise to look for explanations and subsequently finding them (tampering). This exercise results in adding complexity (and wasted time), making things worse. If this embedded, routine time-wasting could be freed up, then that time could be devoted to organizational transformation.

A key principle in QI is the Pareto principle, or 80/20 rule (explained more thoroughly in Chapter 5). Here I apply it to the statistical knowledge needed by boards, executives, and managers: *20 percent of statistics will solve 80 percent of your problems.*

**EXHIBIT 2.1** ▪ **Typical Data Presentations I Have Encountered**

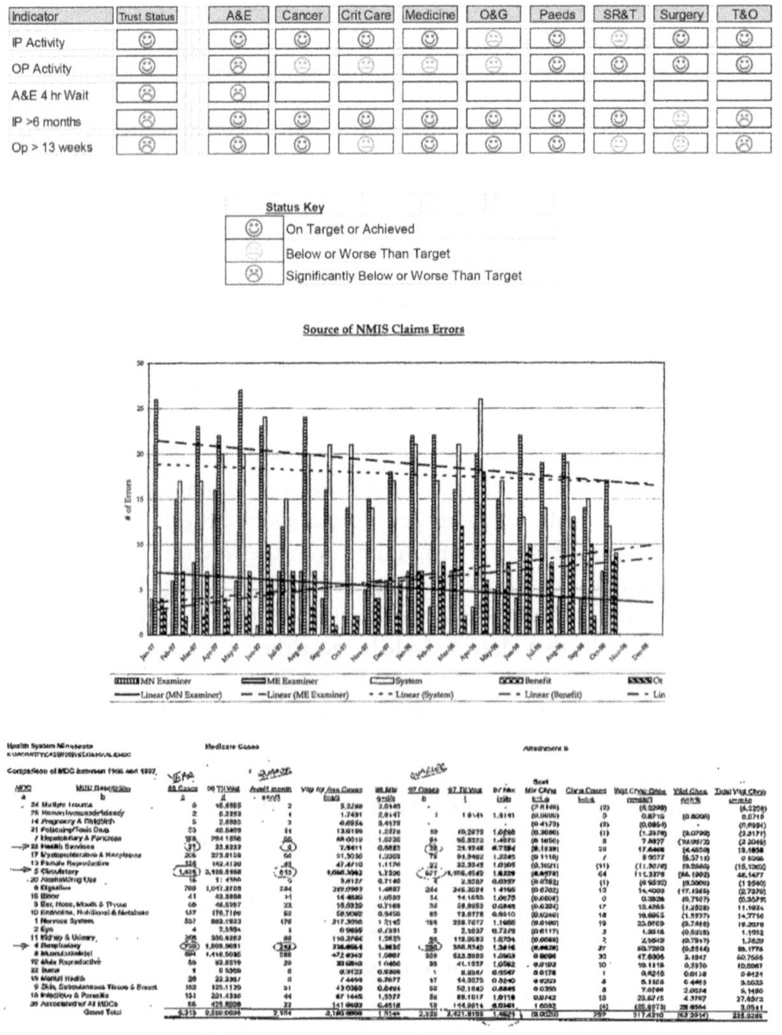

This interpretation of the rule is an example of the *language of statistical thinking*, which needs to cross all organizational barriers. It will cause a quantum leap in your improvement efforts (and routine daily management).

After a brief introduction and scenario, I present 10 lessons to demonstrate the basic concepts of statistical thinking and methods. I hope these concepts will motivate you to begin a dialogue with your improvement facilitators or QI personnel for more effective organizational data use. Further, I hope these give you the background to *teach* this language and these methods to your entire organization (see the stages of organizational transformation in Exhibit 1.2) through your management and leadership behaviors.

Any of these concepts can be immediately implemented into everyday organizational management. I guarantee that their use will catalyze the improvement process toward transforming organizational performance, as well as liberating precious time to move forward with such efforts.

One technique in particular, the common cause strategy of the Pareto matrix (see Lesson 3 and Chapter 5), may have the potential to *solve several of your long-standing organizational issues* that have resisted any efforts to improve them, causing countless routine meetings that have added nothing but organizational complexity and frustration.

### Is This Déjà Vu?

The following scenario is based on some data a friend of mine once gave me on a guideline compliance initiative: "Improve compliance from 50 percent to at least 70 percent short term and 75 percent longer term." I have summarized it in a form I typically encounter and no doubt you do as well. I revisit this scenario in the next main section and apply to it additional enlightening analyses.

### Basic Scenario

Executives are always trying to impress upon me how busy they are. Because they have so many things to manage, many of them like traffic light systems as a quick intuitive summary.

For this guideline compliance scenario, given the current goals, let:

≥70 percent = light (represents green);
65–69 percent = **medium** (represents yellow); and
<65 percent = **bold** (represents red).

The actual performances are given in the following list. The graphical summary in Exhibit 2.2 consists of three groupings of three bar graphs each (current goal of 70 percent drawn in):

1. Far left: Your current quarter's three monthly results for October = **66.67 percent**, November = **63.89 percent**, December = **69.44 percent** (first set of bars in time sequence);
2. Middle: This month/last month/same month last year, adding December one year ago (**33.33 percent**) (second set of three bars in time sequence); and
3. Far right: Comparing this fourth quarter's average with the third quarter's average with the fourth quarter's average last year, the results are respectively **48.15 percent**, 69.44 percent, and 66.67 percent (third set of bars in time sequence).

EXHIBIT 2.2 ■ Bar Graph Analysis of Quarterly Guideline Compliance (Goal: >70%)

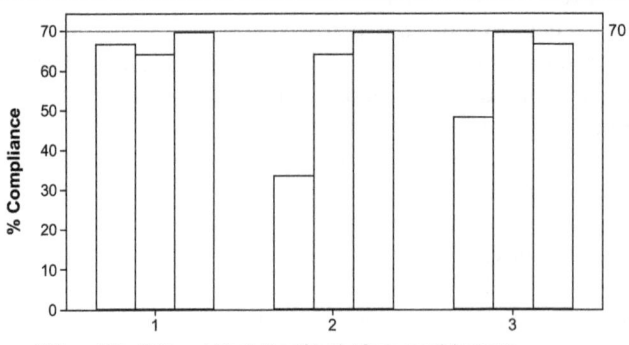

1) Current Qtr., 2) Current Month / Last Month / Same month last year,
3) This qtr. / last qtr. / Same qtr. last year

EXHIBIT 2.3 ■ Trend Analysis of Guideline Compliance (Goal: >70%)

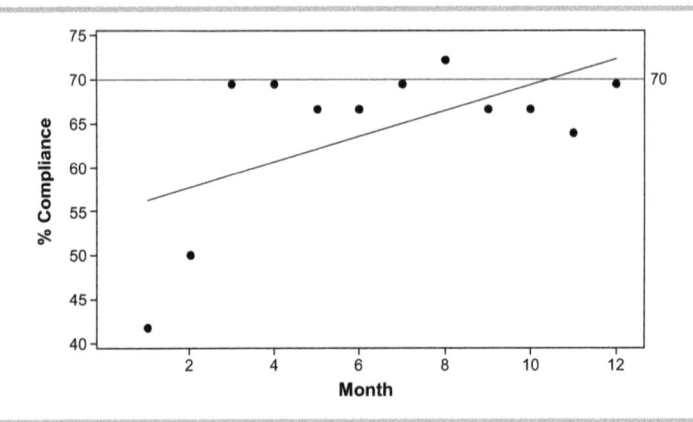

The graph in Exhibit 2.3 shows a trend analysis of the past 12 months' results with the goal superimposed. Given this typical graphical presentation, how would you conclude that the organization is doing relative to the short-term goal of greater than 70 percent?

Just for the sake of completeness, and because this project was a specific agenda item, Exhibit 2.4 is a summary of the project history, which includes all the intervention data plus baseline with the 65 and 75 percent targets drawn in.

How much time do you spend in meetings like this, which usually also include tables showing percentage change and variance to goal (perhaps even similar to the table in Exhibit 2.1) for each key organizational index? How much are the additional paper, ink, and color copying costs?

## THE LENS OF STATISTICAL THINKING

My favorite graphic tool for initially analyzing a set of data is the *run chart*. It is a simple plot of data in its naturally occurring order with the *median* of the data drawn as a

### EXHIBIT 2.4 ▪ Guideline Project History Trend

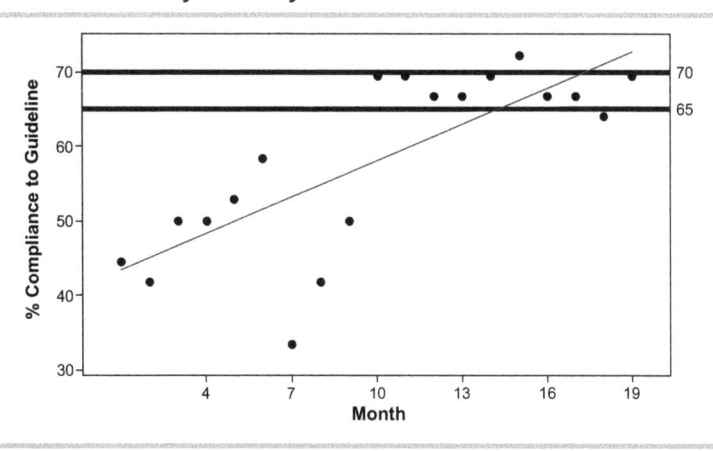

### EXHIBIT 2.5 ▪ Statistically Defining a Trend

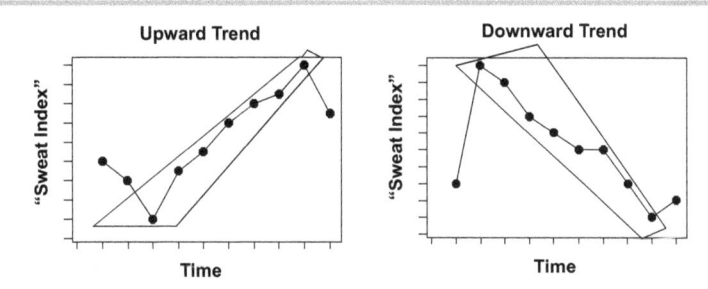

Special Cause — A sequence of *seven* or more points continuously increasing or continuously decreasing (or six successive increases or decreases) indicates a trend in the process average.

Note 1: Omit entirely any points that repeat the preceding value. *Such points neither add to the length of the run nor break it.*

Note 2: If the total number of observations is *20 or less,* *six* continuously increasing or decreasing points can be used to declare a trend (or five successive increases or decreases).

Note 3: This test is good until you have 200 data points, where the test now becomes *eight* continuously increasing or decreasing points (or seven successive increases or decreases).

This rule is to be used only when people are making conclusions from a tabulated set of data *without any context of variation for interpretation.*

---

reference line. Exhibits 2.5 and 2.6 show graphical representations of run charts, and they demonstrate two basic statistical rules for determining special causes:

1. *Trend,* which is a sequence of seven or more points continuously increasing or decreasing, *that is,* six *consecutive* increases or decreases; and
2. *Clump of eight,* which is a run of eight consecutive points either *all* above or *all* below the median.

**EXHIBIT 2.6** ■ Defining a Process Shift: The "Eight in a Row" Rule

Plot the dots — Rule 2: The "Clump of Eight"

Special Cause: A run of 8 consecutive points either *all* above or *all* below the median

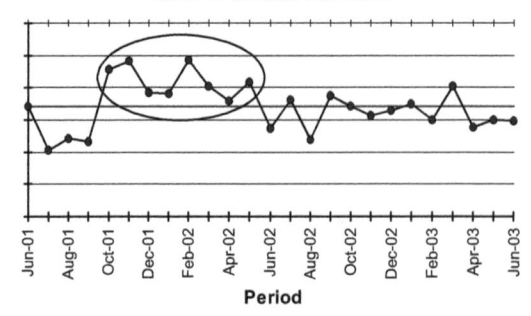

- A *run chart* is a simple, time-ordered plot of a set of data in its naturally occurring order with the *median* of the data (the value where half of the data are literally larger and smaller) drawn in as a reference line.
- A *run* consists of a set of points either *all* above or *all* below the median. It is "broken" and begins a new "run" when a data point crosses the median; any data point *on* the median *neither* breaks *nor* adds to the current run.

If this test occurs, it indicates that during the time period plotted, there has been at least one significant process "shift."

---

Let's now return to the guideline scenario and apply this simple analysis. The data given to me are shown in Exhibit 2.7. My friend had implemented a guideline in December 1997 and wanted to know whether it had worked. At the time, I was given the data only through December 1998.

I phoned her and asked, "Vera, how many times have you heard me speak? What do you think I'm going to do?" She knew immediately and replied sheepishly, "Plot the dots?" Exhibit 2.8 shows the data sorted to determine the median and the resulting run chart. Because the quantity of numbers is even, the median is the average of the two middle values *in this sorted sequence. Note the clumps of 8 or more points, that is,* observations 1–9 and observations 10–19. You would need *only one* of these as a signal to conclude a "change." Because the later data has a higher compliance percentage, one can conclude Vera's intervention was effective.

Also note the initial three increasing data points immediately after her intervention in December 1997. Even though our other rule showed a special cause, the process changed too fast to trigger the trend rule of six consecutive increases (there are only three). That doesn't matter. The other rule detected the change; only one signal is needed to declare a special cause. These two rules work together.

To a point, the initial intervention was successful. One can see that the process has leveled off to approximately 68 percent. (Vera changed her inputs, and the process *transitioned* to what it was perfectly designed to get given these new inputs. The result was still short of the goal.) If 75 percent compliance is desired, there will need to be an additional intervention to move the process further using a common cause strategy.

Things were fine for a while, then, as you see, compliance seriously dropped for January and February 1999. I received a panicked phone call. I told Vera to show the clinics the entire plot to date. Given this feedback, as you can see, the process recovered in March 1999.

*Run charts* are not only powerful for analysis, but can also become a common organizational language to give powerful feedback and provide direction for further improvement.

Consider the hypothetical difference posed as the last two data points of each graph in Exhibit 2.9 in the context of its (usually unplotted) history.

Typical of many board meetings, participants are not even provided a graphical summary (see Lesson 4). It has become increasingly common to have important issues summarized in the traffic light format shown in Exhibit 2.10. This type of display greatly inhibits practical application (see Lesson 6).

A run chart is the most important initial analyses of a set of data. One can then easily calculate the common cause limits as well as the difference between two *consecutive* points that is truly special cause (an example is given in Appendix 2A). These calculations are remarkably simple and easy to make during a boring meeting, and they represent your chance to stop the data insanity and start more productive conversations.

With this brief introduction and the two simple special cause tests, the following 10 lessons will further demonstrate the incredible power of these tests.

**EXHIBIT 2.7** Diabetes Guideline Compliance Data

| Month | % Compliance |
|---|---|
| 6/97 | 44.44 |
| | 41.67 |
| | 50.00 |
| 9/97 | 50.00 |
| | 52.78 |
| | 58.33 |
| 12/97 | 33.33 |
| | 41.67 |
| | 50.00 |
| 3/98 | 69.44 |
| | 69.44 |
| | 66.67 |
| 6/98 | 66.67 |
| | 69.44 |
| | 72.22 |
| 9/98 | 66.67 |
| | 66.67 |
| | 63.89 |
| 12/98 | 69.44 |
| | 55.56 |
| | 50.00 |
| 3/99 | 69.44 |

## DATA SANITY: 10 LESSONS TO SIMPLE, ENLIGHTENING, AND PRODUCTIVE ALTERNATIVES TO ROUTINE DATA PRESENTATION

In my years of working within organizations and teaching data analysis and QI, I've identified many lessons on how to present data so that it can be properly interpreted and acted on. I've also seen how leaders and organizations tend to overreact to improperly presented information. I believe that the following lessons are key takeaways for anyone reading this book. Lesson 1 sets the stage for several recurring key themes the rest of the lessons will cover.

### Lesson 1: Two or Three Points Do Not Make a Trend

At the close of a fiscal year, many organizations have an annual review, which is usually some variation of "trending" the three-month performance of the fourth quarter and comparing those results to last year's fourth quarter and this year's third quarter to some goals. The misguided theory is that one can look at overall trends, percent changes, and variances from goals and/or budgets, then make projections and establish the next fiscal year's goals.

It is usual practice to use some combination of three numbers to predict (alleged) trends. Did you realize that given three different numbers, there are six distinct ways they

**EXHIBIT 2.8** ■ **Determining the Median and the Resulting Run Chart of the Audit Data**

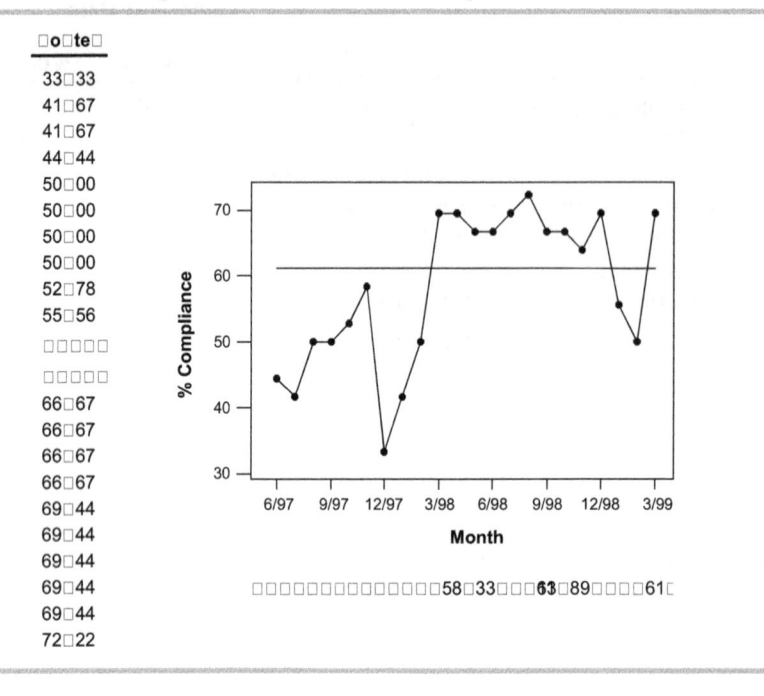

| Rate |
|---|
| 33.33 |
| 41.67 |
| 41.67 |
| 44.44 |
| 50.00 |
| 50.00 |
| 50.00 |
| 50.00 |
| 52.78 |
| 55.56 |
| 58.33 |
| 61.11 |
| 66.67 |
| 66.67 |
| 66.67 |
| 66.67 |
| 69.44 |
| 69.44 |
| 69.44 |
| 69.44 |
| 69.44 |
| 72.22 |

**EXHIBIT 2.9** ■ **Interpreting a Two-Point Difference in the Context of Its History**

Does it look like this? (Different process)
*Special cause*

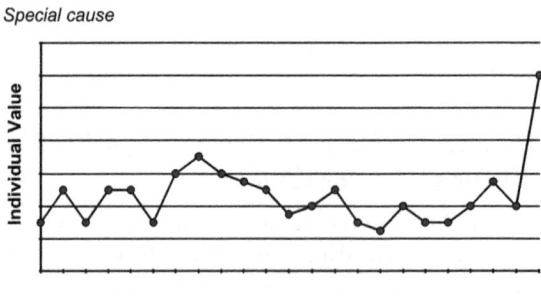

Or this? (Same process)
*Common cause*

EXHIBIT 2.10 ■ Weekly Traffic Light Performance Report

| Period | Region 1 | Region 2 | Region 3 | Region 4 | Region 5 |
|---|---|---|---|---|---|
| 4/6/2003 | 85.1% | 96.4% | **83.5%** | 88.0% | 86.6% |
| 4/13/2003 | **83.9%** | 94.7% | **84.3%** | 89.0% | 85.4% |
| 4/20/2003 | 85.1% | 94.6% | **81.4%** | **84.0%** | 86.0% |
| 4/27/2003 | 85.2% | 92.2% | **84.0%** | 85.6% | 84.8% |
| 5/4/2003 | **84.9%** | 93.9% | **82.3%** | **83.9%** | 86.0% |

| | | | | | |
|---|---|---|---|---|---|
| 8/31/2003 | **88.0%** | 96.1% | **86.5%** | **84.5%** | 90.9% |
| 9/7/2003 | 91.4% | 92.1% | **85.7%** | **85.5%** | 93.5% |
| 9/14/2003 | 90.0% | 94.4% | **88.2%** | **89.9%** | 91.6% |
| 9/21/2003 | **89.6%** | 92.9% | **86.3%** | 91.0% | 92.1% |
| 9/28/2003 | **89.6%** | 94.1% | **89.1%** | **89.2%** | 92.2% |

In an actual traffic light table, each cell is coded in green, yellow, and red to indicate relative values. For the purposes of this book, colors are represented by typeface weight.

For this table, the following key is used:
≥90 percent = green = light weight
85–89 percent = yellow = **medium weight**
<85 percent = red = **heavy weight**

EXHIBIT 2.11 ■ Six Graphs

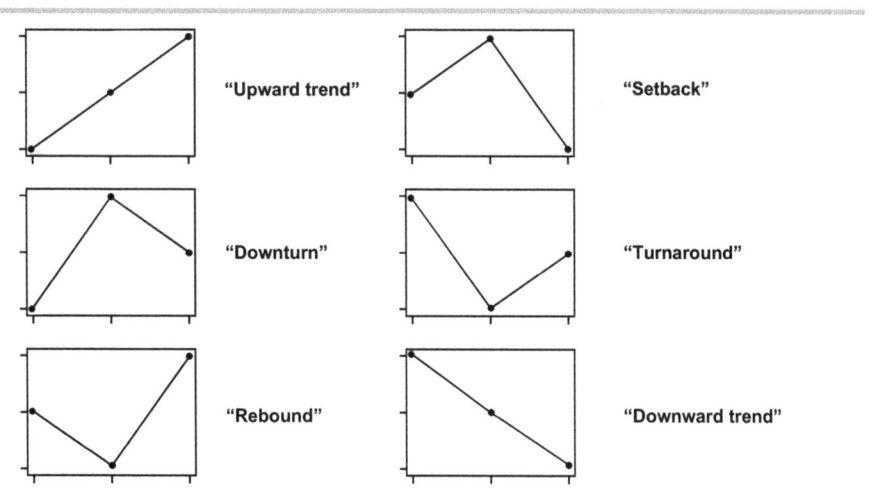

"Upward trend"

"Setback"

"Downturn"

"Turnaround"

"Rebound"

"Downward trend"

Source: Davis Balestracci Jr., MS, *Quality Digest*, February 2005. www.qualitydigest.com. Reprinted with permission.

can appear? The graphs in Exhibit 2.11 show the possibilities, along with several familiar terms used to explain them as special causes.

The question isn't whether the numbers differ from one another. The deeper question should be, "Is the process that produced the third number the same as the process that produced the second and first numbers?"

I've developed an analog of W. Edwards Deming's famous red bead experiment. Let's say I have an audience of 50 people. I hand out coins and set a goal. For 50 people, the goal is to get a number greater than or equal to 20. I call this performance "green." Similarly, 15 to 19 is "yellow," and fewer than 15 is "red." I then ask them to flip their coins. Only for those who obtain "heads," I ask them to flip it again, then I count the number of "double heads." I compare it to the goal and calculate a variance. At the end of three such flipping sequences, the group has one of the six patterns. I ask the group how they would prepare a quarterly report of their performance vs. the goal. At this point, there would be as many interpretations as there are people in the room.

I then demonstrate an easy calculation to show the expected range for double heads, given the number of participants in the room. For 50 people, this expected range (common cause) is approximately 3 to 21, and the average of the three flips is usually around 12 to 13.

The key point is that as long as the participants' three numbers lie within the statistically calculated limits (which they always do), they are indistinguishable from each other and the process average because the process didn't change. Each of the three times, it was 50 people flipping a coin and counting double heads.

To calculate month-to-month percent changes, vary the goal, attribute a trend, or explain the sequence of three using any of the six special cause terms is totally inappropriate. This is treating common cause as if it were special.

Note that the common cause variation of 3 to 21 encompasses the range of the red, yellow, and green endpoints; arbitrary assignment to colors is treating common cause as if it were special. The average is what you would expect for 50 people flipping a coin and counting the double heads, the probability of which is $(\frac{1}{2} \times \frac{1}{2})$ = 25 percent – 12.5. Also, the goal is within the common cause range of variation (also known as context of variation). Players will occasionally "meet" the goal just by virtue of random chance. After just three data points, it is clear that this process is perfectly designed not to meet the goal.

### What Does "Trend" Really Mean?

Looking at the six patterns in the coin-flipping exercise, it's really just simple math; calling a sequence of three observations that all either increase or decrease a "trend" *without a context of variation* has a 33 percent risk of being random, *that is*, two out of the six random possibilities. For my audience of 50, let's say their three results were in order 11, 12, and 17. Statistically, this would not be an upward trend because they lie between the common cause context of 3 and 21 that I calculated.

From statistical theory, it takes a sequence of six *consecutive* increases or decreases to declare a trend (with 20 data points or fewer, you may use five). In my experience, this is rare. The importance of this rule is to remind people to stop declaring trends when shooting from the hip in reaction to a table of numbers, as is the case in many managerial meetings.

And using the concept of process, should one observe this rule, it indicates only that there is a new process because of changed inputs. What is perceived as a trend is many times only a transition to a new level (known as a *step change*).

The quicker, statistically accurate way to declare a new process (special cause) is to determine whether a data point falls outside the context of variation of the data, *that is*, its common cause limits. In the case of the coin flip, suppose I now had the same 50 people flip the coin *only once* and counted the number of heads. Let's say we obtained 25 (a reasonable assumption). Notice that this is greater than the previously calculated upper limit of common cause (21) and was produced by a different process, which is flipping once instead of twice. We can declare 25 as a special cause. Note that it didn't trigger the trend rule; 11, 12, 17, and 25 are only three increases. Calculating common-cause limits increases your power of detecting a difference.

### An Introduction to Ranking

After the three flips, each participant has achieved the double-heads zero, one, two, or three times. As tempting as it might be to compare individual performances, there is actually *no difference* between zero percent (zero out of three, which is about one-third of the audience) or 100 percent (three out of three; usually, there is one). This kind of comparison is discussed extensively in Lesson 10 and the case study, which are about rankings.

### Key Points

- Any sequence of numbers needs a context of variation within which to be interpreted.
- This variation is not based on intuition or what someone "thinks" it should be, which many times is either an arbitrary number ending in zero or five or an arbitrary percentage (ending in zero or five) of the average.
- This variation is inherent to the process and must be calculated from process data.
- This technique applies to managerial and operational data as well as production product data or clinical outcomes. There is no distinction; everything is a process.

Lessons 2 and 3 are among the most important in both this chapter and the book.

## Lesson 2: From Reactive Strategies to Deeper-Fix Strategies

### The Accident Data

In manufacturing, safety is paramount and there are routine meetings on accident occurrences. A manufacturing plant had 45 accidents one year and set a goal for the next year of reducing them by at least 25 percent. The subsequent total was 32, which was a 28.9 percent decrease. In fact, a well-meaning (but inappropriate) trend analysis (Exhibit 2.12) showed the decrease was more on the order of 46.2 percent (4.173 vs. 2.243; obtained by using the beginning and ending points of the trend line).

This *seemed* to reflect well on the hard work of the safety committee during its monthly safety meetings, where *each individual* accident was dissected to find its root cause. That is, each undesirable variation (or accident) is treated as a *special cause*.

Note that there are three months with zero events. The reasons for these were also discussed and used to evaluate the effects of previously recommended solutions, which is another example of applying a special cause strategy to explain common cause variation. Based on these data, 80 actions (reactions to 77 accidents plus three months of zero) have been implemented during the past two years, which included new policies, reporting forms, awareness posters, additional visual safety alerts in dangerous places, and plant safety meetings.

The key question from the beginning should have been: "*Is the **process** that produced 32 accidents different from the **process** that produced 45 accidents?*" From what you've previously learned, if the answer is yes, one should be able to create a run chart of individual monthly results and see at least one of three things: (1) a trend of six consecutive decreases and/or (2) a run of eight consecutive points above the median in the first year and/or (3) a

**EXHIBIT 2.12** ▪ Regression Analysis of Accident Data

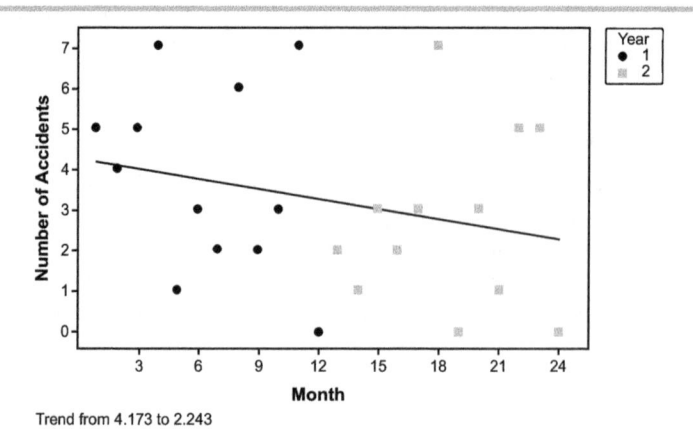

Trend from 4.173 to 2.243

Source: Davis Balestracci Jr., MS, *Quality Digest*, September 2005. www.qualitydigest.com. Reprinted with permission.

**EXHIBIT 2.13** ▪ Run Chart for Accident Data

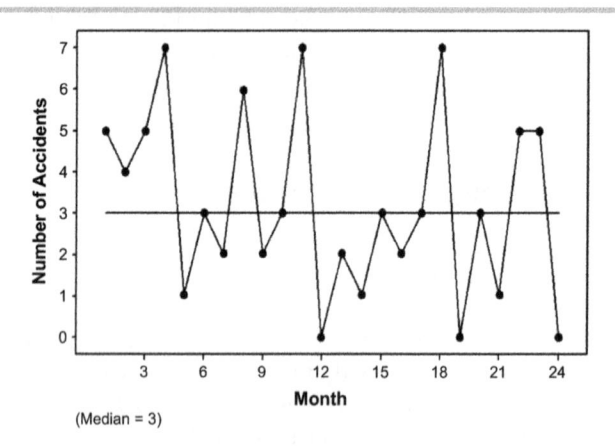

(Median = 3)

Source: Davis Balestracci Jr., MS, *Quality Digest*, September 2005. www.qualitydigest.com. Reprinted with permission.

run of eight consecutive points below the median in the second year. Look at Exhibit 2.13. What do you see? Or more importantly, what don't you see? (Chapter 5 contains a more detailed look at this data.)

Exhibit 2.13 shows common cause. This run chart does not trigger either basic special cause test.

The special cause strategy of looking at each accident individually is well meaning, but misguided, which the chart confirms. *The process has not improved* and remains perfectly designed to produce accidents. And more complexity has no doubt been added during the two years.

It is important to note that although the plot demonstrates common cause, it does not mean you have to accept the current performance. It means that the typical special

EXHIBIT 2.14 ■ Medication Errors

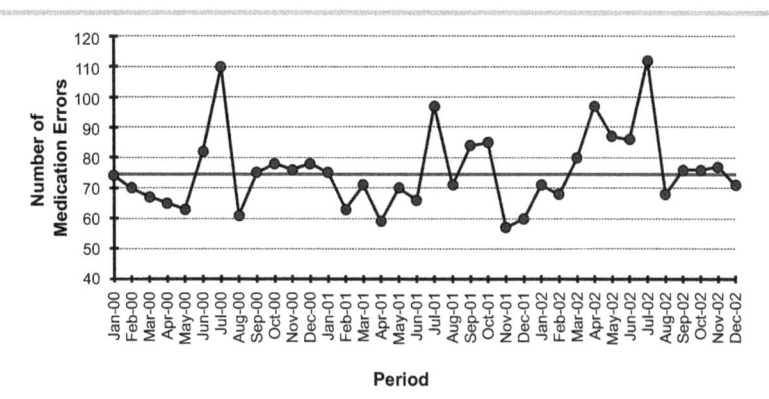

Source: Davis Balestracci Jr., MS, *Quality Digest*, September 2005. www.qualitydigest.com. Reprinted with permission.

cause strategies of investigating the *individual* months people dislike, comparing *individual* months to each other, or investigating *individual* accidents would most probably be wasted effort.

To quote a favorite saying of W. Edwards Deming, "Statistics on the number of accidents don't help to improve the occurrence of accidents." One must dig deeper. There are common cause strategies that aren't well known but provide a logical method to improve common cause variation.

The most useful initial common cause strategy is to expose hidden special causes that are unknown, yet aggregating predictably to create the *appearance* of common cause. Using the underlying structure of how data were collected sometimes allows *stratification*, a "sorting," if you will. One particularly powerful form of stratification is shown in Lesson 3.

Meanwhile, here's a simpler form of stratification that is useful in some cases in conjunction with the run chart.

### The Medication Error Data

I once consulted with a medical center and attended its monthly meeting on medication errors. They gave me the monthly reports from the past two years, and at the top of each report was the number of errors for *this month, last month, and same month last year*. Ignoring all the comments and discussion about finding the trend, I used the reports to sketch a quick run chart of the past three years of performance (Exhibit 2.14). Using the two rules, it demonstrates common cause.

Many times, knowing how the data were collected allows one to somehow "tag" each data point on a graph by some input criterion. The purpose is to help see whether there is a clustering pattern to either *all* the high values or *all* low values; when they occur it is *always for the same reason*.

For this example, it is as simple as using "month." Do you see a *pattern to the months with high values*? I stopped the meeting dead in its tracks by asking, "What happens in July?" Besides a lot of vacations, that's when the new residents start. Do you *think* that might be the reason for the noticeable spikes in medication errors?

So there's a separate process for July and then there's the process for all other eleven months of the year. Because we can predict what's going to happen in July, might it be prudent to see how that could be *prevented*?

Also, because July has its own unique process, its error pattern is probably different from a more typical month; July's errors should *not* be mixed in with other months' errors. If this special cause hadn't been found, it could have seriously clouded the powerful technique of Lesson 3.

When charts exhibit common cause, labeling the points is sometimes a good initial strategy.

### Key Points

- A run chart can exhibit common cause, but that does not mean you must accept the current level of performance. There are common cause strategies to identify ways to proceed in the improvement process.
- You cannot treat data points or incidents individually.
- Special causes could still be hidden in common cause variation. As you will see in Lesson 3, they can predictably aggregate to create the appearance of common cause.
- Sometimes, labeling the data points will expose special causes that are present because there is a pattern to either all the high or all the low values; they always occur for the same reason. This was true in the medication error data and is also demonstrated in the Real Common Cause example in Chapter 6 on page 202.
- Exposing these patterns is important because they could compromise the powerful stratification analysis in Lesson 3.

### Lesson 3: Process Stratification via the Pareto Matrix

*Using the Pareto principle is a powerful common cause approach to focus a vague situation, especially if you can use it in two dimensions.* A classic technique is from Joseph Juran's writings on QI. It's a Pareto matrix, the purpose of which is to isolate the "20 percent of the process causing 80 percent of the problem." Many people have told me that this has been by far their most useful diagnostic tool. One group from the upcoming Lesson 6 scenario applied it and went from 90 percent conformance to 98 percent conformance to a crucial target.

In Lesson 2, it was shown that despite meeting an aggressive 25 percent reduction goal (i.e., 45 accidents during the first year and 32 the following year), the process that produced the 32 was no different from the process that produced the 45. It was common cause. Now what?

One advantage to the common cause nature of the problem is that *all 77 incidents were produced by the same process.* There is no value in looking at individual accidents, but rather, all the accidents can be combined (aggregated), which is perfectly designed for using the Pareto matrix. The matrix is simply a visual presentation of common cause data that invites deeper discussion. Theories can then be brainstormed for factors by which this aggregate can be "sliced and diced" (stratified) to reveal hidden special causes. For example, look at "event type" and "unit" in Exhibit 2.15.

Note the advantage of looking at the data in two dimensions: The usual Pareto analysis applies. Two units account for most of the events (accidents), and two event types

EXHIBIT 2.15  Matrix of Adverse Events

| Event Type | Unit | | | | | | Total |
|---|---|---|---|---|---|---|---|
| | A | B | C | D | E | F | |
| 1 | 0 | 0 | 1 | 0 | 2 | 1 | 4 |
| 2 | 1 | 0 | 0 | 0 | 1 | 0 | 2 |
| 3 | 0 | 16 | 1 | 0 | 2 | 0 | 19 |
| 4 | 0 | 0 | 0 | 0 | 1 | 0 | 1 |
| 5 | 2 | 1 | 3 | 1 | 4 | 2 | 13 |
| 6 | 0 | 0 | 0 | 0 | 3 | 0 | 3 |
| 27 | | | | | | | |
| 28 | | | | (less than 6 each) | | | |
| 29 | | | | | | | |
| Totals | 6 | 19 | 7 | 3 | 35 | 7 | 77 |

account for many of the accidents. However, look at the power of the matrix presentation when the high numbers are investigated further.

Unit B, despite its many accidents, has excellent performance except for event type 3. Also, because no one else is having trouble with this event type, the odds for rectifying this situation are quite good because it's isolated to a single unit and knowledge might already exist in the system. However, *it might not reflect departmental competence* but merely *a different input* to the work process (e.g., people, methods, machines, materials, measurement, and environment) that is *unique* to that department and makes its work environment inherently more dangerous. A plant-wide safety seminar on event type 3 would accomplish absolutely nothing. *It would treat a special cause* (that only applies to *one* unit) *as if it were a common cause* (applying to *all* units) and waste a lot of people's time and the organization's money in the process.

Unit E, conversely, has no such clear, localized action. For whatever reason, its *entire safety performance* is suspect because it's experiencing all the event types. This will take further investigation of Unit E's events, which, although not a pleasant thought, has focused the issue to one department and not all six.

Seeing the lack of any pattern for event type 5, it becomes obvious that it's a problem for the entire plant because everyone is experiencing it. It's not as simple as saying, "Be more careful." *The plant is perfectly designed to have this type of hazardous situation.*

If appropriate action could be taken on these three significant sources of undesirable variation, there's the potential to reduce events (accidents) by approximately 40 to 50 percent. The current special cause strategy of concentrating only on the monthly total and overlooking this common cause strategy means that Unit B *would continue* to have event type 3, Unit E *would continue* its poor safety performance, and event type 5 *would continue* unabated, making it perfectly designed to continue its current level of performance for the past two years.

If a process exhibits common cause variation, it is much more productive to have people brainstorm ways to stratify data rather than wasting energy to explain why this month's result is different from last month's. It also helps to focus subsequent, more detailed diagnosis on only the 20 percent of the process causing 80 percent of the problem. *Isn't this more effective than starting a vague project with a vague question such as, "What causes accidents?"*

***Key Points***

- Some problems continue to be frustrating because they're being treated as special causes when the process exhibits common cause behavior.
- Pareto analysis is one of the most powerful tools available for improvement because it focuses a vague situation, which can sometimes result in even deeper focus.
- Pareto analysis finds unwitting hidden special causes that are coming together to produce the appearance of common cause on a run chart.
- Data from any common cause period can be aggregated to stratify by process input.
- It is usually better to try to stratify in two dimensions whenever possible.

## Lesson 4: When Processes Moonlight as "Two Point" Trends

My experience is that governing boards always have the vague objective of "knowing how we're doing," which is then passed on to an analyst who gladly and dutifully complies by diving into organizational databases. These vague objectives lead to vague analyses, which always lead to vague conclusions and vague follow-up actions.

The following is a true story and typical of what I see played out in boardroom after boardroom — comparing the past 12 months of performance to the previous 12 months (many times via two bar graphs with some kind of "trend" line). The board was presented with a report from an emergency medicine environment focusing on a particular activity, in this case, responding to cardiac arrests.

The report stated: "We're running a slightly higher number of cardiac arrests per month. The total amount of cardiac arrests has risen from a mean of 21.75 (January to December 2011) to 22.92 (January to December 2010). This is an increase of 14 cardiac arrests in the last 12 months."

The report continued:

> Next, we interpreted the data relating to [ventricular fibrillation (Vfib)] cardiac arrests. ...This could be *significant* to our outcome, and...indicates a need for more sophisticated statistical analysis. It was already shown that the number of cardiac arrests has increased by a mean of 1.17 per month. Now we're adding to that increase a decrease of times we're seeing Vfib as the initial rhythm. From January to December 2010, we arrived on scene to find Vfib as the initial rhythm with an overall mean of 6.75 times. That gave us a capture rate of 32.03 percent. This last year, January to December 2011, we're arriving to find Vfib as the initial rhythm with an overall mean of 5.92, and a capture rate of 25.81 percent. This obviously means that during the last year, we've responded to more cardiac arrests and found them in more advanced stages of arrest.

Let's test these conclusions. "Total arrests responded to" is an important organizational number. It's also clear that the proportion of these arrests in Vfib is important, so I created it as a new response, *for example*, for January 2010, it is 6 out of 18, or 33.33 percent. I then plotted the dots to produce two run charts (Exhibit 2.16).

As you see in both cases, there are neither "six consecutive increases nor decreases" nor any "run of eight consecutive points either all above or below the median." The conclusion is that *nothing* has changed in two years, which everyone in the room would have concluded in about 10 seconds had the data been presented in this way and had they

**EXHIBIT 2.16** Arrests and Vfib Run Charts

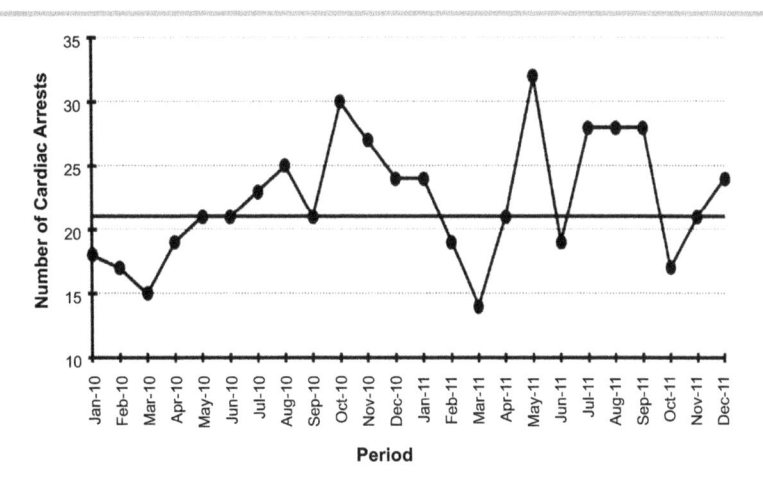

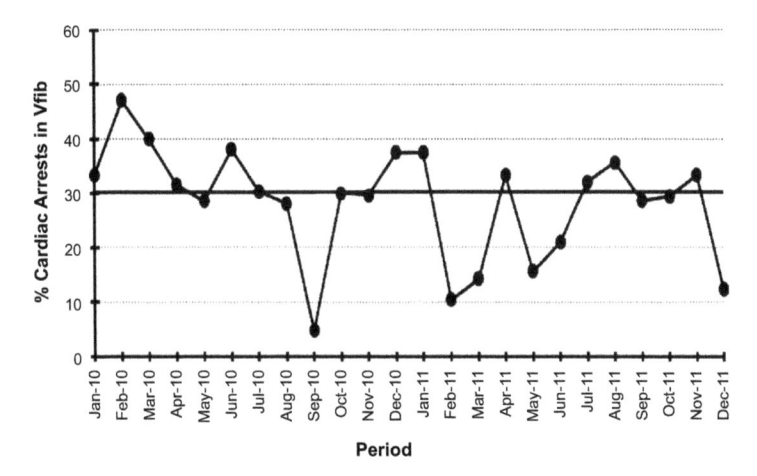

Source: Davis Balestracci Jr., MS, *Quality Digest*, June 2005. www.qualitydigest.com. Reprinted with permission.

known the simple statistical theory of run charts. Moreover, it could have saved precious meeting minutes of empty discussion and hours of subsequent searches as people looked for explanations and found them.

It is important to ascertain whether *the process that produced the current number is the same as the process that produced the previous number.* New results are produced only by new conversations. Never underestimate the power of looking at a situation as a process and plotting the dots even with administrative data.

The analyst who gave me this data came up to me after the seminar and said, a bit embarrassed, "Thank you for showing me what to do differently." Analysts are valuable resources; help make their jobs more interesting and you will achieve results beyond your wildest dreams.

### Key Points

- Plot the dots!
- These plots and their common theory of interpretation will reduce the human variation of peoples' perceptions of data and get them to agree on a situation easily within seconds.
- Plotting the dots results in less time treating common cause as special and creates new, more productive conversations about a situation.
- More time for patient care is produced by less frontline distraction from explaining numbers.

### Lesson 5: Bar Graphs Are Not Welcome

Exhibit 2.17 shows three graphs of the same data (percent computer uptime). The top bar graph uses an origin of zero. The middle bar graph lets the program default to a scale.

Contrast the bar graphs with the run chart analysis at the bottom of Exhibit 2.17. There are no trends, no runs of eight, and nothing unusual about achieving 100 percent (probably just luck). Can we use the common cause strategy of a Pareto matrix, aggregating all 19 months downtime, then using the common cause strategy of stratification to improve?

Exhibit 2.18 shows a stacked bar graph with 19 potential "dots" that can, with little effort, be converted to a run chart (Exhibit 2.19). The run chart tells the story quite well. Nothing's changed for ***five years*** (it's all common cause variation and one quarter is no different from another quarter), despite a lot of well-meaning improvement efforts. Wouldn't a Pareto matrix analysis of *all 150 bacteremias* be helpful?

When speaking at conferences, I'm always intrigued when I visit the poster sessions. I encounter countless aisles of bar graphs, especially the displays with two bars, "before" and "after." (Remember the lesson from Chapter 1: "Given two different numbers, one will be larger.") I've noticed that the "two-scale" syndrome seen in Exhibit 2.20 is also routinely used. Note the differing left and right vertical axes (hence, the description two-scale). The horizontal axis is "time." This poster touted a profound change.

I discreetly extracted the data by hand and sketched a run chart of the *rate* (infections per patient) in Exhibit 2.21. The run chart shows otherwise (common cause); note how you agree with me within 10 seconds. I have no doubt that these people worked very hard and probably did 149 root cause analyses, treating *each* infection as a special cause because they were unexpected events and "shouldn't" have happened. And I'm sure a lot of changes resulted, which only added complexity but not value. As Brian Joiner loves to say, "Vague solutions to vague problems yield vague results."[1]

What if they did a Pareto matrix on the aggregation of *all 149 infections* — a root cause analysis of their root cause analyses, if you will? When I show this to improvement practitioners in my seminars, I'm usually met with a stunned silence.

The time has come to speak up and stop tolerating meetings where useless displays like bar graphs result in destructive managerial actions or well-meaning, but ultimately ineffective, team actions.

### Key Points

- Plot the dots!
- All the hard work in the world won't improve performance.

EXHIBIT 2.17  Chart of Percentage Computer Uptime vs. Month

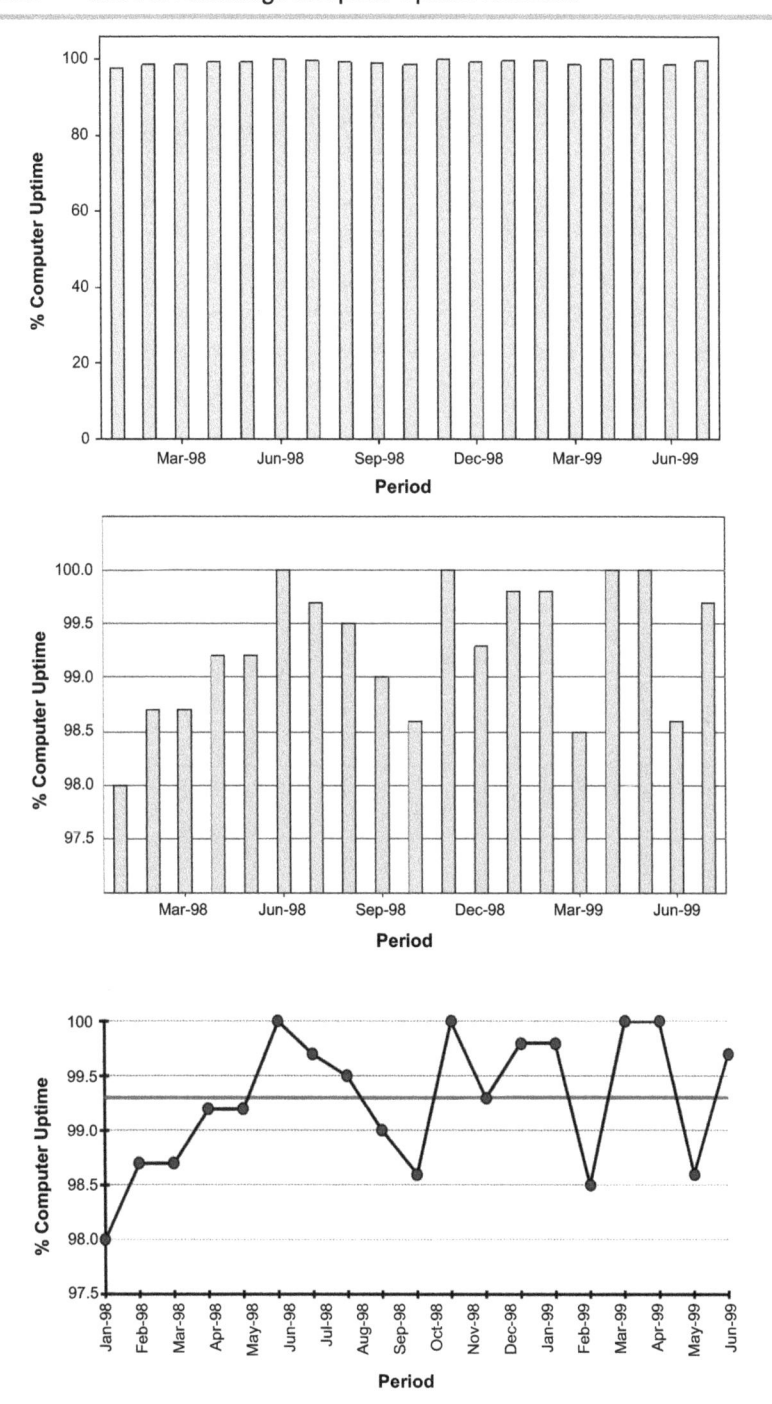

Source: Davis Balestracci Jr., MS, *Quality Digest,* June 2006. www.qualitydigest.com. Reprinted with permission.

**EXHIBIT 2.18** ■ MRSA Bacteremia 2001–2002 to 2005–2006

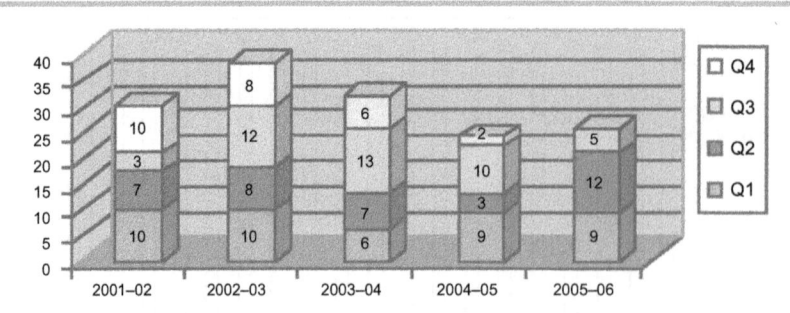

Source: Davis Balestracci Jr., MS, *Quality Digest*, June 2006. www.qualitydigest.com. Reprinted with permission.

**EXHIBIT 2.19** ■ Quarterly MRSA Bacteremias

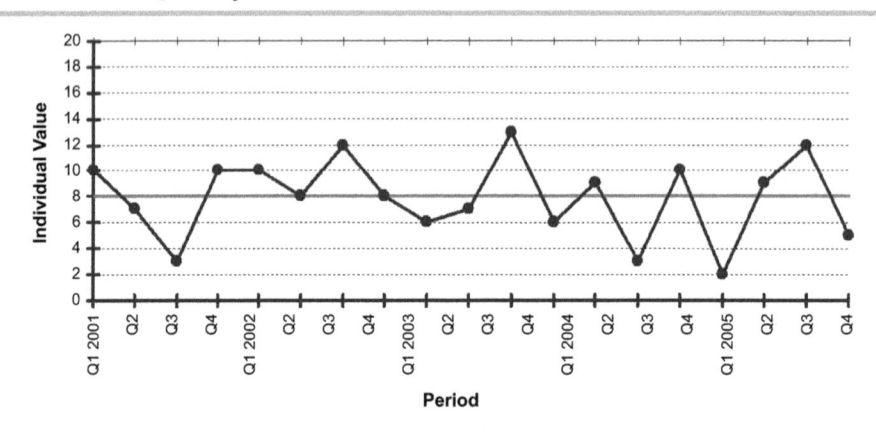

Source: Davis Balestracci Jr., MS, *Quality Digest*, June 2006. www.qualitydigest.com. Reprinted with permission.

- The chart is the proof!
- Looking at an aggregate produced by the same process is far more powerful than considering incidents one at a time.
- Common cause situations are more common that people think.

## Lesson 6: It's Time to Ignore the Traffic Lights

It has become increasingly routine to have executive data summaries prepared in the traffic light format with green representing figures that are within an acceptable range, yellow in a range of concern, and red showing data that is beyond what is considered acceptable. The problem with traffic light charts is that the intended audience of the chart responds to the colors rather than the underlying process producing the data and causes of variation.

In 2003 the United Kingdom was in the middle of a significant QI effort regarding its healthcare system. The government set 50 arbitrary targets to be met by each of 28

EXHIBIT 2.20 ■ Number of Infections and Number of Patients

Source: Davis Balestracci Jr., MS, *Quality Digest,* June 2006. www.qualitydigest.com. Reprinted with permission.

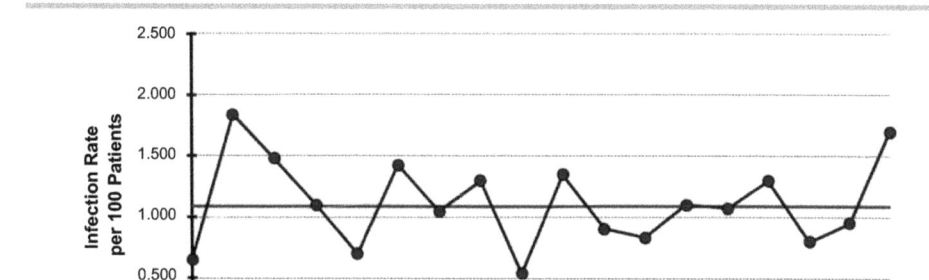

EXHIBIT 2.21 ■ Infection Rate

Source: Davis Balestracci Jr., MS, *Quality Digest,* June 2006. www.qualitydigest.com. Reprinted with permission.

regions. One particularly important target was the wait time at hospitals' accident and emergency (A&E) departments with a universal goal that patients must wait no longer than four hours at least 90 percent of the time. Exhibit 2.10 is an example of the weekly report sent to the government related to this target. If the performance was greater than 90 percent, it was reported as "green," while a performance between 85 percent and 90 percent was reported as "yellow," and a performance less than 85 percent was reported as "red."

The results frequently were debated for endless hours in meetings during which administrators would react to their hospitals' latest daily result, especially if it was red. It was customary on red days for managers to descend on the A&E department to expedite things, then hold meetings to go over every individual target breach to determine what

**EXHIBIT 2.22** ■ Region 28

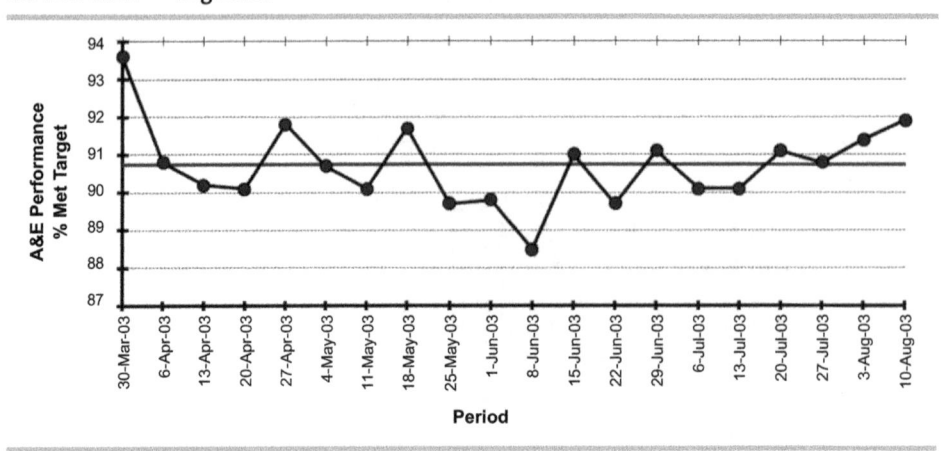

[Run chart: A&E Performance % Met Target vs Period from 30-Mar-03 to 10-Aug-03, with values ranging approximately 87 to 94, centerline around 90.7]

should have been done differently. In other words, every individual target breach (i.e., undesirable variation) on a red day was often treated as a special cause.

What if the administrators had simply assessed the true process behavior and/or variation by plotting the dots? The run chart for one of the 28 regions is shown in Exhibit 2.22 (median = 90.75). It shows no trends of six increases or decreases and no individual runs of eight or more. Therefore the data demonstrate common cause.

To further confirm common cause, (1) the common cause limits could easily be calculated as 87.6 to 93.8 (see Appendix 2A), between which the data fall and (2) any week can differ from its immediate predecessor by as much as 3.9. The largest week-to-week difference in this data is 2.8. Thus any number in that range cannot be given a traffic light interpretation and is indistinguishable from the average of 90.7. In fact, given a process-oriented definition of "meeting target" (*averaging* 90 percent), *this region was meeting it all along*. Also, despite all the time and energy being spent to improve this process, *there has been no change from April through August*.

*Red, yellow, and green is a plague on process.* There is zero value in looking at individual breaches, comparing week-to-week performances, or making breaches on red days special causes, as is done by many managers. In this wait-time example, red days are no different from target breaches on a yellow or green day. Nearly all the administrators had been responding to common cause results with special cause tactics.

Could the administrators apply a Pareto matrix to the last two weeks of breaches? Should they have investigated whether time of day or the day of the week influenced the process? Should they have asked whether the patient needed a laboratory test or X-ray or what percentage of patients ultimately required hospitalization?

I long for the day when red, yellow, and green tabular reports are replaced by solid theory, run charts, and charts with common cause limits. The math skills required include the ability to count to eight, subtract two numbers, and sort a list of numbers from lowest to highest, and use of simple addition and multiplication. These are easily done by hand during a meeting when people are wasting your time explaining tables of red, yellow, and green numbers.

The actual calculation of the common cause limits and the maximum difference between two consecutive data points for these data are shown in Appendix 2A.

### Key Points

- Using traffic light interpretation of literal current performance is wrong. The focus should be on the average of the most recent stable period as the process performance indicator.
- Red, yellow, and green targets are arbitrary and offer no concept of the process's common cause variation. They open the door to rampant inappropriate actions.
- "Is the difference from the goal common cause or special cause?" is the most important question to ask.
- In the case of percentage indicators, what percentage compliance is your process perfectly designed to attain, which also means, what percentage of the time is your process perfectly designed not to be compliant?
- Any target breach can be considered variation. "Is this breach due to a common cause or special cause?" is the deeper question.
- If a process is common cause, a breach on a red day is no different from a breach on a yellow day and is no different from a breach on a green day. You can aggregate all breaches to apply Pareto analysis.

### Lesson 7: Are You Perfectly Designed to Have Complaints?

*Even if events "shouldn't happen," your medical group practice might be perfectly designed to have them and keep having them.* Common cause strategies can help you analyze your processes, the variation within them, and the results.

I was at a hospital presenting to an audience of 150 people. All of a sudden, one board member stood up, interrupted me, and demanded that something be done about complaints. I took the organization's data (number of complaints and percentage of them resolved within 20 days) and projected the run charts shown in Exhibit 2.23.

In Exhibit 2.23a, you will note a run of eight above the median (observations 2–9) in the graph for total complaints. I looked at the date where this sequence ended and asked the audience, "What happened?" The two people responsible for collecting these data answered sheepishly, "We changed the definition of 'complaint.'"

After the change, however, things look pretty stable; they are perfectly designed to have complaints (common cause). And typically, each complaint was handled individually (Level 1 fix — special cause strategy; see Chapter 1). The run chart tells the story; there was no improvement. The person hired to deal with individual complaints will continue to be gainfully employed for as long as he or she wishes.

Over this time period, Exhibit 2.23b shows that the hospital has improved the rate at which it resolves complaints within 20 days. The beginning of the run chart shows it to be in a transition. It eventually levels off to what the new process is perfectly designed to get given the inputs that changed, which is around 75 to 80 percent. It can now be compared with any desired performance.

It is now perfectly designed to resolve 75 to 80 percent of complaints within 20 days, but it is also perfectly designed *not* to resolve 20 to 25 percent of complaints within 20 days. If the goal requires further improvement in that rate, the organization can now aggregate reasons for complaints not being resolved within 20 days. It can now do a

**EXHIBIT 2.23** ■ Run Charts of Total Complaints and Percentage Resolved Within 20 Days

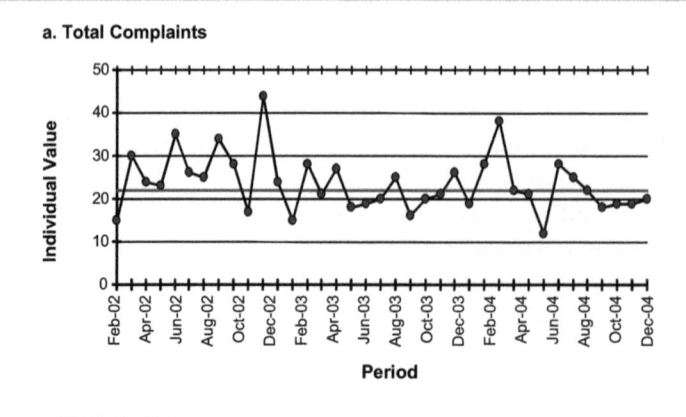

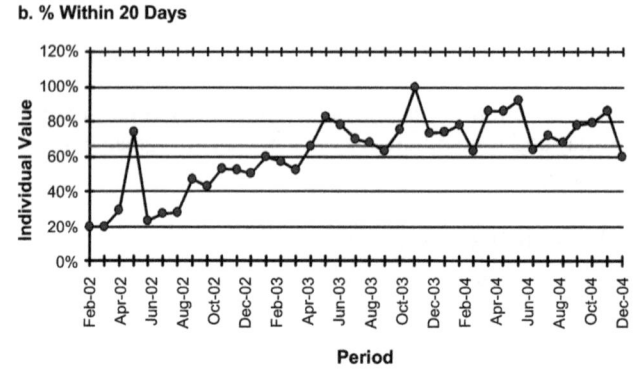

a. Total Complaints

b. % Within 20 Days

Pareto matrix of these reasons to see whether there might be any additional, currently hidden, opportunities to improve. What would *not* be helpful as a strategy is if a manager demanded, "You got 100 percent resolutions one month, so why can't you do it consistently? I'm giving you a short-term goal of at least 90 percent" (treating common cause as special cause).

When I created the control chart for total complaints (Exhibit 2.24), it was one of the few times I heard a collective gasp from an audience.

Even though the hospital is averaging about 22 complaints per month in any one month, the actual number will come in somewhere between 2 and 42 complaints, *and* one month can differ from the previous month by as many as 24. No wonder things *seemed* so chaotic. However, despite this wide variation, there is a saving grace: The process is *stable*, which allows the application of a common cause strategy. As a result, one can aggregate as many complaints as possible from the stable period to look for patterns. Because the organization is averaging around 20 complaints a month, maybe it should do a Pareto matrix of the most recent, say, seven to eight months, which would likely result in 150 to 200 complaints.

Are you becoming convinced of the power of this common cause strategy and how opportunities to apply it are virtually everywhere?

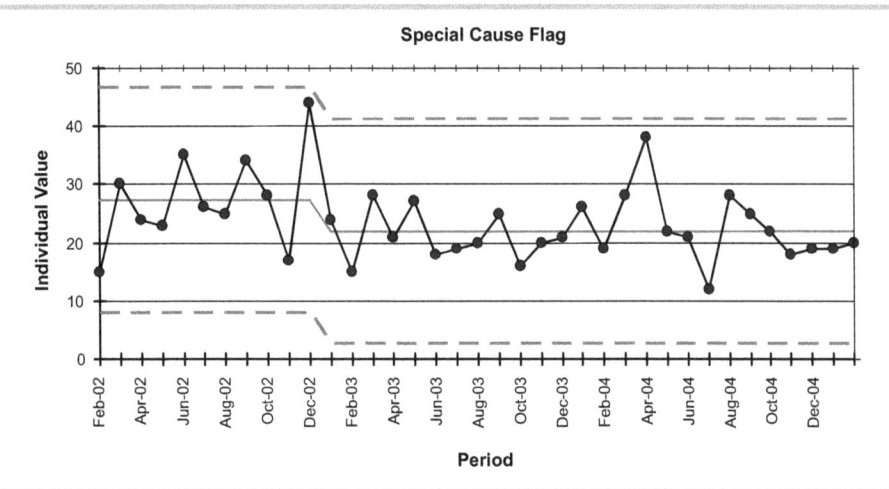

EXHIBIT 2.24 ■ Control Chart of Total Complaints (Monthly)

*Key Points*

- Complaints (unacceptable process variation) are yet another example of unexpected events that are perfectly designed results of a process.
- The intuitive Level 1 fix of treating every complaint as a special cause will not prevent future complaints.
- Not all process special causes are due to the methods input; many times, the measurement definition is the culprit.
- In spite of wide common cause variation that is intuitively unacceptable, common cause strategies for improvement can easily be applied because of the process's stability.

### Lesson 8: Budgeting as a Process?

How much executive and management time is spent on creating, then managing (and revising), the organization's budget? Is it 20 percent? 30 percent? All managers know what they should do come forecasting time; with best intentions, they put on rose-colored glasses. But how often has it happened that your best intentions get sidetracked, especially with unexpected expenses (which are typically treated as special causes)? Don't let yourself or your management get sidetracked on meaningless charts that treat actual vs. budgeted performance differences as special causes. Instead think of it as another opportunity to understand and apply the additional power of common cause strategies.

*Spending Patterns Don't Lie*

The organization's current processes are usually perfectly designed to consume what's being consumed, even if we wish differently.

A friend of mine had to attend meetings every two weeks to account for how she was doing vis-à-vis her budget. You all know these meetings. The manager goes around

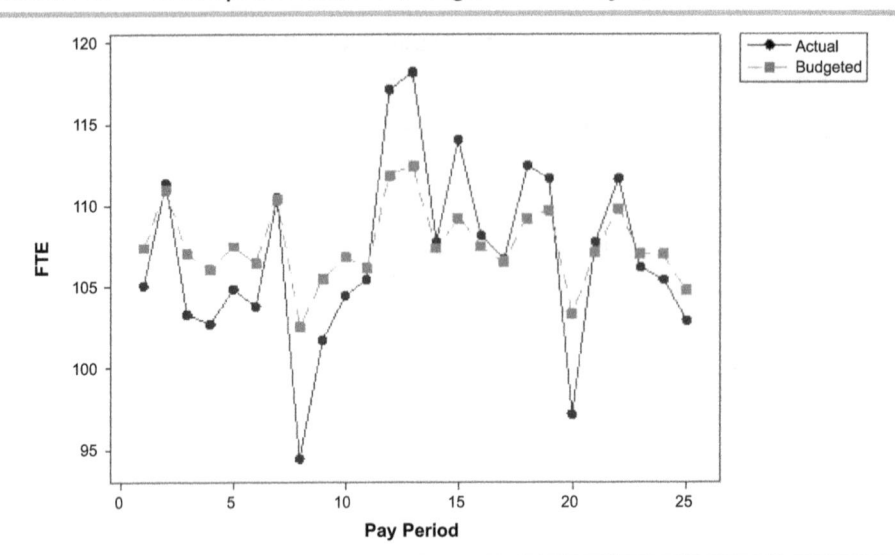

**EXHIBIT 2.25** ▪ Scatterplot of Actual FTE, Budgeted FTE vs. Pay Period

the table, asks why you're either over or under your budget (usually the former), and demands, "What are you going to do about it?"

A graph I repeatedly see is the simultaneous plotting of actual performance vs. budget, which I call a "mating earthworm plot." Exhibit 2.25 shows my friend's budget performance regarding her paid full-time equivalent (FTE). Note the recent string of 10 out of 11 periods above budget, although she received kudos during the most recent meeting because the last three periods are below budget.

How much of your time is spent at meetings where performance-vs.-budget graphs like this are presented? Or are they bar graphs, stacked bar graphs, or tables titled "This Month," "Variance to Budget ($)," "Percent Variance," "Last Month," "12 Months Ago," "Year-to-Date," and "Year-to-Date 12 Months Ago"? The little circles, finger-pointing, and excuse-making thrive in this data environment.

These routine meetings were driving my friend crazy, and she wanted me to help extract some sanity out of the situation. I asked her for the data, resulting in the two run charts seen in Exhibit 2.26. The one on the top is a run chart of her actual performance, and the other is a run chart of this actual performance minus the budgeted performance.

*The results show that her process was perfectly designed to get the results it has always gotten.* How can this make sense? What about the special cause in the graph on the bottom (observations 12–19 above the median)? There was a process change of sorts, and it wasn't my friend's methods of managing her money. The manager noted her initial history of coming in under budget and **cut her budget!** How could this change the results of the spending process she's currently perfectly designed to get?

It becomes even more dramatic when one does a control chart of the variance, as seen in Exhibit 2.27. As seen from the average of my friend's process *since the budget change, she's currently perfectly designed to settle approximately one FTE above budget* (the average). Yet her variance as calculated every two weeks will be in the range of –7 to 9, and one

## STATISTICAL THINKING AS A CONDUIT TO TRANSFORMATION

**EXHIBIT 2.26** ■ FTE and Variance to Budget

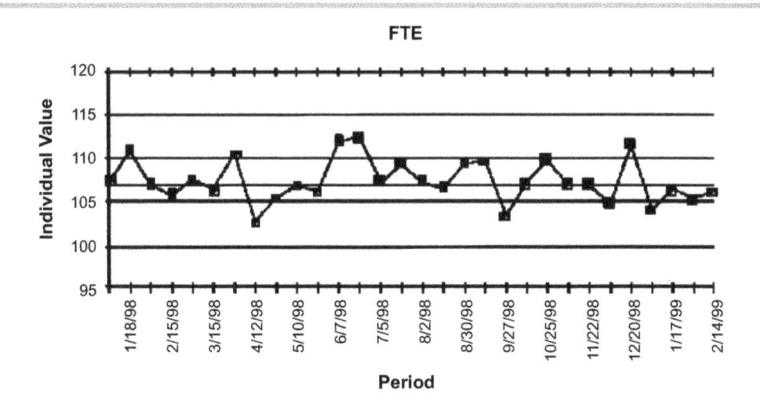

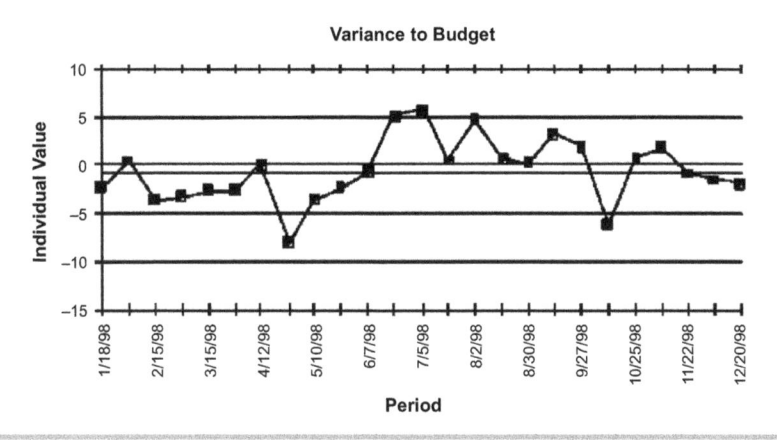

**EXHIBIT 2.27** ■ Variance to Budget

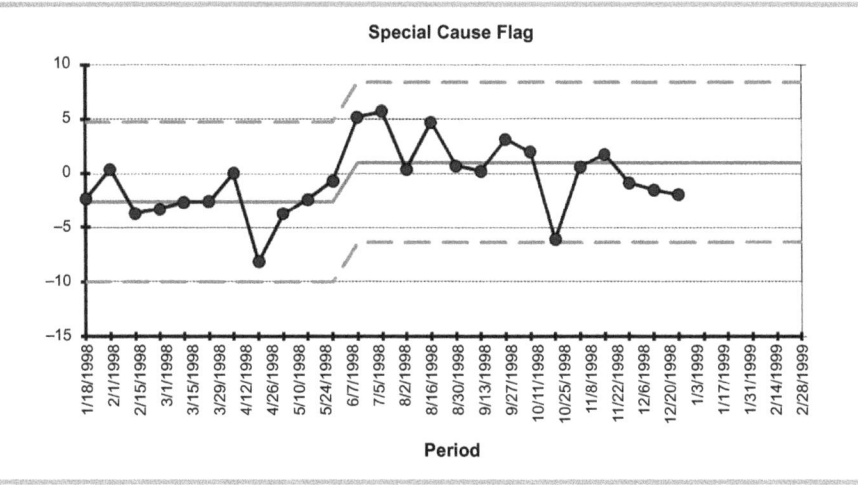

period can differ from its predecessor by as much as 10.1. The process has spoken, and it isn't as crazy as it many times feels.

The biweekly meetings looking at the current performance in a special cause fashion are a waste of time, and my friend *will* come in over budget. If the new budget is so important, why don't her managers do a Pareto matrix analysis of where the currently perfectly designed spending process's aggregated dollars have gone over this stable period?

*Key Points*

- Your budget process might be more perfectly designed than you think.
- Budgets are just arbitrary goals. The actual spending is what the process is perfectly designed to obtain.
- Variances are not necessarily special causes.
- It's not about managing the individual numbers, but the overall process producing the average.
- Common cause strategies could be very useful.

### Lesson 9: A Common Financial Technique Is Wrong and Invalidates Run Charts

There is a routine technique of rolling previous data that is used to calculate some key organizational financial figures. This method could lead you astray. It creates the appearance of special causes even when only common causes are present.

When given a set of data never seen before, two questions should become routine:

1. How were these data defined and collected?
2. Is any analysis appropriate, given the way the data were collected?

With that in mind, how would you analyze the three processes shown in Exhibits 2.28, 2.29, and 2.30?

Actually, despite appearances to the contrary, these are three plots of the *exact same data*. How were these data defined and collected? First, I generated 61 random, normal observations. Then I ran three processes:

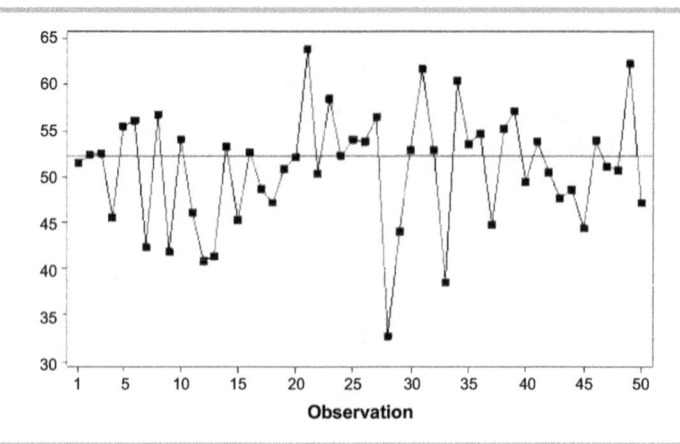

**EXHIBIT 2.28** ■ Run Chart of Process 1

**EXHIBIT 2.29** ■ Run Chart of Process 2

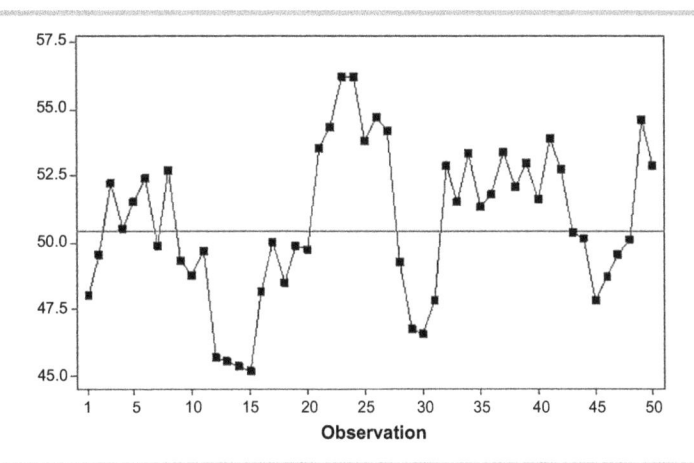

**EXHIBIT 2.30** ■ Run Chart of Process 3

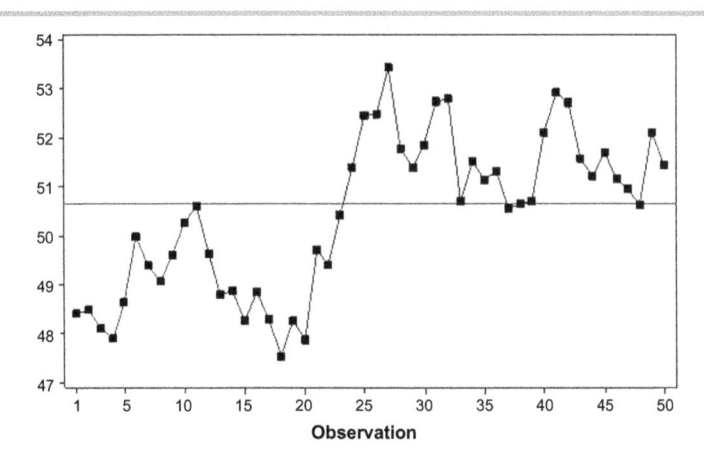

- *Process 1* is a run chart of observations 12–61, which are the last 50 observations. As you see, there are no special causes if you apply the trend rule and eight-in-a-row rule.
- *Process 2* is the same data except I rolled three previous observations into each data point then took the average. This is similar to a routine technique used in financial data, the *four-quarter rolling average*. The first data point is the average of observations 9–12, the second data point averages observations 10–13, and the final data point averages observations 58–61. Each data point has three points of "memory" from the previous data point. So it is indeed a plot of observations 12–61.
- *Process 3* is similar to the preceding process except that 11 previous observations have been rolled into each data point, then the average taken. This is comparable

**EXHIBIT 2.31** ■ Run Chart of Process Data Combined

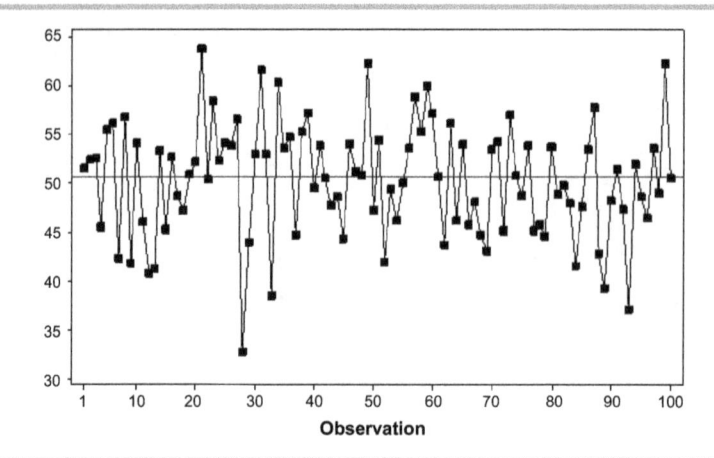

to the *12-month rolling average* (many times used to calculate days outstanding for accounts receivable). The first data point is the average of observations 1–12, the second data point averages observations 2–13, and the final data point averages observations 50–61. Each data point has 11 points of "memory" from the previous data point. Once again, it is a plot of observations 12–61.

As you see in these latter two plots, the two standard statistical run chart analysis rules have multiple violations; however, because of the memory inherent in each data point of these latter two processes, the usual runs analysis for taking action is *inappropriate for the way these data were defined and collected*: The observations are not independent. Control charts and any calculation of common cause would be equally invalid.

Next, I generated 50 more observations from the same process as Process 1, which were then appended to its chart (see Exhibit 2.28). The resulting run chart for these combined 100 observations is shown in Exhibit 2.31.

As expected, because of the nonoccurrence of the two run chart special cause rules, this plot confirms the process stability of the two combined sets of data. I then proceeded as before to generate and plot the rolling averages of 4 and 12, respectively, by appending the second set of data to the first and continuing the previous rolling calculations (Exhibits 2.32 and 2.33).

Note that the behavior in the second half of both of the rolling average graphs (see Exhibits 2.32 and 2.33) is totally different from the first half and equally incorrect. Even though the underlying process is stable, rolling the numbers creates the appearance of rampant instability all in the name of innocently trying to reduce variation through (allegedly) "smoothing" them. W. Edwards Deming was fond of using a quote from a Mobil Oil Company ad from 1972: "For every problem there is a solution: simple, neat, and wrong."[2]

This also creates extra, non-value-added work in an organization when explanations for these artificially created special causes (no doubt called "trends") are demanded, found, and acted upon.

Trying to smooth variation to make it go away does not make it disappear and creates special causes that aren't even there. Every process exhibits variation. So find the variation

EXHIBIT 2.32 ■ Run Chart of Combined Data Rolling Average of 4

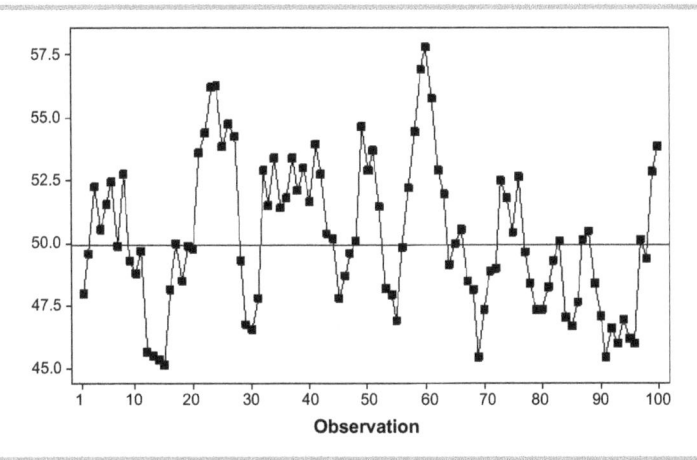

EXHIBIT 2.33 ■ Run Chart of Combined Data Rolling Average of 12

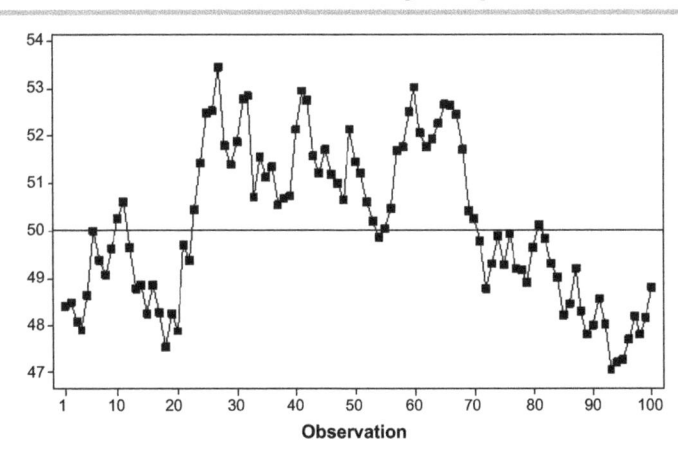

and understand it so that appropriate action can be taken. People don't like variation, but it can be easily handled (refer to Lesson 7). Ultimately it is not as difficult as you think, but to say that it is initially counterintuitive is a vast understatement.

### Key Points

- Well-meaning attempts to reduce variation do not make it disappear and can actually make it appear worse.
- Rolling average techniques can create appearances of special causes when there is only common cause.
- It is better to know what the actual common cause variation is to be able to react appropriately to improve a situation.

## Lesson 10: Understand the True Definitions of Above Average and Below Average

Ranking has become increasingly important as motivation for higher payment such as physician pay for performance and/or punishment for imposing harsh penalties. Benchmarking databases have categories such as above average or below average, quartiles, and 90th percentile performance. Organizations become concerned when one year's ranking drops 10 places from the previous year.

Can we bring some sanity to these processes through statistical thinking? Lessons 8 and 9 just scratch the surface of the power of truly understanding above average and below average. But remember, "20 percent of statistics will solve 80 percent of your problems." Moreover, it will stop the unintentional, unwitting, demotivating "crazy-making" that I've seen from misunderstanding this important concept.

It is routine for leaders to look at their data just to determine if they are above or below average or where they rank compared to other departments or organizations. The following examples demonstrate the dangers in some familiar ranking schemes.

### Comparing Performances

Suppose I had 30 people each flip a coin 50 times. How many results of heads would you expect each person to get? Your immediate tendency is to say 25. But ask yourself if every single person can get 25. From my experience, most people say, "Okay, probably between 20 and 30." Note that many prefer nice round numbers, usually ending in 0 or 5. Maybe some of you would say 15 or 35, but I doubt it; your intuition cannot accept that much variation. Exhibit 2.34 shows some simulated results of this scenario presented as a bar graph comparison.

How do we compare these 30 performances? Who is above average? Who is below average? Some people might mentally draw 20 and 30 on Exhibit 2.34. That yields two below-average performers and three above-average performers.

Some people might say, "Let's look at the top and bottom 10 percent." Others will say, "Let's look at the top and bottom 15 percent" (choose an arbitrary percentage ending

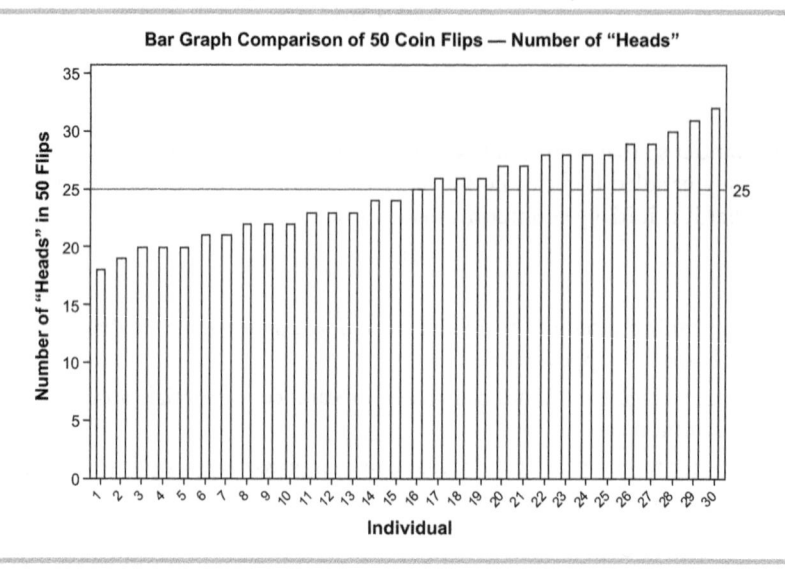

**EXHIBIT 2.34** ■ Bar Graph Comparison of Individual 50-Coin-Flip Performances

EXHIBIT 2.35 ■ Bar Graph Comparison of 30 Coin Flip Performances — 25th and 75th Percentiles Drawn in with the Average

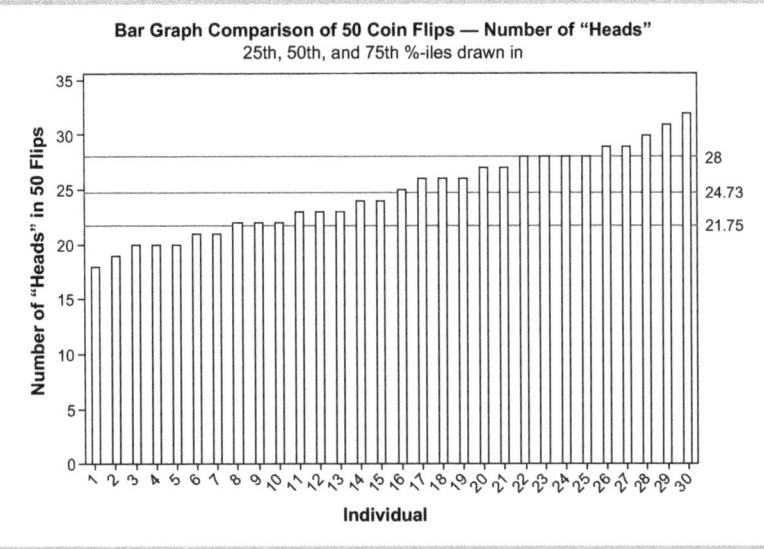

**Bar Graph Comparison of 50 Coin Flips — Number of "Heads"**
25th, 50th, and 75th %-iles drawn in

*[Bar graph showing Number of "Heads" in 50 Flips for Individuals 1-30, with horizontal reference lines at 28, 24.73, and 21.75]*

in 0 or 5). Some people want to be more statistical, so they say, "Put in the quartile lines to find the top and bottom quartiles of performers." I'm happy to oblige (Exhibit 2.35).

Some people might ask, "Are the data normally distributed?" I answer, "Yes, the *p*-value is 0.408."

They then dig way back into their brains and remember something about using the normal distribution and "two standard deviations" to declare outliers. And because they cannot afford to be so conservative, they say, "Put in one and two standard deviation lines around the average." Once again, I'm happy to oblige (Exhibit 2.36).

### *Mentally Drawing Little Circles: WAGs and SWAGs*

These attempts to reconcile the coin flip data are all variations on drawing little circles. There is diversity in how people are perceiving this variation: It represents a mixture of WAGs (wild a** guesses) and SWAGs (statistical wild a** guesses).

### *The Appropriate Analysis*

Exhibit 2.37 shows the only appropriate analysis for these data (I will spare you the math for now). Note that *there are no differences*. The line limits of 14 and 35 are calculated *from the data*, where LCL is the lower control limit and UCL is the upper control limit. Statistically, this means that any performance between 14 and 35 are no different from the average value. No evidence appears of any differences in performance, which also means there are no quartiles.

It can be seen as a different view of a control chart. However, the horizontal axis does not reflect time. It represents the distinct categories of comparison, so ordering is actually arbitrary. In this case, the comparison is being made by "individual." I chose to put the data in ascending order.

**EXHIBIT 2.36** ■ Bar Graph Comparison of 30 Coin Flip Performances — One and Two Standard Deviation Lines Around the Average

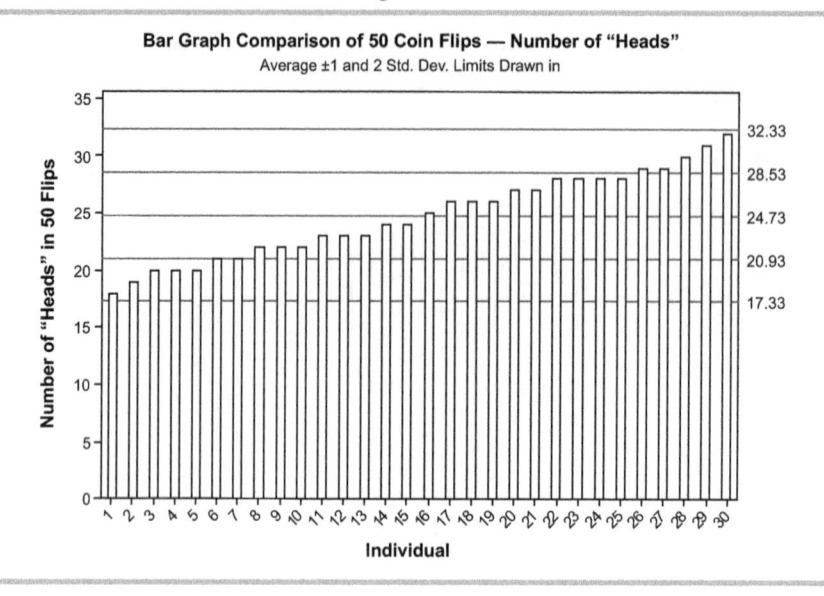

Bar Graph Comparison of 50 Coin Flips — Number of "Heads"
Average ±1 and 2 Std. Dev. Limits Drawn in

*[Bar graph showing 30 individuals with values increasing from ~18 to ~32. Reference lines at 32.33, 28.53, 24.73, 20.93, and 17.33.]*

**EXHIBIT 2.37** ■ Proper Analysis of Coin Flip Data via Analysis of Means

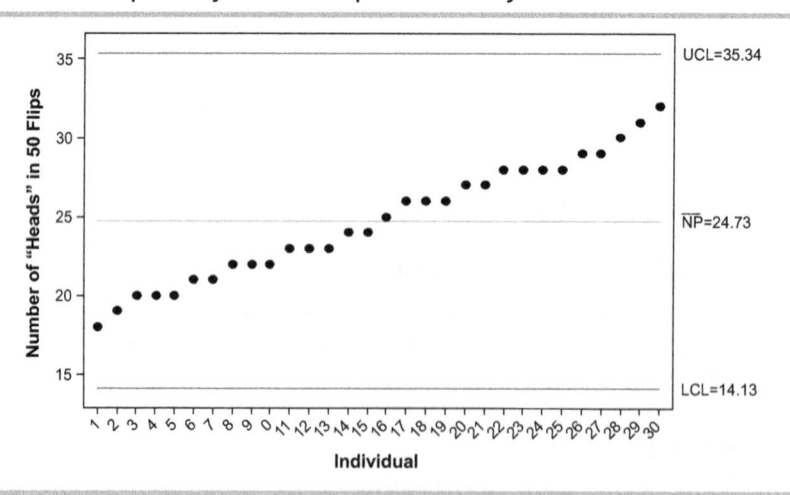

*[Dot plot showing 30 individuals with values from ~18 to ~32. UCL=35.34, $\overline{NP}$=24.73, LCL=14.13.]*

### What If This Situation Were a Group Practice Indicator?

Suppose these data represented some important aspect of performance of 30 group practices. One assumes valid reasons exist for this common grouping; their "processes" from carefully considered criteria (actually, process inputs) should be similar. Because such a comparison is considered a fair one, the practices are also assumed to be performing at the entire peer group's average (the process average) unless the data tell us otherwise. In other words, "Is any individual performance merely statistical variation on the average?"

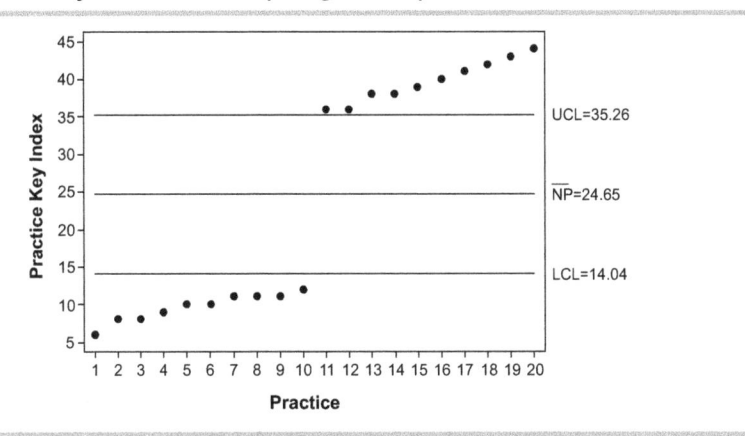

EXHIBIT 2.38 ■ Analysis of Means Comparing 20 Group Practices

*Back to Flipping Coins*

The process of flipping a coin 50 times and counting the number of heads is perfectly designed to get a number between 14 and 36. And in a roomful of people, no one can tell ahead of time who will get either the 14 (or the lowest number greater than or equal to it) or the 36 (or the highest number less than or equal to it). And if the coin flip is done again, different people will get those numbers. In essence, it is a lottery.

In comparing performance, why should people be penalized for poor performance if it could have been obtained randomly? Similar to the control chart, this type of comparison, referred to as analysis of means (ANOM), to be explained extensively in Chapter 7, calculates a band of common cause variation around the average. This common cause is used as a yardstick to declare special causes. It is only when data points are outside the common cause limits that they can be considered truly above or below average.

It is not unusual, as with this coin flip data, for there to be no above- or below-average performances. And it is important to note that there is no preset amount of outliers, such as "top 5 percent," "top 10 percent," "top quartile," "bottom quartile," "bottom 10 percent," and so forth.

So we arrive at another nugget of statistical wisdom: Given a set of numbers, 10 percent will be the top 10 percent. But are they truly above average?

I once obtained a graph comparing some group practices on a survey item that looked something like Exhibit 2.38. None of the practices was even "average" (between the UCL and LCL lines). It was originally thought that these 20 practices represented a fair comparison peer group. Obviously, they did not. What it did suggest was a fundamental difference between these two clusters, and looking at the practices as defined by these clusters found an underlying process factor of which they were unaware.

*Common Cause Calculations for Percentages Are Different*

Using ANOM is one of the few valid ways to compare percentage performances. The common cause calculations are different from those for a time-ordered control chart.

Even though these analyses involve the concept of standard deviation, they do not use the traditional calculation most people are taught in introductory statistics courses. This

EXHIBIT 2.39 ■ Stacked Bar Graph for Survey Result "Recommend the System?"

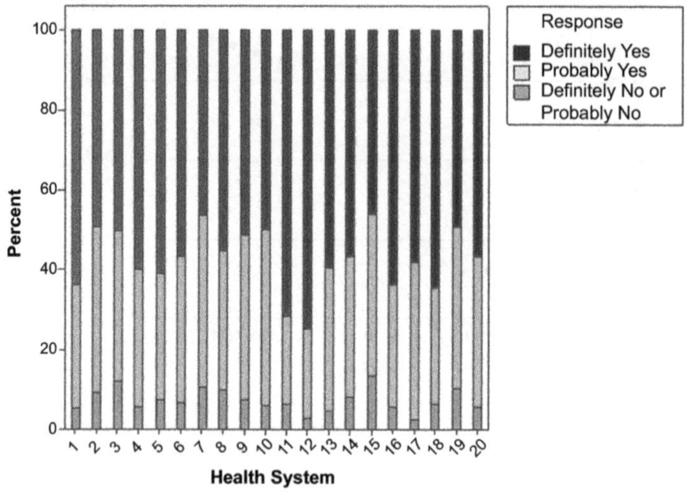

Source: Davis Balestracci Jr., MS, *Quality Digest,* March 2006. www.qualitydigest.com. Reprinted with permission.

particular calculation will be discussed in Chapter 7; my goal in this chapter is to show that what is important is not the mechanics of getting the graph, but its interpretation.

### Demanding These Presentations from Your Analysts

For board members, executives, and managers reading this book, some of you may not feel the need to know how to calculate these charts. Perhaps that is a valid attitude, but I hope you will be motivated to *demand* that data presentations be in this format; it would be a much better use of analysts' time and your own.

The important thing to realize is that a set of performances has an inherent common cause band that must be known to make fair comparisons. Many performance indicators are expressed as percentages, and the common cause band is dependent on how many events are in the denominator.

### Applying Analysis of Means to Patient Satisfaction Comparisons

To demonstrate once again the broad applicability to everyday data, the next example shows an application to a newspaper's published patient satisfaction comparison. This is a topic that makes most people — especially board members, executives, and middle managers reading this — perspire, and it is probably one of your organization's "vital 20 percent" of indicators.

The local paper published an article rating the 20 health systems in my metropolitan community. It used the graph in Exhibit 2.39 to chart responses to the question: "Would you recommend your clinic to adult friends or family members?"

I happened to work at System 19 and we were flagged in the dreaded bottom quartile. I was asked to investigate the data and was able to obtain them from the source (Exhibit 2.40).

EXHIBIT 2.40  System 19 Chart

| System | Definitely Yes | % Definitely Yes | Probably Yes | % Probably Yes | Pr / Def No | % Pr / Def No | Total Respondents |
|---|---|---|---|---|---|---|---|
| 1 | 158 | 64.0 | 76 | 30.8 | 13 | 5.3 | 247 |
| 2 | 121 | 49.6 | 101 | 41.4 | 22 | 9.0 | 244 |
| 3 | 125 | 50.6 | 92 | 37.2 | 30 | 12.1 | 247 |
| 4 | 147 | 60.0 | 83 | 33.9 | 14 | 5.7 | 245 |
| 5 | 151 | 61.1 | 78 | 31.6 | 18 | 7.3 | 247 |
| 6 | 138 | 56.6 | 89 | 36.5 | 16 | 6.6 | 244 |
| 7 | 114 | 46.7 | 104 | 42.6 | 26 | 10.7 | 244 |
| 8 | 138 | 55.4 | 86 | 34.5 | 25 | 10.0 | 249 |
| 9 | 125 | 51.7 | 99 | 40.9 | 18 | 7.4 | 242 |
| 10 | 124 | 50.2 | 108 | 43.7 | 15 | 6.1 | 247 |
| 11 | 176 | 71.5 | 53 | 21.5 | 16 | 6.5 | 246 |
| 12 | 186 | 75.3 | 55 | 22.3 | 7 | 2.8 | 247 |
| 13 | 146 | 59.6 | 88 | 35.9 | 11 | 4.5 | 245 |
| 14 | 139 | 57.0 | 85 | 34.8 | 20 | 8.2 | 244 |
| 15 | 113 | 46.1 | 99 | 40.4 | 33 | 13.5 | 245 |
| 16 | 156 | 63.9 | 74 | 30.3 | 14 | 5.7 | 244 |
| 17 | 144 | 58.3 | 97 | 39.3 | 6 | 2.4 | 247 |
| 18 | 159 | 64.6 | 71 | 28.9 | 16 | 6.5 | 246 |
| 19 | 120 | 49.4 | 97 | 39.3 | 25 | 10.3 | 243 |
| 20 | 140 | 56.9 | 92 | 37.4 | 14 | 5.7 | 246 |
|  | 2,820 (Total) | 57.4% (Average) | 1,727 (Total) | 35.2% (Average) | 359 (Total) | 7.3% (Average) | 4,909 (Total) |

Source: Davis Balestracci Jr., MS, *Quality Digest*, March 2006. www.qualitydigest.com. Reprinted with permission.

It is a classic customer satisfaction survey on a 1–4 scale, where 1 = definitely not; 2 = probably not; 3 = probably yes; and 4 = definitely yes. Note that Exhibit 2.39 combines the "definitely not" and "probably not" responses.

Rather than calculate a weighted score (which has a shaky basis), re-ranking and using the Ouija board to interpret the 20 numbers, I decided to do two analyses via a percentage chart ANOM: the first for the "definitely yes" data and the second for the combined "definitely not" and "probably not" data.

As you can see from Exhibit 2.41, the overall average of the 20 systems is 57.4 percent of the people answering "definitely yes." So the real question should be, "Given the overall average of 57.4 percent, is our system's difference from the overall average common or special cause?" or, put another way, "What range of percentages is expected if a process has an average of 57.4 percent, 250 surveys are sent out, and no one is a special cause?"

Looking at the common cause limits, which are the two horizontal lines on either side of the average, any results between 48 and 66.9 percent are statistically *indistinguishable* from each other as well as from the overall average of 57.4 percent.

Another obsession with data like these is to rank the 20 systems via quartiles. In this case:

- Quartile 1 (i.e., best): 1, 11*, 12*, 16, 18
- Quartile 2: 4, 5, 13, 17, 20
- Quartile 3: 3, 6, 8, 9, 14
- Quartile 4 (i.e., worst): 2, 7**, 10, 15**, 19

EXHIBIT 2.41 ■ Analysis of Means for "Family and Friends Recommendation": Comparison by System "Definitely Yes"

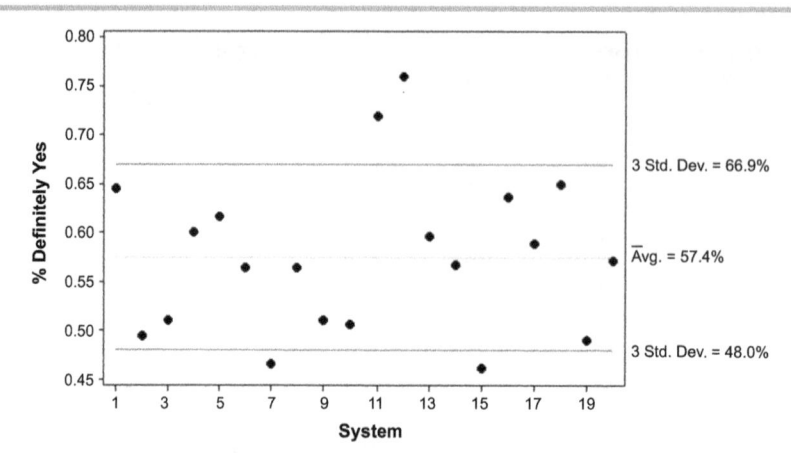

[Chart: % Definitely Yes by System (1-20); Avg. = 57.4%, 3 Std. Dev. = 66.9% (upper), 3 Std. Dev. = 48.0% (lower)]

Source: Davis Balestracci Jr., MS, *Quality Digest*, March 2006. www.qualitydigest.com. Reprinted with permission.

Using the statistical criteria, Systems 11 and 12 are truly above average (*) and Systems 7 and 15 are truly below average (**).

Based on this data, System 19 happened to lose the lottery. I'm sure Systems 1, 16, and 18 were no doubt quick to take advantage of their lottery win and design new marketing materials saying, "We are in the top quartile of clinics recommended by family and friends."

Similarly, for people answering "definitely no" or "probably no," the system average is 7.3 percent. A similar analysis was performed in Exhibit 2.42, except this system's average of 7.3 percent was used. Any results between 2.3 and 12.3 percent are statistically indistinguishable from each other as well as from the overall average of 7.3 percent.

Using quartiles (given the nature of the question, a higher number indicates poor performance):

- Quartile 1 (i.e., worst): 3, 7, 8, 15*, 19
- Quartile 2: 2, 5, 6, 9, 14,
- Quartile 3: 4, 10, 11, 16, 18
- Quartile 4 (i.e., best): 1, 12, 13, 17, 20

Using the statistical criteria, no system is truly above average (good performance) and System 15 is truly below average (*) (poor performance).

Based on this data, System 19 once again happened to lose the lottery. But it's just a matter of time. Maybe System 19 will win next year or maybe another survey done by someone else will exonerate them.

How many hours are you spending in meetings looking at data like this? Wouldn't you rather have new, different, productive conversation? Maybe you don't know or even want to know how to make these relatively simple calculations, but I'm willing to bet that you have someone in your organization who can or would be absolutely delighted to learn.

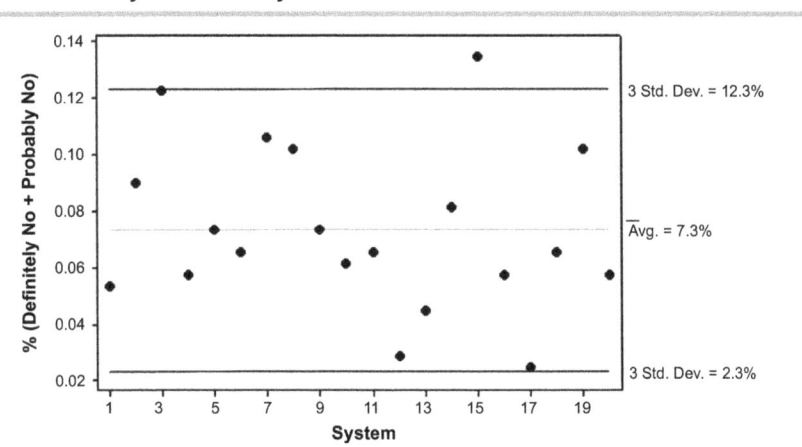

EXHIBIT 2.42 ■ Analysis of Means for "Family and Friends Recommendation": Comparison by System "Definitely No + Probably No"

[Chart: scatter plot of % (Definitely No + Probably No) vs System (1–19), with 3 Std. Dev. = 12.3%, Avg. = 7.3%, and 3 Std. Dev. = 2.3%]

Source: Davis Balestracci Jr., MS, *Quality Digest*, March 2006. www.qualitydigest.com. Reprinted with permission.

### Key Points

- Given a set of numbers, 25 percent will be the top quartile and 25 percent will be the bottom quartile (and 10 percent will be the top 10 percent and half will be above average).
- Even ranked performance comparisons need to take common cause into consideration as a yardstick for exposing true differences and special causes such as "above average" and "below average."
- The process will tell you what the common cause is.
- There is no preset arbitrary percentage of either good or poor performers.
- It is not unusual for a set of ranked numbers to have no outliers, such as the preceding "definitely not + probably not" analysis in which there were no exceptional performers.

If this example has piqued your interest, I highly recommend that you read an article called "Can Chance Make You a Killer?" and try out its simulator (www.bbc.co.uk/news/magazine-10729380).[3] I hope you will become outraged at the games being played with your data that result in arbitrary rewards but, more often, arbitrary punishments...*that take time away from improving patient care.*

### Case Study: Even a World Leader in Quality Doesn't Get It

After 20 years of teaching statistical principles, I'm still amazed at the fierce resistance I get from leaders. It is inconceivable to me how any leader with a true passion for excellence would refuse to understand simple variation, especially given the enormous power such understanding would unleash in an organization. Deming himself said, "If I had to reduce my message for management to just a few words, I'd say it all had to do with reducing variation."[4]

This case study uses rankings. Often, when people are trying to make comparisons, they will rank groups on several factors and then use the sum of their respective ranks to come to a conclusion.

I attended a talk given by a world leader in quality (WLQ), and most of you know of him. He presented the data in Exhibit 2.43 as a bar graph, as shown in Exhibit 2.44, without any context of variation for interpretation. Each number is the sum of rankings for 10 aspects of 21 counties' healthcare systems. (Lower sums are better: minimum = 10; maximum = 210; average = $10 \times 11 = 110$.) He talked quite a bit about quartiles, which of course aroused my suspicion.

I wrote and asked him for the data including the individual rankings (see Appendix 7A for actual data), and he graciously complied.

There is a surprisingly simple (for a statistician) statistical analysis using the combined individual sets of rankings as responses. This is known as the Friedman test (explained in detail in Lesson 1 of Appendix 7A using data from this chapter). In this case, its $p$-value is 0.001, which means if I conclude that there are differences in the scores of these 21 counties, there is less than one-in-a-thousand chance that I'm wrong, which are pretty good odds.

**EXHIBIT 2.43** County Healthcare Rank Sum

| Rank Sum | County |
|---|---|
| 42 | 1 |
| 76 | 2 |
| 84 | 3 |
| 87 | 4 |
| 92 | 5 |
| 99 | 6 |
| 101 | 7 |
| 102 | 8 |
| 105 | 9 |
| 105 | 10 |
| 107 | 11 |
| 108 | 12 |
| 112 | 13 |
| 113 | 14 |
| 114 | 15 |
| 121 | 16 |
| 128 | 17 |
| 131 | 18 |
| 145 | 19 |
| 157 | 20 |
| 181 | 21 |

Source: Davis Balestracci Jr., MS, *Quality Digest*, September 2006. www.qualitydigest.com. Reprinted with permission.

There's little doubt that differences exists among counties. Two standard calculations can determine how much of a difference between counties' scores is considered too much. On the conservative side, I will say a difference of greater than 91 between two counties is significant. If I am willing to take a risk, a second calculation would declare a difference of more than 51 between two counties to be significant.

**EXHIBIT 2.44** Bar Graph of Sums Ranked by County

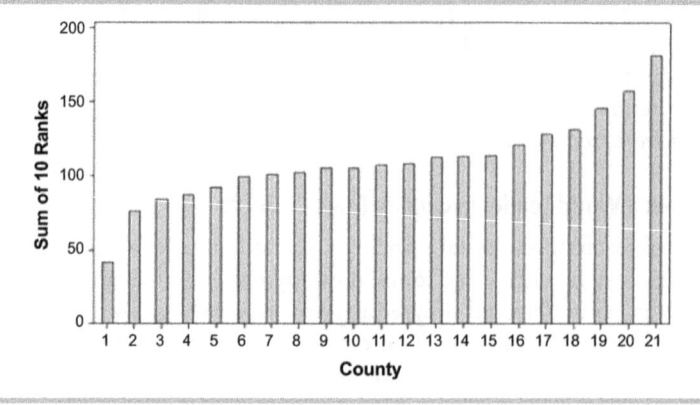

# STATISTICAL THINKING AS A CONDUIT TO TRANSFORMATION

**EXHIBIT 2.45** Analysis of Means Comparing 10-Score Rank Sums: Comparison by County

[Chart: Overall $p = 0.05$ & $p = 0.01$ decision lines shown. Y-axis: 10-Rank Sum. X-axis: County (1-21). Reference lines at $+3.5SL=174.6$, $+3.1SL=165.9$, $\bar{X}=110$, $-3.1SL=54.1$, $-3.5SL=45.4$.]

Source: Davis Balestracci Jr., MS, *Quality Digest*, September 2006. www.qualitydigest.com. Reprinted with permission.

Given the table of these scores and the two criteria for declaring differences, I could present this data at a meeting and there would still be a lot of human variation in interpretation.

### *What Is the Data Sane Alternative?*

We can also use a variation of ANOM similar to the application in Lesson 10; in this case, establishing common cause limits around the average of 110. This results in the graph shown in Exhibit 2.45. The two sets of horizontal lines on either side of the average (±3.5 SL [sigma limits] and ±3.9 SL) are, respectively, criteria for overall 5 percent and 1 percent risks of declaring something significantly different from the average when it is not. Note that two counties (No. 1 and No. 21) fall outside the wider limits (<1 percent risk of being wrong).

Given this graph, the statistical interpretation would be that there's one truly outstanding county (No. 1) and one county truly below average in performance (No. 21). The other 19 counties are, based on these data, indistinguishable and *cannot be ranked*. Note that the largest difference between the common cause counties (No. 2 and No. 20) is 81, which is within the conservative criterion of needing to be more than 91 to be declared significantly different.

I shared this fascinating analysis with WLQ, and our e-mail correspondence follows:

> WLQ. A subtle issue you did not tackle is the political-managerial issue of communicating such insights to [the two special-cause counties] and the counties that thought they were "different" but, statistically, aren't. I wonder what framework one could use to approach that psychological challenge.
>
> DAVIS. Hey, I'm just the statistician, man! ...I think the issue is how people and leaders like *you* plan to facilitate these difficult conversations, which will be profoundly different and more productive. This is the leadership that quality

gurus keep alluding to and which seems to be in such short supply. I'd be a willing participant in these discussions, but my job is first to keep you all out of the "data swamp." Although I'd love to pilot some of these conversations with you or other leaders, we must first figure out what this process should be. What we decide could help the quality improvement movement take a quantum leap forward and that prospect is exciting. ...[This] "language" must be a fundamental piece of any improvement process. People who understand the language and who are promoted because of it must lead the process. If this trend could become culturally inculcated, then the defensiveness would stop. The discussion would then focus, as it should, on process. I've seen far too much concern about "hurting people's feelings." This new focus would change that, as well as support conversations that could lead to appropriate action. ...We need new conversations, and this could be a key catalyst.

WLQ. Nope. I don't buy it. Yes, I am a leader and need to carry the message. But I know you too well to let you off the hook. I'd love to see you try to lead these conversations and experiment with approaches. You're a leader, too.

DAVIS. Give me an opportunity, and I will do my best to lead that conversation (and feel that we could begin by co-facilitating it). *Have you fathomed the potential of this?*

That was in 2006 and I'm still waiting for a reply and/or opportunity. I haven't received a response to further e-mails.

Can you see the potential implications of this simple example? Please accept my challenge to wean your cultures from (1) drawing circles around numbers; (2) looking at smiley faces, bar graphs, trend lines, and traffic light data interpretations; (3) comparing numbers to goals and throwing tantrums; or (4) thinking that the patronizing platitudes sold in airport bookstores are leadership substitutes.

### Key Points

- Even for a comparison approach that is intuitive, in this case, summing up a series of rankings, variation still exists and its magnitude could be surprising.
- The process always tells you what this variation is.
- When comparing a group of things that "should" be similar, treat them as a system with a common average. Anything falling in between the common cause limits around the average cannot be ranked and are indistinguishable from each other and from the overall average.

## SUMMARY

This chapter was intended to create an eye-opening awareness of the importance of integrating good data skills based in process-oriented thinking into everyone's daily work. It will transform your organization and create the time for quality improvement.

A key change in management thinking is the realization that everything is a process and that leaders are managing processes. It is only by studying process variation and reducing inappropriate and unintended variation that organizational progress on key goals is made, especially if you dare apply it to the budgeting process.

To summarize the chapter's key concepts:
- Plot the dots. A lot of questions need to be asked before you can get a run chart: What exactly should be plotted? How should the number be defined? How often should it be collected? Where should it be collected? Who is going to collect it? What is the proposed action? Is it collected in such a way that you can take the proposed action?
- The two *basic* statistical rules of run charts are (1) the statistical definition of trend (and its rare observance) and (2) the eight in a row, either all above or all below the median.
- A context of variation to interpret *any* sequence or list of numbers is needed.
- Beware of rolling averages; averaging out variation does not make variation disappear and will even create special cause patterns that are not there.
- Recognize common cause vs. special cause by thinking of the 50 coin flips and the resulting range of 14 to 36 heads outcomes and remembering that summed rank data can be analyzed statistically.
- Commit to more routine use of common cause strategy, especially the Pareto matrix.

For transformation to take root in a culture, all levels of management, supervision, and informal culture leaders should initially become proficient in the skills listed in Exhibit 2.46 and display their behaviors.

### EXHIBIT 2.46 ▪ Management Skills Required for Improvement and Transformation

- Resist the tendency to treat every problem (i.e., undesirable variation) that walks into one's office as a special cause and immediately solve it. Facilitate the employees who work in the situation to understand the sources of variation and address root causes. React with questions, not necessarily action. Get some data if at all possible.
- Facilitate the conversion of anecdotes about perceived problems into data; design a data collection on work in progress or a flowchart to document the process (or lack of a process) within which the anecdote is occurring. Good data are helpful in stripping the emotion out of a situation and getting a helpful preexisting measure of the problem's extent.
- Take a good, hard assessment of current data collections and reports. Question the objective of each: how it is collected and measured, and whether it adds any value to the organization. (Is it answering the question that it really needs to answer?)
- Avoid overuse of written surveys. Organizations tend to make written surveys amorphous in objectives and overload them with excess baggage. Instead, substitute routine talking to customers, both internal and external, through focus groups and help clarify perceptions of troublesome situations. When necessary, this will focus the objectives of any subsequent data collection and result in simple, efficient surveys that can be meaningfully analyzed (see Chapter 10).
- Do not react to numbers alone, whether presented in tables or individually. Instead, use graphical displays (run charts, control charts, analyses of means) to understand and react appropriately to variation. Insist that data reports be presented in a similar format.
- Use the time saved by implementing data sanity to conduct walk-arounds and educate the culture to the need for process-oriented thinking; data sanity; and simple, ongoing displays of process performances.

These skills should become routine. Simultaneously demonstrating their use to the culture through your behavior creates an atmosphere in which transformation has a chance to flourish and succeed. The fact that these are tangible skills to be immediately applied will accelerate comprehension of their subtleties. People must obtain core competency skills to become process oriented in evaluating a situation (reduce inappropriate and unintended process variation for better prediction), data oriented for understanding vague situations (use Pareto analysis to isolate major opportunities; be aware of common cause vs. special cause strategy), and chart oriented in displaying and analyzing data (keep in mind process baselines for all key organizational indicators, the effects of interventions and holding gains, and a nontampering response to variation). Ask appropriate questions in reaction to variation, ask more questions and verify with data, and avoid arbitrary numerical goals and the tendency to treat *any* variance from a goal as special cause.

## APPENDIX 2A: CALCULATING COMMON CAUSE LIMITS FOR A TIME-ORDERED SEQUENCE

Exhibit 2A.1 shows the data used in Lesson 6. I now use them to show how to obtain the calculated common cause performance range of 87.6 to 93.8 on the resulting control chart.

Column 1 contains the weekly time stamp of the data, and column 2 contains the data in their natural weekly time order.

In column 3, I calculate what is statistically called the *moving range*. It is formed by taking the absolute value of the difference between two consecutive numbers in the natural sequence.

For example, the first two moving ranges are (90.8 − 93.6) = −2.8 (absolute value = 2.8) and (90.2 − 90.8) = −0.6 (absolute value = 0.6); the process continues down to the last two numbers: (91.9 − 91.4) = 0.5.

In column 4, these moving ranges are then sorted so that the *median moving range* ($MR_{Med}$) can be found. It is the key number for all subsequent calculations.

For these data, 20 data points yield 19 moving ranges. To determine the median, use the number of numbers, [(19 + 1)/2] = 10. This means that the 10th *sorted* moving range is the $MR_{Med}$.

For these data, $MR_{Med}$ = 1.0, and it is used in the following two calculations.

One month can differ from its *immediately preceding* month by as much as:

$$3.865 \times 1.0 = 3.9$$

As observed from the table, none of the moving ranges exceeded 3.9.

For the expected range of performance:

$$90.7 \pm [3.14 \times 1.0] = [87.6 - 93.8]$$

The values 3.865 and 3.14 are constants derived from statistical theory. They are always used with any time sequence of data from which a median moving range has been calculated. They never change.

From statistical theory, the maximum difference between two consecutive data points in a time sequence is:

$$(3.865 \times MR_{Med})$$

The naturally occurring variation to be expected from a process, if the run chart shows no special causes, is:

EXHIBIT 2A.1  Accident and Emergency Conformance to Goal Data

| Date | Region 28 | Moving Range | Sorted Moving Ranges |
|---|---|---|---|
| March 30, 2003 | 93.6% | — | 0 |
| April 6, 2003 | 90.8% | 2.8 | 0.1 |
| April 13, 2003 | 90.2% | 0.6 | 0.1 |
| April 20, 2003 | 90.1% | 0.1 | 0.3 |
| April 27, 2003 | 91.8% | 1.7 | 0.5 |
| May 4, 2003 | 90.7% | 1.1 | 0.6 |
| May 11, 2003 | 90.1% | 0.6 | 0.6 |
| May 18, 2003 | 91.7% | 1.6 | 0.6 |
| May 25, 2003 | 89.7% | 2.0 | 1.0 |
| June 1, 2003 | 89.8% | 0.1 | 1.0 (Median) |
| June 8, 2003 | 88.5% | 1.3 | 1.1 |
| June 15, 2003 | 91.0% | 2.5 | 1.3 |
| June 22, 2003 | 89.7% | 1.3 | 1.3 |
| June 29, 2003 | 91.1% | 1.4 | 1.4 |
| July 6, 2003 | 90.1% | 1.0 | 1.6 |
| July 13, 2003 | 90.1% | 0 | 1.7 |
| July 20, 2003 | 91.1% | 1.0 | 2.0 |
| July 27, 2003 | 90.8% | 0.3 | 2.5 |
| August 3, 2003 | 91.4% | 0.6 | 2.8 |
| August 10, 2003 | 91.9% | 0.5 | |

$$\text{Average} \pm (3.14 \times MR_{Med})$$

In this case, only because the run chart showed no special causes, you can calculate the average of all the data, which is 90.7. Noting the range of common cause, overlap appears between the weekly "green" performance and the "**yellow**" performance goals.

The resulting control chart is shown in Exhibit 2A.2.

This further confirms the initial run chart analysis that no significant change has taken place in this process in almost five months despite multiple daily efforts to improve it. And note that the three weeks in a row of **yellow** performance (items 9–11) cannot be distinguished from random variation.

However, you do *not* have to accept this level of performance. Chances are that improvement efforts have been using *special cause strategies* (reacting to every data point or incident that was felt to be an aberration or didn't meet the standard). It is most likely that a *common cause strategy* will be more productive — most likely, a Pareto matrix to start with.

**EXHIBIT 2A.2** ▪ Control Chart of Accident and Emergency Weekly Performance

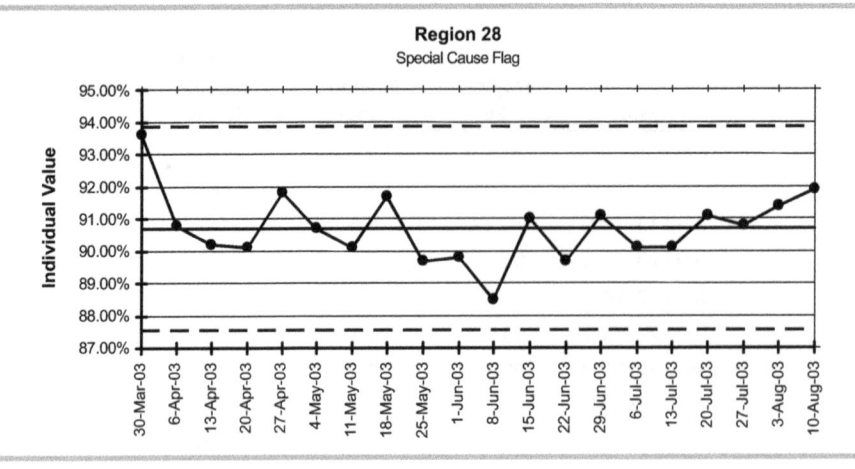

## REFERENCES

1. Joiner, Brian L. 1994. *Fourth Generation Management: The New Business Consciousness.* New York: McGraw-Hill.
2. Deming, W. Edwards. 2000. *Out of the Crisis,* 388. Cambridge: MIT Press.
3. Blastland, Michael. July 23, 2010. "Can chance make you a killer?" *BBC News Magazine.* www.bbc.co.uk/news/magazine-10729380.
4. Neave, Henry R. 1990. *The Deming Dimension,* 57. Knoxville, TN: SPC Press.

## RESOURCES

American Society for Quality (ASQ) Statistics Division. 2000. *Improving Performance through Statistical Thinking.* Milwaukee, WI: ASQ Quality Press.

Conover, W.J. 1998. *Practical Nonparametric Statistics,* 3rd ed. New York: Wiley.

McCoy, Ron. 1994. *The Best of Deming.* Knoxville, TN: SPC Press.

Ott, Ellis R., Edward G. Schilling, and Dean V. Neubauer. 2005. *Process Quality Control: Troubleshooting and Interpretation of Data,* 4th ed. Milwaukee, WI: ASQ Quality Press.

Wheeler, Donald J. 1993. *Understanding Variation: The Key to Managing Chaos.* Knoxville, TN: SPC Press.

CHAPTER 3

# A Leadership Belief System: Basic Skills for Transforming Culture

*Faced with the choice between changing one's mind and proving there is no need to do so, almost everybody gets busy on the proof.*
— *John Kenneth Galbraith*

---

### KEY IDEAS

- Most quality improvement efforts have had disappointing results because of overemphasis on internal education focusing on "process," "tools," and "data." They are only the tip of an underlying seven-layer organizational pyramid, of which the underlying "human" process is actually more important.
- Success will require dealing effectively with the *natural* cultural resistance to being changed.
- People's stated reasons for resisting change may not be what they really mean; *all* change is a perceived threat to basic needs.
- A culture rich in feedback will be required for true transformation.
- Feedback needs to be results based, in the moment, and focused on specific *behaviors* that are not demonstrating commitment to organizational results.
- Feedback needs to be given with genuine concern for individuals' organizational success.
- A simple, practical model based in cognitive psychology applies both to individuals' behaviors and tolerated organizational behaviors and subsequent results.
- New results will require new organizational and individual "beliefs."

---

### FEELING STUCK?

It all seems so logical, doesn't it? Focus on processes, improve your management and clinical processes and decision making through using quality improvement (QI) tools, give people good technical and administrative information, and the organization should get better. As I alluded to in the introduction, it is tempting, more interesting, and dramatic to lead in the vein of *Star Trek* Captain Jean-Luc Picard: "Make it so." However, in more than 25 years of facilitating QI, I have learned one thing: Change would be so easy if it were not for all the people.

Before delving deeper into data and process analysis, we must first look at the process of introducing change in organizations. Without understanding how people and organizations react when faced with change, none of the QI efforts will be successful.

The learning organization is here to stay. Yet adult learners are a particularly ornery breed, and it is delusional to expect that intensive in-house seminars will somehow allow participants to attain anything even close to mastery when comfortable old habits are threatened. Further, leadership carries a naive assumption that employees will, upon being trained in such seminars, subsequently choose to act on the knowledge when back at their jobs, which they perceive to take up more than 100 percent of their time. So, we need to keep in mind some timeless classic wisdom from more than 70 years ago that is just as applicable today: "When we are dealing with people, let us remember we are not dealing with creatures of logic. We are dealing with creatures of emotion, creatures bustling with prejudices and motivated by pride and vanity."[1]

## Your First Two Leadership Mantras

Here is some other wonderful leadership wisdom I very recently encountered: It's in the interval between stimulus and response where the leader emerges. In other words, the leader emerges as a result of intense interior work that allows him or her to transcend ingrained, automatic past responses. My goal in this chapter is to help you cultivate this interval and leverage it to full advantage. I begin by giving you two mantras I have shared with many audiences to help them calm down and redouble their efforts to overcome, as you will see, "disgustingly predictable" (said tongue in cheek) resistance to *any* change.

Learn this as leaders right up front. It is a given that people don't object to change; they just hate being changed themselves. When you are explaining the reason for a needed change and people respond in anger, telling you why they cannot do it, telling you why it applies to everyone else but them, or asking you to explain it yet again and you want to throttle them, take a deep breath and say to yourself, with a smile in your heart: "Those darn humans, God bless 'em. They are acting just like 'people.'"

Now, take on this further challenge: Recognize that staff members have the luxury of acting like people, whereas you, as a leader, do not. You now have to ask yourself (leadership mantra 2), "How do I change to get them to want to volunteer to change?"

Management consultant Peter Block says it so well: "Most important human problems have no permanent solution." That is another given.

As you build leadership skills in yourself and your team, here is some further insight from Goleman, Boyatzis, and McKee. It also alludes to the adult learning issue mentioned in the previous section:

> When it comes to building leadership skills that last, motivation and how a person feels about learning matters immensely. People learn what they want to learn. If learning is forced on us, even if we master it temporarily…it is soon forgotten. …So when a company requires people to go through a one-size-fits-all leadership development program, participants may simply go through the motions — unless they truly want to learn. In fact, a well-established principle of behavior change tells us that when a person has been forced to change, the change will vanish once the browbeating ends.[2]

## The Human Process

Recall Exhibit 1.1, the "universal" process flowchart and Jim Clemmer's brilliant "process" paragraph quoted in Chapter 1. The processes Clemmer describes are inhabited by people, who are good, decent, honest, hardworking folks all trying to do their best and all very human.

The everyday process breakdowns needing improvement are happening to these stressed, very human people and to your customers. Formal organizational efforts will be needed to expose and deal with the emotional fallout of poorly designed processes. Improving them will require accurate, timely, useful, nonthreatening interpersonal feedback both to management and among the employees. It will also require unprecedented cultural cooperation, support, and collaboration. More proactive customer feedback and involvement will be a part of improving everyday processes as well.

At a recent conference, I heard Stephen Mayfield, former senior vice president of quality and performance improvement for the American Hospital Association, state that top management is aware of only *4 percent* of daily ongoing operational problems, middle management is aware of only *9 percent*, supervisors are aware of 74 percent, and the frontline employees are fully aware of *100 percent*. Given the way organizations are currently designed and managed, leaders have little knowledge about true process performance and the effects of system interactions.

Organizations are experiencing unprecedented stress, which creates a flourishing environment for symptoms of what Faith Ralston[3] calls "corporate craziness" (Exhibit 3.1), which are frenetic behaviors mired in crisis orientation, cost cutting, meetings, and more meetings to usually account for lack of desired results.

As I have already said many times, one's current processes are perfectly designed to get the results they are already getting, and this includes corporate craziness. Reactions to its elements become ingrained in current process inputs, create dysfunctional feedback (or none at all), and infiltrate the organizational culture, with inevitable effects on interpersonal relationships, interdepartmental relationships, and ultimately, relationships with customers.

EXHIBIT 3.1 ■ Symptoms of "Corporate Craziness"

- Lack of focus or direction
- Frenetic behaviors
- Obsession with technology
- Too busy working to care
- Judgmental attitudes
- Indirect or vague communication
- Excessive number of closed-door conversations
- Too many and/or unproductive meetings
- Crisis orientation
- Blame in reaction to mistakes
- Reactive budget processes
- Secretiveness about decisions

Source: Faith Ralston, professional speaker and author of *Play Your Best Hand* and *Emotions@Work*. Used with permission.

## The Quality Pyramid

### The "Engine" of Quality Improvement

Let us consider the logical elements of QI as its "engine" forming the top of a pyramid. Exhibit 3.2, a graphic suggested by Grinnell,[4] displays this concept.

The engine levels include:

- Level One: Quality of doing, which is the processes employees use to do their jobs, directly yielding an organization's results (key: context of process-oriented thinking);
- Level Two: Quality of thinking and decision making that supports the doing (key: statistical thinking and quality tools); and
- Level Three: Quality of information that influences employees' thinking (key: high-quality technical and administrative information).

The main result of the flurry of organizational quality training efforts during the last 30 years has been creating a good awareness of these concepts, but ultimately, with disappointing results. Refining thinking skills through many of the traditional quality tools and frameworks such as Six Sigma and Lean should sharpen the decision-making capability. However, as a history of failed programs has shown, focusing just on the tools and using them through, generally, projects not directly related to deeper organizational strategic issues is not enough to ensure improvement.

All these efforts give cursory attention to the most nontrivial task of creating and attaining the significant cultural behavior changes at many levels that are required for true success.

### The "Fuel": Information Flows through Relationships

To feed the need for the engine's "fuel," the pyramid widens (Exhibit 3.3) to include:

- Level Four: Quality of information that influences employees' behavior (personal feedback);
- Level Five: Quality of relationships through which this information flows; and
- Level Six: Quality of perceptions and feelings that influences employees' relationships with others, including coworkers, other departments, and management (organizational culture).

Ultimately the base of the pyramid (and its interaction with Level Six) is the bottleneck (Exhibit 3.4).

- Level Seven: Quality of individual mind-sets, which is the personal operating beliefs and values, and resulting emotional baggage. *Every* employee brings to work processes that are shaped by the unique experiences of each individual's first 20 years of life.

In most organizational environments, people have neither been trained to give feedback appropriately nor manage their ego's reactions to feedback in necessarily healthy ways. Fear and defensiveness tend to be the rule within most organizations, and long-standing cultural patterns are ingrained. Emotional blockages caused by bad relationships will determine the amount, quality, and timeliness of information flow between people.

Every good book on QI makes a key point that being successful in transforming an organizational culture will require feedback and lots of it both up and down the organization. In fact, in the best-led cultures, leaders will aggressively seek honest feedback on their performance, realizing that feedback is *a perception being shared and not a truth being*

# A LEADERSHIP BELIEF SYSTEM

**EXHIBIT 3.2  The "Engine" of Quality**

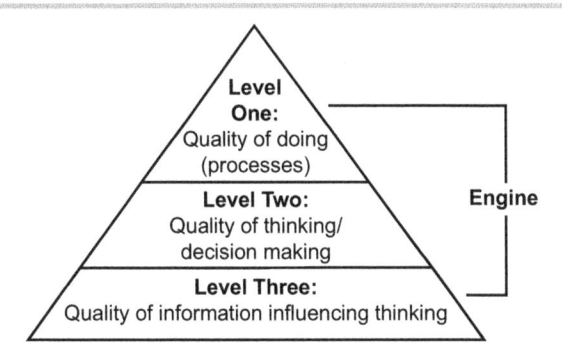

- **Level One:** Quality of doing (processes)
- **Level Two:** Quality of thinking/decision making
- **Level Three:** Quality of information influencing thinking

(Levels One–Three = Engine)

Source: Adapted from John R. Grinnell Jr., "Optimize the Human System," *Quality Progress*, November 1994, pages 63–67. Grinnell Leadership (Chapel Hill, NC 27514) provides executive team and organization development for hospitals.

**EXHIBIT 3.3  The "Fuel" of Quality**

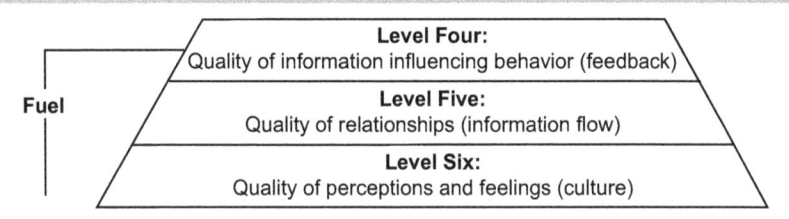

- **Level Four:** Quality of information influencing behavior (feedback)
- **Level Five:** Quality of relationships (information flow)
- **Level Six:** Quality of perceptions and feelings (culture)

(Levels Four–Six = Fuel)

Source: Adapted from John R. Grinnell Jr., "Optimize the Human System," *Quality Progress*, November 1994, pages 63–67. Grinnell Leadership (Chapel Hill, NC 27514) provides executive team and organization development for hospitals.

**EXHIBIT 3.4  The Base of the Pyramid: Those Darn Humans**

- **Level Seven:** Quality of individual mind-sets (personal beliefs and values)

Source: Adapted from John R. Grinnell Jr., "Optimize the Human System," *Quality Progress*, November 1994, pages 63–67. Grinnell Leadership (Chapel Hill, NC 27514) provides executive team and organization development for hospitals.

*declared*. The culture's perception is the leadership's reality, and it allows leaders to ask themselves three important questions in response:

1. Is that a perception I would like the culture to have?
2. If that perception continues, will the organization be able to attain its desired results?
3. If the answers to questions 1 and 2 are "No," how do I have to change to create a different perception?

This leads to leadership mantra 3: "As a leader, I must learn to swallow my ego 10 times before breakfast and another dozen times before lunch."

Organizational commitment is needed to depersonalize issues and create a culture where feedback can flourish (and the answer is not "360-degree feedback," as discussed later in this chapter, in the section by the same name). As mentioned in Chapter 1, immediate expectations of both blaming processes — not people — and zero tolerance for blame as a cultural norm will cause a much-needed quantum leap in cultural morale that will allow this commitment to happen.

Now the truly hard work begins: Despite establishing such norms, an inevitable element of individual, personal accountability will be needed to show these expected behaviors and desired organizational values (from your mission, vision, and values) for purposes of obtaining desired organizational results. A harsh reality is that regardless of the best efforts to improve Pyramid Levels Four through Six, ultimately, the behavior process of the person standing in front of you is also perfectly designed to show the behavior he or she is displaying because of his or her already established personal values and resulting belief system (Level Seven). And it is unconscious, automatic, and unintentional. *Everyone* is going to need to change some aspects of his or her behavior.

And another harsh reality is that regardless of the best efforts to improve Levels Four through Six, ultimately your current organizational culture (Level Six) is also perfectly designed, because of its established (unconscious) values and resulting belief system, to *tolerate* the behaviors it is exhibiting. And these are unconscious, automatic, and unintentional. Again, everyone is going to need to change some aspects of his or her behavior.

The last sentence of the previous two paragraphs may not be a comfortable thought, but it will be necessary if your wish is to attain truly unparalleled quality. And in the right context, it is much more easily accomplished than many past uncomfortable efforts *everyone* has no doubt experienced.

## The Pyramid's Base

There is a results-based psychology known as cognitive therapy (sometimes called *rational therapy*) that can serve an organization well. Psychiatrists Albert Ellis and William Glasser have been particularly influential in applying these ideas to everyday life. It has a deceptive simplicity that is easy to learn and apply. With persistence, you *will* attain desired results. The key is keeping a context of an intense focus on organizational results to drive cultural change through changing underlying *belief systems* — both organizational and individual.

Imagine a pane of glass similar to a car's windshield in front of one's face that is filtering one's own unique view of the world. This windshield is sometimes called a "belief window." It is made up of literally thousands of individual beliefs shaped by one's own unique experiences of approximately the first 20 years of life. Many of these beliefs relate to one's sex, ethnicity, and decade of birth.

Adult behaviors result from ongoing patterns of reinforcement and learning what behaviors got us rewarded or punished in terms of getting the following four basic needs met:

1. To survive
    - To be viable
    - To be profitable
    - To be strong
    - To be in control
    - To be safe

2. To love and be loved
   - To have good relationships
   - To have friends
   - To be admired
   - To be trusted
   - To be helpful
   - To be part of a group or team
3. To feel important (self-esteem) and have power
   - To be valued
   - To be a leader
   - To play an important role
   - To make a difference
   - To be successful
   - To have meaning in our lives
4. To experience variety, fun, and autonomy to choose
   - To be challenged
   - To have excitement
   - To grow in competence
   - To be innovative
   - To interact with others
   - To learn new things

This resulting belief system results in unconscious, predictable adult behavior patterns, which are unique individual patterns *everyone* brings to work. And herein lies the power of this model: People's behavioral patterns can also be easily analyzed to intuit the underlying belief system.

Research has shown that 90 percent of one's belief system is formed by age 12 and that it undergoes an unconscious "final lock" at age 20. These well-entrenched beliefs are then changeable only by significant emotional events, either personal (birth, death, illness, near-death experience, marriage, losing a job), societal (the Great Depression, World War II, the Kennedy assassination, September 11), or the sudden realization (through appropriate feedback) that some of the displayed behaviors from this belief system are ultimately detrimental to a successful personal life (e.g., potential for a marriage breaking up or loss of a friendship) or one's organizational success (e.g., potential to lose one's job or not get promoted). Such stress is a powerful motivator for *considering* changing an unintentional self-defeating belief, but then again, we are all "darn humans." Making such changes takes *incredible* energy.

Once one's belief system locks, instead of being open to letting experiences further shape beliefs, the tendency now is to filter experiences to *conform* to beliefs. At this stage, a danger exists to initially *perceive* any experiences contrary to one's belief system as a potential threat. Luckily, most perceived threats are relatively benign. Usually, being the humans that we are, we just ignore them and stay feeling comfortably superior in our belief system and its view of the world.

However, if the freedom to ignore an experience is not an option, stress is created that upsets the balance and temporarily and immediately diverts all available energy to meeting the need perceived to be in danger, usually guaranteeing the very behavior that will ensure it ultimately does not get met. This energy typically manifests as defensive behaviors, which are somewhat irrational, potentially alienating, but predictable, defensive behavior patterns that loosely manage to get the threatened need met in the short term. Now, however, the potential exists to do long-term damage to relationships because of how the other people involved experience this behavior and choose to respond, or not.

A common pattern I have observed is when tension has the potential to create conflict, such as when a nurse is fearful of appropriately confronting a physician's bullying behavior. People on the receiving end of such behavior, especially in a healthcare culture, often simply avoid the conflict by doing nothing. This reaction is essentially putting all of one's current energy into survival or fear of not being loved (going along to get along). It may extricate the person from the situation in the short term, but the dysfunction has actually been reinforced. This result virtually guarantees that the person doing nothing will have to face a similar situation with this physician or another physician. It does not resolve the long-term situation for either the nurse, the physician, or the organizational culture, and it *will affect achieving organizational results.* Further, in not addressing the situation, an opportunity has been lost to create long-term personal inner peace for both the nurse and the physician; each has self-defeating beliefs.

In physicians' defense, the brutal internship and residency process has the very real danger of ingraining the physician cultural belief (of their teachers) that "I must always be right and I am right." This belief also manifests in physicians perceiving a threat to feeling important, their autonomy, or possibly even the fear of being sued (survival). Note that I'm not judging the belief. It is institutionalized in the culture of physician education. The choice available now is in how to deal with it. Will continuing that belief allow an organization to achieve its results? Several more examples are given in the rest of this chapter to test this issue.

The ultimate goal for all of us humans is to get the four needs in balance. As I have experienced (and am still learning), when every issue becomes a conscious choice and the urge to display defensive behavior is resisted, an inner sense of personal control and peace emerges.

## Expanding the Model

Ellis was dissatisfied with the dominance of Freudian thought in the practice of psychiatry in the 1950s. He saw the need for healing through changing what he called "critical self-talk" (this concept applies to Pyramid Level Seven). He called his new therapy "rational therapy," which later evolved and opened into the field of what is now called *cognitive-behavioral therapy.*

One could almost say that Ellis's approach is as simple as ABC.

- **A** is the **a**ctivating event (or adversity) that you experience;
- **B** is the **b**elief(s) that you have about that event or adversity, filtering it through your belief system to see how it pertains to your four needs; resulting in
- **C**, which is the **c**onsequence of those beliefs (observed behavior), including emotional consequences to all relationships involved with the person and the activating event.

The flow of cognitive therapy, like the alphabet, is:

A → B → C

Ellis tried to help his clients see that C follows B, not A. In other words, the consequences of a situation follow one's beliefs, not the original activating event.

The activating event is a trigger for a belief system and is filtered through its "rules" with the four needs in mind, producing the resulting (automatic, conditioned) behavior virtually immediately. This behavior could be described objectively and nonthreateningly, as could the consequences it ultimately created in the given situation.

As an example, two people can experience the same activating event (e.g., a rainy day). But because they have different belief systems, they will end up with completely different emotional consequences. The person who believes that "rainy days are depressing" will experience the day as depressing. The person who believes that "rainy days are delightful" will experience delight. One has *choice* in how to respond.

This model works very well for behaviors and interpersonal interactions. Its wonderful simplicity can be further adapted to an organization's culture and observed employee work behaviors. In this context, one more piece needs to be added — the R, or **r**esults experienced by the organization from the consequential behaviors (actions) of its employees:

$$A \to B \to C \to R$$

This startling realization emerges: If the consequences of employees' behaviors are not producing the desired organizational results, then the organizational cultural beliefs are holding them back.

To model my contention that your current processes are perfectly designed to get the results they are already getting,

$$A_1 \to B_1 \to C_1 \to R_1$$

Obviously, you would not be reading this book if you did not want to achieve new, better results, $R_2$. However, the current organizational culture's belief system, $B_1$ (which is perfectly designed to yield the current employees' behaviors, $C_1$), is perfectly designed to attain $R_1$.

When new results are desired, the tendency is to use an activating event (A) where people *describe* the $C_2$ actions needed by the employees to produce these $R_2$. Recalling Ellis's comment that C does not follow A, unless the A can create a changed $B_2$, it will be filtered through $B_1$, virtually guaranteeing the continuation of $R_1$ results. This idea supports my earlier contention that logic virtually never changes behaviors: One must address the underlying belief system driving the status quo $C_1$ or be virtually guaranteed that the organization will continue to produce $R_1$.

From Ellis's explanation and experience, a common $B_1$ belief about training — "Logical explanation produces changed behavior" — is false. One possible new $B_2$ belief is, "Continuing the $A_1$ activating event of presenting logical information expecting it to change current $B_1$ beliefs is wasted time and effort."

This belief, then, might yield the following $B_2$ belief system about training:

- Because logical explanation does not work, a different activating event ($A_2$) is needed.
- Information must be presented in such a way to change the current $B_1$ belief system to $B_2$ beliefs that will drive $C_2$ consequential behaviors to produce desired $R_2$ results.

- We will need to experiment with various $A_2$ to test which ones work more successfully.
- If we begin to attain $R_2$, we are successful.

So the questions for leaders and change agents teaching improvement now become:

- How do leaders create different activating events, $A_2$, to motivate new and changed beliefs in employees, $B_2$, which will have desired behavioral consequences, $C_2$, to drive the desired organizational results, $R_2$?
- How do leaders stop recreating old activating events, $A_1$ (or even *perceptions* of old activating events), that will inevitably reinforce old, unhealthy beliefs, $B_1$, that will then have undesirable behavioral consequences, $C_1$, that will tend to result not in $R_2$ but, most probably, previous $R_1$?

*New results will require new beliefs* both as an organization and as employees working for the organization. Whether it is motivating employees' individual behaviors to show the desired organizational values or attaining needed organizational results, dealing with belief systems is at the core of making behavioral change.

### Those Darn Humans

People tend to recognize experiences that reinforce their existing $B_1$ beliefs rather than those that promote the new $B_2$ beliefs. As leaders, you must recognize that most experiences will need to be interpreted for people to help them form the $B_2$ beliefs you want them to have.

The deeper challenge as leaders is how do you create an organizational atmosphere where employees would be able to replace self-critical, self-defeating beliefs with self-accepting (and *other-people-accepting*) beliefs so as to experience a strong improvement in morale? In other words, how will leaders' actions contribute to improving the quality of employee mind-sets, the vital Level Seven base of the quality pyramid?

One of Ellis's favorite refrains was:

- "Practice USA — Unconditional Self-Acceptance!
- But that's not enough. You also need UOA — Unconditional Other-Acceptance!
- And ULA, too — Unconditional Life Acceptance!"[5]

### Changing Self-Defeating Beliefs

Ellis worked tirelessly for decades to help people change their beliefs, especially self-condemning beliefs. In his psychotherapy practice, he focused diligently on the $B_1$ beliefs that were holding clients back from happy lives. As leaders, not only do you have to work on this (for yourselves and your employees through ongoing coaching) but you also need to work diligently on the organizational cultural $B_1$ — the beliefs that are holding it back from attaining its desired $R_2$ results.

Consider the following as part of your new leadership $B_2$: "Our culture will focus on replacing critical, resentful thinking with forgiveness, acceptance, and love (hence, blaming processes and zero tolerance for blame)." Such a belief would ultimately benefit your customers more than you could ever imagine, especially if they had an $A_2$ activating event of experiencing such a culture.

The next section sheds further insight on utilizing this model to see through the lens of learning more about the influence of belief systems.

## A DEEPER CULTURAL CONTEXT FOR UNDERSTANDING RESISTANCE TO CHANGE

Joseph Juran's insights into what he coined "cultural resistance to change"[6] in his book *Managerial Breakthrough* were a startling revelation to me in the late 1980s. He likened an organization to a "culture" with unique "tribes" (in the case of medicine, examples include physicians; different specialties among physicians; nurses; other clinical personnel, such as laboratory and X-ray technicians; executives; middle management; finance; housekeeping; and cafeteria), each with its own unique belief system of unwritten rules (including ingrained perceptions about "those other tribes"). Any new member of a tribe quickly intuits these rules, which he or she had better absorb if expecting to get along or be accepted. And each tribe contributes in its unique way to a larger overall organizational culture set by the executive tribe.

Each subculture tribe, like individuals, has a belief system and a cultural "windshield" through which it views the organization, resulting from its professional culture, degree of status to which its members feel entitled, and the organization's perceptions about it. The same powerful forces are at work generating the desire to get the four basic needs met (survive, love and be loved, feel important, achieve variety and autonomy).

Similarly to individuals, these groups will exhibit defensive behaviors when they perceive a need being threatened. So every person coming to work temporarily adds yet another filter dictated by professional and organization cultures to their unique windshield when they walk through the door. This results in an intriguing interaction between Levels Six and Seven of the pyramid to create a "work persona."

Any proposed change has two parts: the change itself and the social consequence of the change. Juran pointed out that this social consequence is the real troublemaker, an uninvited guest, if you will, that parasitically appends itself to a seemingly logical solution. He developed "rules of the road" for dealing with this behavioral phenomenon, which I have ultimately found more valuable for dealing with specific project interventions (see Chapter 8). Now that you are aware of this aspect of cultural behavior, what can you as leaders can do every day as you try to align your culture to mission, vision, and values?

Juran also noticed that people's stated resistance to changes, even those that would have obvious benefit, were often puzzling. What he eventually realized was that these reactions were just superficial, masking much deeper issues, usually *perceived* threats to deeply held tribal professional $B_1$ values; fears of tribal survival; and, sometimes, conflicts with individuals' personal values. Many of these threats relate to feeling that survival (job security, identification with the tribe), job importance and status, organizational respect, or autonomy might be threatened. Notice that I am emphasizing "perceived."

A large part of dealing with resistance is understanding the deeper reasons beyond what people initially explicitly state in opposition to a change. Juran called these the "stated reasons" (immediate reactions to create gratification or a distraction, or defensive behavior creating short-term benefit) vs. the "real reasons" (the underlying threatened deep, unmet, personal or group need, which is filtering improperly through a dirty belief system windshield and needs healing and/or changing).

Part of organizational and individual growth will be replacing faulty $B_1$ beliefs and personal biases that would compromise an individual's, a work group's, and the organization's long-term successes. In essence, given the premise in the previous section that any change is perceived as a cultural threat, *everyone's* belief system windshield needs to clean away its self-defeating beliefs to achieve needed growth (ultimately leading to personal and organizational inner peace).

Thus, depending on how this defensive behavior is handled, satisfying individual stated reasons, usually to short-term benefit, can result in serious long-term destruction to the organization. A threatened culture or tribe will unintentionally do its best to distract and divert precious energy from the needed change: There is a strong pull for a culture to keep things predictable.

When a very strong reaction is experienced to a proposal, an unrelated, deep-seated issue and very strong attachment to it is unwittingly trying to sabotage communication. It is fruitless to either argue with or redouble your effort to find logical explanations to convince a person or a work group otherwise when they are in this hot-button mode: Their energy is currently totally committed to the status quo and getting that threatened need met, albeit in a dysfunctional manner.

Regardless of whether the perception is true or not, *if the threat is real to them, it is real to you as a leader.* How you will change to get them to want to change is your challenge. Can you create an $A_2$ activating event that might get them to consider changing their current $B_1$ belief about a situation with the hope that you can *eventually* have them exhibit $C_2$ behaviors to drive your $R_2$ results? In other words, how will you intuit and address the perceived threat and its underlying driving $B_1$ so that it can be defused?

You cannot personalize the situation. It has nothing to do specifically with you, although it could be caused by a *belief* about you, unrelated to the proposed change that past experiences in dealing with you have created. That possibility is worth examining, and then changing that belief about you before moving forward.

How then do you keep your hot buttons insulated? Time and time again, I hear that a major barrier to proceeding with a QI effort is "lack of physician support," which may or may not be true. (It might be interesting, if you have that belief, to examine what might be the real reasons underlying that stated reason.)

Usually, an ongoing or repeating conflict requires both sides to examine their individual belief windows as being contributors. As I have learned from humbling personal experiences, if you tend to find yourself in the same frustrating situation in different guises, there is a good chance that a self-defeating belief is lurking in your belief system.

The following are two scenarios regarding physician behavior, which I will use to make some universal points. As a leader, people will throw all sorts of stated reasons at you for not wanting to change, and your everyday reality — your given — is the real reason that people hate being changed. Further, they are going to act like darn humans. So how do you deal with that?

Scenario 1: A physician in a one-on-one meeting tells you that he or she is in agreement with a practice guideline, yet, when you present to the peer group, your supporter is as vehemently trashing your proposal as is his or her colleagues. You feel betrayed. Why did the physician not support you in the peer-group forum? Perhaps he or she was attending to values of loyalty to the tribe and did not want to be perceived as an outsider. Perhaps peer professional collegiality carries more immediate benefit to his or her daily work life than does yours. Perhaps he or she is weighing those referrals from colleagues that pay the mortgage and college tuition bills (survival).

Scenario 2: Consider those times when practice guidelines are presented to physicians. The initial immediate reaction, almost universally, is "cookbook medicine!" At least that is the stated reason. What could be the real reason? They may perceive that implementing the guideline could threaten their survival (job security); make them seem less important (professional esteem); make them perceive a loss of respect in the culture at large (self-esteem); or make them feel that their much-desired autonomy is being taken away.

At this point, any logical argument will fall on deaf ears because all of their energy is now being spent defusing your threat. And physicians tend to be strong personalities; they may make it their goal to make sure your proposal is not implemented, either through overt sabotage or classic stonewalling.

If you allow that to happen, in the short term, they have shown you how "important" they are and that need has been met for them. However, consider the long-term consequences to the organization and your patients:

- The organization's success has been compromised, especially if the guideline is key to mission, vision, and values (assuming you made sure of that beforehand).
- Ill will has been created in your relationship, especially if the blocking of the proposal is taken personally by the executives.
- If you react by exerting your need to feel important at the physicians' expense to "show them who's boss," their resistance may now go "underground." I *guarantee* that it will not disappear.
- Negative beliefs the two groups have about each other in their ongoing power struggle have been reinforced, and possibly, new ones are created.
- A situation like this will inevitably be created again.
- To carry the scenario to its extreme conclusion, the more overt saboteurs might ultimately be dismissed (a destructive long-term consequence to them of getting their short-term need to feel important met). My experience has shown this result to culminate in fear-inducing consequences for those who stay. They will keep their heads down and emotionally check out, which is a disastrous cultural consequence reinforcing the $B_1$ belief of the inevitability of the physician–executive power struggle.

As I have been emphasizing, the usual result of defensive behavior is short-term benefit, but long-term destruction. Bad beliefs are contributing to the situation, and belief windshield cleaning is needed by one or, usually, both sides.

Knowing from past experiences that this reaction is a given and that you are perfectly designed to have resulting beliefs that physicians have about you, consider changing the established dynamic (and their $B_1$ beliefs toward motivating the right actions). What if you were to initially act through the $B_2$ belief? "If the guideline implementation is going to be effective this time, I need to consider how I have to change to get them to want to change." How might this affect your subsequent actions (activating events) in your planning? Compare the following $A_2$ with what you may have done in the past ($A_1$):

1. Before even presenting this proposal to the physicians, did you do your homework in thoroughly communicating the organization's mission, vision, and values? Did you ask yourself if what you are proposing is truly vital to the organization's future? If not, the culture will most probably "eat it for lunch."
2. Can you keep your hot button insulated in response to the inevitable resistance?
3. Will you be able to anticipate stated reasons to intuit the real reasons and the underlying need(s) being threatened?
4. Can you create genuine assurance that the underlying need(s) will be met with the suggested change?
5. Are you willing to subsequently listen to their concerns (they will get creative during this disarming process and offer more stated reasons) and explain the proposal in the context of mission, vision, and values yet again?

> **EXHIBIT 3.5** ■ Facilitation/Dialogue Process: Separating Facts from Feelings
>
> 1. Acknowledge the presence of strong feelings.
>    - Understand the past.
> 2. Clarify individual feelings and needs.
>    - What expectations have not been met?
>    - What disappointments have we experienced?
>    - What mistrusts have developed over time?
>      – Each side shares its own perspective, *uninterrupted by others,* except for clarifying questions.
> 3. Separate personal needs from business needs.
> 4. Identify and respect the needs of the business.
> 5. Be willing to change based on what you learn.
> 6. Believe that a win-win solution is possible, for you, for others, and for the organization.
> 7. Be truthful and compassionate in the process and its follow-up.
>    - Peer coach to results by depersonalizing issues and focusing on specific behaviors that could compromise organizational success and/or individual success.
>    - Seek feedback on progress *and act on it.*
>      – Recognize whether your behavior has truly changed.
>      – If your behavior has changed and the group with whom you had the formal dialogue hasn't noticed (or pretended not to notice), ask what they would need to observe to "make it right" and reinforce it when you do.

6. If either a long-standing history of hostility with this group or excessive emotion is present, consider taking a time-out to use the process described in Exhibit 3.5. Or use this model as a vehicle in conjunction with the initial presentation.[3]
7. In the context of identifying and respecting the needs of the organization (and patients), can you engage them in dialogue to create a win-win solution?
8. Are consequences to the physicians for not complying with the proposal clear and reasonable? Can you get their agreement?
9. Can you suggest a follow-up process both to receive and give feedback? Can you ensure through your subsequent $C_2$ actions that the feedback you get will be that you have kept your promises?

I suggest that this process has a chance of motivating desirable $B_2$ for your audience.

In any person, organization, or tribe, the four needs *will* make themselves known one way or another. All behavior seems to be geared to getting them met every second people breathe. And patterns of behavior do not lie; they can be read to intuit threatened needs and underlying belief systems.

It is a new leadership responsibility to create through the appropriate $A_2$ activating events, a more productive $B_2$ alternate belief in the resisting group that will drive desired behaviors toward desired $R_2$ results. And you might have to change some of your beliefs in the process. Look around you every day: There truly are no secrets. And relax, *everyone* will eventually need belief window surgery (yet another given).

The elegant simplicity and practicality of the cognitive-behavioral framework has probably been the most useful knowledge of my career for enhancing overall change agent effectiveness, in myself and others. The needed wildcard missing from past transformation efforts is to create, through one's own behavior, the expectation and facilitation of people to voluntarily manage their ego reactions to change in healthy ways so as to pursue organizational goals in a manner that identifies and respects the needs of the business.

## The Need for Clear $R_2$

The preceding nine questions could actually be used for any proposed change as a powerful new style of activating event ($A_2$). However, to be truly effective, $R_2$ organizational results must be *clearly* defined so there is (1) strong motivation for trying to create new beliefs as well as (2) measurable endpoints to use as further feedback. Otherwise, the inherent inertia of the current culture, with all of its vested interests, is just too difficult to overcome.

Most cultures are all too familiar with the usual annual vague goal-setting process, which is perceived as an $A_1$ — "more of the same." In other words, those darn humans will probably put their hands over their hearts, pledge to the new goals, and get back to the real work, producing $R_1$. Just the typical $A_1$ of saying "These $R_2$ results are important" and the follow-up of "But this time we mean it" is hardly inspiring. I can guarantee that the culture still perceives this as an $A_1$ experience; the group has heard *that* before and probably successfully stonewalled it, and the culture has tolerated it.

An example of this process was one very large group practice with which I worked. They went from a physician chief executive who was considered visionary and passionate about QI to a chief executive who was not a physician but a classic bean counter. He also believed in using arbitrary numerical goals with draconian accountability to motivate. When asked how he planned to deal with a physician culture used to having a physician chief executive, he answered, "Easy, it's like giving my dog obedience training and using the choke chain liberally."

Two years into this administration, I ran into a friend of mine who was a physician at the practice and said, "Wow, it's been a big change at your practice. I can only imagine what you physicians are going through! How is it? How are you coping?" to which he smiled and answered, "Davis…I come in, I see patients, I go home." And such is the power of culture. The frontline healthcare workers are already, in their eyes, doing the best they can and working as hard as they can. They are jaded and have seen it all. Unless they are given a very good reason to do otherwise, they are just going to "come in, see patients, and go home." This is yet another given for executives (who, you recall, are aware of only 4 percent of the everyday frontline issues) and change agents.

One must create the infrastructure that allows leadership to say, "Yes, Dr. X, I understand. But I need you to see patients in such a way that you move these five indicators in these directions. If we together can do that, our patients will benefit, our purchasers will benefit, and we will have a long future together here. We are going to display these five indicators to you every month so you and we can see how we are doing." If the mission, vision, and values statements are strong and clear, and if they have been thoroughly communicated and agreed to, there is a good chance that Dr. X might consider changing his belief system. The belief that "I am being treated like a dog" would not result in Dr. X considering such a change.

If you are confused about what $R_2$ you want, then your staff is confused, and they will keep producing $R_1$, which you are already perfectly designed to get. If you are clear about the $R_2$ you want, then they will then *act* confused and:

- Interpret the $R_2$ results through their current $B_1$ beliefs and mildly tweak their $R_1$, but the results will still be, in essence, $R_1$;
- Give you stated reasons why they cannot do it, hoping you will go away; or

- Like they have usually done in the past, ignore them, put their heads down, and keep working hard to "come in, see patients, and go home," driven by the naive $B_1$ belief and stated reason, "How can hard work like this not be rewarded?"

Juran felt strongly that there was no such thing as "improvement in general" and believed in specifically targeted projects. Similarly in a culture of continuous improvement, it is only through targeting specific results within a coherent mission, vision, and values that a culture can be aligned and guided. And clear results deriving directly from clear mission, vision, and values statements are crucial to attaining unprecedented levels of improvement.

The clearly stated and thoroughly communicated $R_2$ results then become an anchor from which to view your leadership role: to create the appropriate $A_2$ activating events to motivate the needed $B_2$ beliefs while giving needed personal feedback through the espoused *values* to reinforce and drive needed $C_2$ consequential behaviors.

## 360-Degree Feedback

My definition of *insanity* is doing things the way you have always done them and expecting different results. Many of you reading this, I am sure, have gone through a 360-degree feedback process. Did it really change anything long term? In my experience, it usually does not. So be careful about trying it again in this newfangled context you are learning here unless some clear $B_2$ beliefs about values and feedback are established and anchored to clear $R_2$ results.

As you have no doubt guessed, I am no fan of the 360-degree feedback process. I have found it to be an excuse for people to passively aggressively "dump their buckets" with personal hidden agendas thinly veiled as helpful feedback. If your current culture has toxic elements in its $B_1$ belief system (and it does), this feedback process will be toxic, as will its results, unless leaders have the emotional intelligence to look beyond the stated reasons to intuit the real reasons and know how to take action on them, *both* on themselves and the culture at large. But as I have said, we all need therapy, and most people will neither volunteer for it nor ultimately listen to it; this is a given.

As you can imagine, when I was employed as an organizational change agent, I received a lot of criticism regarding my "direct" style, but I was never told who gave that criticism. And despite many efforts to change my style, it was just never enough to satisfy some people; once again, I never knew who.

Maybe, behind the stated reason of "I don't like Davis's style," there lurked, in many cases, the real reason: "I don't want to change, and his style (which makes me uncomfortable reminding me that I have to change) is a good excuse for me not to."

I have a psychiatrist friend who says, regarding feedback, "If they can't say it to my face, it doesn't exist." If you have a culture in which face-to-face feedback cannot comfortably be done, you are going nowhere, which is a very uncomfortable prospect.

However, with proper establishment of mission, vision, values, and clear organizational $R_2$ results, you can now proactively peer coach in the moment to address everyday behaviors not aligned with commitment to organizational results and values. Through leadership mantras 1 through 3, the wisdom can be achieved to be able to view these behaviors as unintentional and most probably caused by a self-defeating belief *in the person's own belief system*. Once-a-year feedback, which is typically practiced, is not enough to change anything.

This was the case with Dr. Rodney Dueck, my mentor. He would always share feedback as soon as he heard it. He would ask for a meeting and frame it with an absolutely sincere, genuine concern for the person's ultimate success, and in my case, some of this feedback was blistering. It would also be delivered without the slightest hint of judgment and with the unstated wisdom that my behavior was probably only mildly related to the actual situation. In looking back, there was always something self-defeating deep within my personal belief system that was involved. My belief window needed surgery if I was going to be successful at work and increase the inner peace in my personal life.

Very difficult feedback through a culturally entrenched peer coaching process will then need to become another cultural norm. An atmosphere of trust allows appropriate and sometimes vigorous addressing of dysfunctional behavior but with nothing less than respect and sincerity and *without attacking the human being.*

Consider how the following example of feedback compares with what you have experienced in the past:

> We believe in treating one another with respect in this company, and I know you hold that belief. But that was not the experience I had in this morning's meeting when you spoke to Jim about the idea he presented. The behavior you exhibited will help neither the organization's success nor your personal success. That proposal is key to our future, and I could hear your colleagues talking about how much your reaction disturbed them, which concerns me about your future credibility in their eyes. Help me understand your strong reaction so we can move forward to repair the damage and be successful in this effort.

Contrast this with the reaction, "You can be a real pain in meetings. Please tone down your reactions and don't you *ever* behave like that again!" Now imagine getting this response fed back several times in the annual 360-degree feedback process ($A_1$). Which is more likely to make you *volunteer* to examine your beliefs and change?

You would most likely seriously consider responding to feedback delivered without judgment and with a sincere concern for your success, especially if you knew that every time it happened, it would be fed back to you in this manner ($A_2$). In the case of my gentle mentor, he also would not hesitate to fire people after repeated helpful feedback because they had, in essence, "chosen to put themselves out of a job."

In this example, behavior is depersonalized and addressed solely as a barrier to desired organizational results. Feedback is given in the spirit of genuine concern for the person's success, building productive relationships with colleagues, and respect for the human being.

"Help me understand" is yet another ongoing mantra to deal with inevitable resistance. (And do use the words "Help me understand" instead of "Why?" As a psychologist friend of mine shared, when asking a stressed person "Why did you do that?" they tend to hear, "Why *the hell* did you do that?" and will respond in a defensive manner.)

The important thing is to know what behaviors are preventing the organization from achieving its (clearly stated) goals and what behaviors are in conflict with its (clearly stated) values. As I have found through using this process, focusing on organizational results allows needed personal growth to come in "through the back door" and fosters an unprecedented feeling of inner peace. I have had seminar participants feed back to me that, despite my emphasis on organizational results, they have used this philosophy to deal with spouses, children, and even church committees. And to their amazement, it worked, and they felt more in control of their personal lives.

## DECONSTRUCTING THE CULTURE

### Back to the Pyramid

Leadership is a very powerful tribe whose behaviors inevitably shape organizational culture. Research suggests that culture at large will (unintentionally) mirror the behaviors and interactions of its leaders. Considering the preceding discussion about belief systems and the power of this simple concept and its accompanying model, you should have a firm grasp of the extent to which the leadership team's collective beliefs about leadership and power contribute to creating an organization's culture.

Some potentially dangerous beliefs can result from being "the boss" because of:

- Egos becoming invested in the roles played and in the trappings of authority;
- The belief that, because one has paid one's dues, it is fair to expect others to do the same;
- Fear of change and letting go of control;
- Fear of failing in the eyes of the world; and
- Developing habits of behaving and thinking that reinforce the "correctness" of the "boss" approach.

In adapting the behavioral model from individuals to organizations, the executive team, through its resulting belief system of leadership and power, is trying to meet four organizational needs analogous to those needs set forth for individuals:

1. To survive — the organization's need to stay in business (financial survival);
2. To love and be loved — the organization's need for respect;
3. To feel important — the organization's need to have a significant market niche; and
4. To achieve variety and fun — the organization's need to innovate.

Leadership is trying to meet all these needs while simultaneously filtering the whole process through each individual executive's belief system to get their personal four needs met. If an individual's four needs are not in balance, this imbalance could cause some inner conflicts, interpersonal conflict, internal executive team conflict, and resulting problems for the organization.

The consequential behaviors (everyday management) resulting from a leadership team trying to meet these needs and the tribal reactions to them yield an organization's culture. Besides being perfectly designed for the current organizational results, the culture is also perfectly designed for the results of the feedback processes inherent in the quality pyramid's Levels Four through Six.

The needs of individuals and work groups (tribes) (workers delivering care) — Pyramid Level Seven — interact with the needs of the business (culture) — Pyramid Level Six, which are intertwined with the needs of individual executives and managers (their individual Pyramid Level Seven) to determine the quality of relationships through which information flows (Pyramid Level Five) and the quality of the individual and personal feedback processes (Pyramid Level Four).

Quality Pyramid Levels Six and Seven need alignment via clear $R_2$. Once this interaction between organizational and individual needs is understood and aligned, both management and the workforce have an obligation to engage in dialogue that is constructive, nondefensive, nonhysterical, nondumping, and focused on identifying and respecting the needs of the business while balancing individual and organizational needs. The organization's cultural windshield and every individual's windshield need cleaning of their self-defeating beliefs.

As with personal behavior patterns, repeated organizational behaviors such as management decisions and daily behaviors tolerated within the culture can be analyzed to intuit the actual $B_1$ beliefs or values. How do leaders treat each other and staff in the pursuit of organizational aims? Do they *formally* dialogue about it? Dr. Dueck has shared with me four levels of dysfunction, which, if present in the executive team, will inevitably filter into the culture at large through osmosis:

1. Ambiguity is not discussed.
2. Inconsistencies are not discussed.
3. Ambiguity and inconsistencies are not discussable.
4. The undiscussability of ambiguity and inconsistencies is undiscussable.

The same potentially destructive phenomenon that arises with individuals also emerges if an organization perceives an external threat to a need and gets obsessively stuck on managing it. How does it feel when the threat of layoffs puts a culture in survival mode or needed truths are sanitized because the executives have an obsessive desire to feed their egos or maintain an image for the sake of respect in the organization and business community? What happens when your market niche suffers by losing a huge customer? What happens when operational pressures become so intense that innovation is essentially neglected? There will be too much energy focused on short-term issues to the virtual destruction of long-term goals and vision.

Once again in the context of the four needs, for both individuals and organizations, the key is getting them in healthy balance simultaneously as:

- Individual workers;
- Members of a work team;
- Individual executives; and
- An executive team.

## The Scary Corollary

From the model, beliefs drive behaviors. The reverse is also true: If you witness a consistent pattern of behavior, you can usually intuit the belief system driving it. And if you know the beliefs, you can predict future behaviors of that person (or organization) in a similar situation, as well as *the results*. Further, examining your belief system allows you to predict your own results.

Every interaction between two employees creates culture, and the executive tribe's interactions are observed especially closely. What is tolerated as a result of these interactions creates culture and it is being created constantly.

Consider the annual executive retreat. The executives go off-site for two or three days and come back excited with yet another new version of the mission statement. The first statement usually has something to do with the value of respect, such as, "We shall be a culture of respect where it will be safe for any employee to confront any other employee appropriately to uphold the values of our organization." (I have generally found this to be code for "It *should* be safe for nurses to confront a dysfunctional physician, despite the fact that it currently is not.")

So, the executive team has deluded itself that it has indeed created an $A_2$ activating event via an announcement that is going to excite the culture and drive $B_2$ beliefs yielding $C_2$ consequential behaviors and, as a result, desired $R_2$. The workforce embedded in this culture, however, has seen this all before and knows it is just another $A_1$. The result is $R_1$. The executives sense the boredom and then say, "But this time, we *mean* it!" and the workforce says to itself and in conversation with each other after the grand announcement, "We've heard that before, too," resulting in $R_1$.

And suppose a relatively new nurse in the culture does decide to test this new mission statement and indeed appropriately confronts a bullying physician. I have seen the result: The physician is outraged, eventually wears down one of the executive team, and the nurse gets disciplined.

### There Are No Secrets

Know this and know it well: There are no secrets. This wisdom comes from management consultant and former Fortune 500 chief executive officer James Autry, who has written a wonderful leadership book called *Love and Profit* that has also been produced as a powerfully moving video (see Resources). There may be confidential information, but other than that, there truly are no secrets in an organizational culture. (If you don't believe me, then visit your front lobby receptionist and ask, "What are the organizational rumors floating around?") In terms of the scenario from the previous section, rest assured, news of the nurse's disciplining is spreading like wildfire in the culture about 30 seconds after it happens. Now, let us use the $A \rightarrow B \rightarrow C \rightarrow R$ model to examine the no-secrets theory.

An attempted $A_2$ by the nurse resulted in the same old $C_1$ by the management, which now inputs as a perceived $A_1$ into the culture. Several ongoing cultural $B_1$ have been reinforced:

- "Nurses are treated like second-class citizens."
- "A physician will always come out on top in a power struggle."
- Physicians: "I'm entitled to do what I want and am not held accountable for my behaviors."
- Nurses: "I need to 'go along to get along' even if it causes me an ulcer and loss of respect."
- "Management hasn't 'walked the talk,' again."

The new mission statement is officially dead in the water, as is management's credibility.

### Code 13

I have a friend who was employed in a situation like the one described here. It was not unusual for a nurse to be publicly demeaned and bullied by a physician in front of family and staff. Individual confrontations with the physician did not result in altering his or her behavior.

So, a group got together and developed "code 13," which signified that if someone saw a physician bullying staff (physician $B_1 \rightarrow C_1$: "I'm entitled to do this"), he or she would call "code 13" over the intercom with the location. Every supervisor who heard the code would then go to the location, fold his or her arms, and just stare at the offending physician ($A_2$). It took calling the code just six times, with no resulting disciplinary action (executive $C_2$) to cure the physicians ($B_2 \rightarrow C_2$). Because a group was involved in enforcement, it was difficult to discipline, as it had been in the past, or ignore the behavior. And pleas from physicians fell on deaf ears ($A_2$ from administration reinforcing $B_2$ for physicians). Now consider some of the new beliefs created:

- "It takes a unified group effort to overcome long-standing cultural handcuffs and get executives to listen."
- "Physicians are not exempt from treating employees respectfully."
- Physicians: "Unlike in the past, I will be held to the value of treating nurses as respected colleagues."
- Nurses: "Our feedback does help to make a difference in improving our work environment."
- Management: "Nurses deserve our utmost support and are just as valued as physicians."
- Culture: "Maybe management is serious this time, but we'll see."

Because a *group* got together to solve the problem, this deep "cultural handcuff" (see Chapter 4) was able to be addressed. This situation is symptomatic of many cultural handcuffs that are long-standing and virtually invisible because they are so ingrained. If these newer, healthier beliefs could be ingrained into the culture, there would be a better chance of attaining desired results.

As self-destructive organizational belief patterns are exposed as cultural barriers, the continuation of which would seriously affect attaining $R_2$ results, we realize that unlocking cultural handcuffs takes:

- Either a group effort or an interdepartmental effort to create $A_2$ events capable of exposing dysfunctional $B_1$ and creating openness to $B_2$;
- Formal management effort in response ($C_2$) to reinforce the $A_2$ activating event that then becomes
- An observed $A_2$ for the culture to begin to create confidence that management is serious about creating $B_2$; and
- Preventing even a whiff of an $A_1$ that could reinforce old $B_1$.

## Taking the Model Further to Audit a Culture

It is sometimes a helpful exercise to look at your desired $R_2$ organizational results and ask, "What are the daily behaviors we observe, the continuance of which will not allow us to attain these results?" I have had groups brainstorm this question and write every individual behavior on a sticky note. It is not unusual for groups to come up with more than 100 behaviors.

I then have them do what is called an "affinity exercise," a tool that should be in every leader's and facilitator's back pocket. The group silently looks at all of the sticky notes and tries to pick out two or three similar ideas. The individual notes are then separated into a group, to which other people can then add ideas of a similar nature. After about 20 to 25 minutes, the seemingly random individual observations have clustered into 8 to 12 groups. Think about what these groups represent: patterns of behavior, with an underlying belief driving each cluster. In other words, you have just done a cultural audit of the current organizational $B_1$.

**EXHIBIT 3.6** ■ A Cluster of Observed Behaviors

| | |
|---|---|
| **Observed Undesirable $C_1$**<br><br>(What is the underlying $B_1$?) | ■ Make all management reports "rosy."<br>■ Don't tell your peers what you really think of their ideas.<br>■ Don't speak up in meetings.<br>■ Wait until you can solve a problem before telling your boss about it.<br>■ Blame someone else when something goes wrong.<br>■ Anyone who speaks up is labeled a "troublemaker" by management and is evaluated as "not a team player."<br>■ Healthily assertive individuals rarely last longer than two years in this department. |

**EXHIBIT 3.7** ■ The Underlying $B_1$ Cultural Belief

| | |
|---|---|
| **Old Belief ($B_1$)** | Honest communication is a career-limiting move.<br><br>**(Driving need: survival)** |

**EXHIBIT 3.8** ■ An Alternative $B_2$ Belief to Achieve $R_2$ Results

| | |
|---|---|
| **New Belief ($B_2$)** | The way you get ahead is by being open and saying what you think.<br><br>**(Individuals balancing four needs to respect the business)** |

What might you conclude about an organizational culture if you saw the clustered patterns of consequential behaviors ($C_1$), displayed in Exhibit 3.6, being displayed and tolerated day in and day out? Regardless of the group with whom I facilitate this exercise, I almost always come across a cluster similar to this. What is the underlying $B_1$ belief?

I would probably conclude that, regardless of what the organization thinks it believes, the true belief is that declared in Exhibit 3.7.

If this is an issue in your culture, I would ask you to consider an $R_2$ result that this $B_1$ has not allowed you to attain.

Now, to motivate the need for a healthier belief, one has to ask the question, Will continuation of this belief allow us to get our $R_2$ results? (Apply it to your $R_2$.) If the answer is "No," that is a powerful motivator to change. Further, it then begs the question, "What might be a healthier $B_2$ belief?" One possibility is shown in Exhibit 3.8.

Now you can predict the results of this new belief by asking if your organization is able to incorporate this into your organizational belief system, then would your organization be able to attain your $R_2$ results. Your answer should be a resounding "Yes."

If that were a deeply embedded cultural value, what $C_2$ consequential behaviors might be observed on a daily basis? Some possibilities are shown in Exhibit 3.9. This table presents a series of nonthreatening behaviors to which you could coach the culture on a daily basis. The behaviors are grounded in organizational results ($R_2$) and the beliefs to

EXHIBIT 3.9 ■ Possible $C_2$ Behaviors Resulting from Healthier $B_2$ Belief

| New, Desired $C_2$ | • Share appropriate bad news proactively.<br>• Offer your peers straightforward feedback related to business results and their personal success.<br>• Everyone must facilitate open dialogue in meetings.<br>• Let people know early when there is a problem.<br>• When things go wrong, ask, "What else can I do?"<br>• Meetings need to be energized vehicles for teamwork and communication.<br>• Engage someone delivering bad news in healthy dialogue. |
|---|---|

drive them ($B_2$). All you need now is the new $A_2$ activating event of peer coaching in the moment to show that you are serious about the need for coaching ($B_2$).

I did this exercise once with a group of about 50 people who had five distinct organizational $R_2$. I assigned 10 people to each result and asked them to brainstorm and write down current observed daily tolerated behaviors that would be barriers to that specific result.

Afterward, while looking for the underlying belief of each cluster they brainstormed, one participant shared her insight with the group, "Looking at this cluster, it is clear that the message sent to our culture is, 'We do not trust our people.'" I asked her whether she thought it was intentional on management's part; she was sure that it was not. I asked her whether allowing that belief to continue would allow the culture to attain that result. She realized, "No!"

Despite brainstorming on five completely different results, each group discovered the *same* organizational $B_1$ as a barrier. The visceral "hit in the gut" could be felt in the room, which was the needed motivation for a new belief system. During the exercise, some people were amazed at how describing behaviors as simple as where people sat in the cafeteria were able to be clustered to intuit an organizational self-defeating $B_1$ belief.

Review the left column of Exhibit 3.10. It contains some common beliefs that, in my experience, seem to reappear regardless of the organization. Consider whether any of these apply to your culture. Think of your crucial $R_2$ results: Has the practice of tolerating beliefs like these every day allowed you to obtain them?

The right column of Exhibit 3.10 contains possible alternative $B_2$. Try to predict if your culture could attain its $R_2$ with these beliefs vis-à-vis the $B_1$ beliefs in the left column. The challenge is how to create appropriate $A_2$ activating events to drive these new $B_2$ into the culture.

The following questions can help you think further about how your cultural belief system surrounds you every day:

- What do consistent patterns of executive behavior and decisions tell you?
- What do schedules and budgets telegraph?
- What elements of Ralston's "corporate craziness" (see Exhibit 3.1) are tolerated?
- What is the extent of Dew's seven "root causes" (see introduction) in your culture?
- What behaviors are promoted?

As I said to one chief executive who was famous for grand announcements without realizing the extent to which he was laughed at behind his back in the culture, "I'm sorry. Your behavior is speaking so loudly, I can't hear what you're saying." Patterns of

EXHIBIT 3.10 ■ Common Dysfunctional Organizational $B_1$ Beliefs That Are Barriers to Transformational $R_2$

| From Old $B_1$ Beliefs | To New $B_2$ Beliefs |
|---|---|
| There's nothing really wrong; we're still in good shape. | We need to start doing things differently or we may not survive. |
| Each of us can just do his or her job well and be OK. | The company must function as a team. |
| Communication is to be avoided; it's useless anyway. | We need to talk honestly with one another. |
| Nobody is really accountable for anything. Accountability is avoided. | People must be and will be accountable for their commitments and performance. |
| Customers still believe in the quality of our care. | We will lose customers if we don't constantly win them. |
| The next technological acquisition will fix things. | Superior customer service is the key to our future. |
| We jump from one management "flavor of the month" to the next. | We learn the solid theory behind improvement and focus on what's important. |
| Corporate leadership has lost sight of what really goes on in individual hospitals and physicians' offices. | We need to work as a team. |
| We don't listen to most of what our key employees have to say. | We need to listen more, and more closely. |
| Pointing out a problem and speaking up have negative performance evaluation implications. | It is OK to disagree with anyone. |
| The economic environment has many people feeling tremendous insecurity about their jobs. | We will build loyalty, keep our people employable, and deal appropriately with poor performers. |
| Our approach should be hands-off and passive. | Our approach must be hands-on, active, and involved. |
| Change is to be avoided. | Change is to be embraced. |

behavior do not lie. And the sooner you are able to name your personal and organizational realities ($B_1$), the sooner you can begin the needed belief window surgery to align your belief systems in a healthier manner ($B_2$) to attain needed organizational results ($R_2$) and increased inner peace.

In addition to the needed $B_2$ to get $R_2$ is a need for an overarching cultural $B_2$ in line with an organizational value of peer coaching: *Every individual is personally responsible to deal with his or her behaviors interfering with organizational success. It is an expectation that every employee will coach and be open to nonjudgmental coaching in the moment.*

### The Issue of Trust

Using the A → B → C → R process, many organizations will come up with barriers relating to issues of trust. The concept is not as simple as saying, "Gee, we obviously have to change the cultural belief that 'We can't trust people' to 'We can trust people.' Poof — done!" That approach is meaningless for individuals and groups in the culture. What are needed are some serious, consistent activating events. Exhibit 3.11 shows you

## EXHIBIT 3.11 ■ Mutual $B_2$ to Create Trust

**Changing a situation:**
- How many windows have to change?
- What is the only window over which you have control?
- Can you create $A_2$ activating events that might make the other party *open to choosing* to change past behaviors?

**The "I can't trust them!" to "I can trust them" $B_2$ dance:**
- "We have both committed to changing the situation."
- "My behavior will demonstrate that I am indeed committed to changing the situation."
- "I will be open to letting their behavior change my belief window about them."
- "I will seek feedback on my behavior."
- "I will give feedback on their behavior."
- "Feedback will focus on specific exhibited behaviors and be given in the context of organizational success and genuine concern for personal success."

---

how to think more deeply about it through suggesting $B_2$ beliefs that will be required by *each* side involved.

## One More Mantra: "Paperboy Wisdom"

As shown in the previous section, besides being perfectly designed to produce your organizational results, you are also perfectly designed to produce your current culture in terms of:

- *Tolerated* organizational behaviors; and
- *Tolerated* individual behaviors.

Dale Dauten, also known as "The Corporate Curmudgeon" (www.dauten.com), once wrote a column giving 10 lessons he learned as a paperboy. Three of them are relevant for this chapter:

1. Every 10th person is a jerk.
2. The other nine are jerks 10 percent of the time.
3. I want to be one of the other nine.[7]

Ninety percent of the staff members in your culture are "just plain folks" who, especially under the stress of change, are going to exhibit 10 percent jerk time. Another leadership mantra during difficult transitions might be, "Allow 10 percent jerk time." Time and time again people have told me that this idea, along with "those darn humans" has been the most helpful piece of advice from my seminars.

It is important to realize as leaders and change agents that those darn humans have the luxury of exhibiting their 10 percent jerk time publicly. *Anyone in a leadership position does not*, because, if he or she does, those darn humans will conveniently use it against him or her as an excuse (stated reason) not to change.

You do have to allow yourself to be human; however, leaders, executives, middle managers, and change agents will need to keep the inevitable 10 percent jerk time, resulting from the sheer frustration of dealing with those darn humans, private, behind closed doors, and only with the most trusted of colleagues. The frustration is yet another given that goes with the territory of organizational transformation. Every so often, go for lunch or a beer after work and get all of your jerk time about the work culture resisting change out of your system with each other. Then, at the end, say to yourself and each other, with the sincere belief of Ellis's unconditional other-acceptance, "Whew, there was our 10 percent jerk time. Those darn humans; God bless 'em! Now, how do we go back and change to try to get them to want to volunteer to change? Let's go get 'em!"

Oh, yes, you leaders *will* have your inevitable 10 percent jerk time among each other in your routine meetings. One technique I have found very effective if someone exhibits his or her 10 percent is to simply tap on your water glasses with your pen (and possibly even have a jar in the middle of the table into which the person puts $1 for charity). Usually, *everyone* has a good laugh, even the "jerk of the moment," who generally realizes that he or she has "lost it." And then, the issue can be reframed in the context of organizational success and the person can be asked, "Help me understand…" or, as to be described in the next section, "What are *you* going to do about it?"

If you do not relish the fact that you will have to deal with this aspect of culture, Autry is adamant in his advice to get out of management.

Let me give you one example of the power of formally naming the 10 percent jerk time factor. Once I was speaking to an audience of 150 people on this topic, and, during the question session, a participant asked me a question in an extremely hostile tone while ranting about how what I presented had no value. Having already explained the concept of 10 percent jerk time, I stayed calm, smiled, looked at him, and gently asked, "Having our 10 percent jerk time, are we?" The whole room laughed, including the person asking the question. I asked him to clarify his hostility, then asked him to reframe his question. The previous hostility vanished, and productive dialogue ensued.

When we can acknowledge our humanity with humor, it can defuse a *lot* of tension. And as will happen occasionally, leaders obtain much more credibility in the employees' eyes when their culture reflects the comfort to feed back to you that you are indeed exhibiting jerk time, and it is accepted with grace and humor.

Now, what about the 10 percent of the people who display close to 100 percent jerk time? Dauten has a wonderful saying: "Jerks are like vampires. You hold up a mirror and they see nothing."[8] However, despite their attempted monovoxoplegia (paralysis by one loud voice) you can quite easily take away their power.

Once again, I invoke Autry's wisdom: There are no secrets. Virtually *everyone* knows who the organizational jerks are, and it is amazing how much power they are given because that behavior is tolerated time and time again and not appropriately confronted. Many jerks have an entitled attitude that gets them promoted in spite of it (a whole other issue regarding your organizational promotion processes). How to deal with jerks so as not to give them so much cultural power is discussed in the next section. The situation can, for the most part, be defused through the same very simple technique that is used to deal with "the other nine's" 10 percent jerk time.

## A New Definition of Accountability

In today's society, you name a topic, and somebody is mad about it. The sense of entitlement is increasing, and it is accompanied by a perception of loss of personal control. There is a toxic perception that something bad that happens is always someone else's fault. It is easy to see that our current societal processes are infected with what Clemmer calls the "victimitis virus." Look at the anger behind many world conflicts, the lack of personal accountability of many political leaders, the ridiculous salaries given to ego-filled athletes, the mindless business budget cuts and layoffs of hard-working people contrasted with the golden parachutes of failed CEOs — past cultural chickens have come home to roost.

This growing sense of entitlement has resulted in all-too-familiar cultural patterns of whining and avoiding responsibility, grandstanding politicians demanding "accountability," and righteously indignant cries of "Who's to blame?" These are enormous, needless energy drains on society, government, organizational cultures, schools, and families.

Given the tough economic times, the old-fashioned concept of accountability seems to be returning, but in an outdated context of adherence to tough organizational goals through draconian enforcement and consequences. "Who's to blame?" is sometimes euphemistically replaced by "Who's accountable?"

Regardless, blame is one of the more serious symptoms of the prevalent victimhood culture in today's society and its organizations. With a deeper understanding of process, I still feel that zero tolerance for blame should be an organizational norm (the odds are at least 85 to 15 in your favor). However, that does not absolve people from being accountable; rather, it redefines the notion.

Accountability should no longer mean either "account for" or "responsible for." And yet so much time is spent in meetings listening to litanies of excuse making, finger pointing, blaming others, confusion, an attitude of helplessness, or carefully crafted stories to explain *lack of* results. A deeper transformation in mind-set must take place, to a sense of reality, ownership, solutions to problems, and determined action. True accountability is powered by commitment and hard work, with a focus on current and future efforts rather than reactive and historical explanations.

*If one does not attain desired results, one should immediately own that fact, offer no excuses, and answer the question, "What else is it going to take?"* The past is used only for learning, especially to expose and deal with the long-standing, ingrained, and mostly unspoken cultural handcuffs.

I have found that, if you wait long enough, someone exhibiting the victimitis virus will eventually ask a generalized question beginning with "Who," "Why," or "When." Using a very simple technique developed by John Miller (www.qbq.com; see also Resources), to change a person's belief about a situation, ask the person to restate the question under the following conditions:

- "Lack of..." is *never* acceptable as a barrier (it is only a barrier because some deep cultural beliefs and resulting actions have made it a barrier);
- Restate the issue via a *question* beginning with the word "What" or "How";
- It must include the word "I" (not "We"); and
- It must contain an action.

Here is a powerful example for using this technique. I was giving a seminar to 150 people in the United Kingdom and had been forewarned that there would be a physician present who had a tendency to disrupt things with angry rants. I proceeded to give my talks on data sanity and culture (including this technique). During the question-and-answer period, a distinguished-looking woman stood up, and I could feel the tension rise in the room — it was obviously *she*. "This is all very well and good, she began. "But, what about Tony Blair and the ministers? Who is going to give this message to them, and why hasn't anyone done so, and it's futile to keep on going the way we're going..." I interrupted her, "Excuse me, Madam, but you were also present at my second lecture?" I could feel the tension rising further. "I would like you to try and reframe what you just said using a question beginning with 'What' or 'How,' have it include the word 'I,' and contain some type of 'action.' Can you do that?"

Facing an icily silent reaction, I said, "Please work with me here and give it a try." She looked at the floor for about 30 seconds, then said, "How could I see to it that a group of influential physicians got you invited to speak to some health ministers with this important message?" to which I replied, "And if you do that, I would gladly speak to them." I could feel the tension in the room virtually dissipate.

The power of using this technique with your organizational jerks is that it commits them to suggesting an action and allows you to make them subsequently accountable for it. And if they do not follow through, they have in essence lost the right to complain in the future. This $A_2$ event, if applied consistently, will send a $B_2$ signal to the culture that no whining will be allowed to go gently unchallenged. The culture is perfectly designed to whine, so you cannot stop it; however, you can deal with it very productively through this technique. Imagine if you could get the $B_2$ belief ingrained in the culture that the application of this technique *will* be the response to their 10 percent.

## Creating an Empowered Culture

Another frustrating situation this technique will help you handle is that encountered many times by managers when people try to get you to take on their problems. The technique is a way of allowing you to make them accountable for solving issues and defining your role properly after you force them to ask the "What" or "How"/"I"/"[action]" question. When they are finished, you then ask, "What will it take from me to make that happen for you?" "How can I help you in that effort?" or "What barriers do you need me to remove to make it easier for you?"

In other words, your job is to remove the cultural handcuffs to their empowerment. If they succeed, you have created a powerful $A_2$ experience to motivate a key $B_2$ cultural belief: Employees are truly empowered to solve their problems.

Regarding the "'lack of' is *never* an option" statement, it was wonderful wisdom from a consultant friend of mine who was emphatic about it, and time has subsequently convinced me of its effectiveness. "Lack of" is only an option because the current culture has made it an option; think about what having that as a cultural $B_2$ belief can motivate.

In such situations, lack of time will frequently be mentioned as a stated reason. In response, I tell people to substitute the word *priority* for *time* and have them answer again, this time with the follow-up question: "What else is it going to take?" Lack of time is thus not an option for either the empowered employee or the manager removing barriers to empowerment.

Three more healthy $B_2$ beliefs are:

1. I can visit "Pity City." I just cannot live there.
2. "Lack of…" is *never* an option.
3. If I cannot change a situation, I probably have to change the way I think about it.

This process works very well with individual situations or when defusing the inevitable 10 percent exhibited in an everyday meeting. However, dealing with group resistance in a formal meeting being used to introduce significant change is a little more difficult. A very useful technique for handling that situation is given in Chapter 4 as part of your leadership and change agent's "handbook."

## EXHIBIT 3.12   What Can I Do as a Leader Starting Tomorrow?

Some key $B_2$ for a leadership belief system (and mantras) whose $R_2$ will be "To create a culture that will produce organizational $R_2$."

- New results = new beliefs
- Zero tolerance for blame
- Given: People hate being changed.
  - Stated reasons vs. real reasons
  - "Those darn humans — God bless 'em."
  - "Us darn humans — God bless us all."
  - "Most important human problems have no permanent solution."
  - "Culture is 'hungry' to eat my best intentions."
  - "How do I change so as to get other people to want to volunteer to change?"
- Allow 10 percent jerk time:
  - Strong reactions are never for the reasons we think.
  - "Help me understand…"
  - "I must insulate my hot buttons": Leaders have no public jerk time.
  - No whining allowed — to go (gently) unchallenged
  - Jerk time: "Who," "Why," or "When" questions convert to, "What" or "How"/"I"/ "[action]" questions
  - Sample response: "How can I help you make that happen?"
- Promotions are not an entitlement; they are earned through exhibiting desired $C_2$ behaviors clearly aligned with $R_2$ results.
- Feedback and personal and cultural growth:
  - Attack the behavior, not human beings.
  - Walk the talk, giving and receiving feedback.
- Seek feedback:
  - "What feedback do you have for me?"
  - Feedback is a perception being shared, not a truth being declared.
  - "Swallow my ego 10 times before breakfast and another dozen more times before lunch."
  - "How can I make that right?"
- Holding ourselves accountable for holding ourselves accountable:
  - *Accountability* does not mean "account for."
  - "The only person I can change and speak for is myself."
  - Relentlessly asking, "What else is it going to take to achieve $R_2$?"
- Eradicating corporate craziness via cultural honesty:
  - Meeting sanity
- Data sanity:
  - Plot the dots.
- People tend to recognize experiences that reinforce their existing $B_1$ beliefs rather than those that promote the new $B_2$ beliefs:
  - Most experiences will need to be interpreted for people for them to form the $B_2$ beliefs you want them to have.

> "Think of it all as entertainment or I'm going to get an ulcer!"

## SUMMARY
### Organizational and Personal Change

Twenty years ago, I learned a wonderfully simple model summarizing the change process, essentially consisting of the following phases:

- Phase 1: Having awareness;
- Phase 2: Achieving a breakthrough in knowledge;
- Phase 3: Choosing a breakthrough in thinking; and
- Phase 4: Demonstrating a breakthrough in behavior.

*Unless thinking (belief system) changes, behavior will not change in the long term.* Applying this model to the discussion in this chapter:

- Awareness is an activating event, $A_2$.
- Breakthrough in knowledge occurs through a description of desired $R_2$ and needed $C_2$ to drive those results.
- Choosing a breakthrough in thinking is represented by $B_1 \rightarrow B_2$, which can take two minutes to 20 years.
  - The nature of the activating event needs to motivate a $B_1$ vs. $B_2$ struggle, which, through cultural reinforcement, $B_2$ will eventually win.
  - Is it perceived as an $A_1$ (more of the same) or $A_2$ (visceral hit in the gut)?
- A breakthrough in behavior is shown when observed $C_2$ consequential behaviors and $R_2$ results are reflected on the organizational balanced scorecard or in changed individual behavior.

Accomplishing improvement in this framework is hard work and most likely results from a visceral wrestling with one's current belief system and the realization that it is a self-defeating belief that has served one well, up until now. The needed breakthrough in thinking generally occurs only after a conscious realization that current behaviors and actions will not produce long-term desired results, and this realization is usually precipitated by an activating event that causes a deep, visceral internal reaction. One is now at a moment where a conscious choice has to be made to change the current belief system to one that will drive the desired results and be subsequently consistently noticed as a breakthrough in behavior.

### What You Can Do as a Leader

Despite the nice logic of the engine of quality, most of the work needs to be spent on its fuel, which is going to require many new $B_2$ cultural and leadership beliefs. These are summarized in Exhibit 3.12. "What can I do as a leader starting tomorrow?" outlines your biggest immediate challenges and the beliefs (and mantras) needed to deal with them effectively for better results, related to both organizational and personal growth.

Changing belief systems is very serious business, but here is a humorous summary and attitude to take as you embark on this exciting and challenging journey:

- Never believe totally in your own B.S.
- Never believe totally in anyone else's B.S.

B.S. means "belief system" and can also mean "balanced scorecard." Of course, wisdom can be found in both definitions. Painting by the numbers will never produce great art. Why should managing strictly by the numbers produce great organizations?

Learning to deal comfortably with the very normal aspects of human behavior will be a wonderful wildcard in your transformational effort and give you high-octane fuel for an engine that you want to have firing on all cylinders.

## REFERENCES

1. Carnegie, Dale. 1981. *How to Win Friends and Influence People*. New York: Simon and Schuster.
2. Goleman, Daniel, Richard Boyatzis, and Annie McKee. 2002. *Primal Leadership: Realizing the Power of Emotional Intelligence*, 99. Boston: Harvard Business School Press. Used with permission of Harvard Business Publishing. All rights reserved.
3. Ralston, Faith. 2002. *Emotions@Work: Get Great Results by Encouraging Accountability and Resolving Conflicts*, 5, 68. Bloomington, IN: 1st Books Library.
4. Grinnell, John R. Jr. 1994. "Optimize the Human System." *Quality Progress* (November).
5. Joseph, Dan. 2007. *Quiet Mind Newsletter* (September).
6. Juran, Joseph M. 1994. *Managerial Breakthrough: A New Concept of the Manager's Job*, 153. New York: McGraw-Hill.
7. Dauten, Dale. April 8, 1994. "Some Lessons Last Long Past Childhood." *Orlando Sentinel*. http://articles.orlandosentinel.com/1994-04-08/business/9404080826_1_people-are-jerks-customers-conformity.
8. Dauten, Dale. August 9, 1998. "Some Common Sense Notions Are Not Common Enough." *Chicago Tribune*. http://articles.chicagotribune.com/1998-08-09/business/9808090338_1_common-sense-facts-trouble-business.

## RESOURCES

American Society for Quality. www.asq.org.
Autry, James A. 1992. *Love and Profit: The Art of Caring Leadership*. New York: Harper Paperbacks.
Autry, James A. n.d. "Love and Profit: The Art of Caring Leadership" (video). Cambridge, MA: Enterprise Media.
Balestracci, Davis. 2012. "Frustrated by Glacial Improvement Process?" *Quality Digest* (January 25). www.qualitydigest.com/inside/quality-insider-column/frustrated-glacial-improvement-progress.html.
Balestracci, Davis. 2012. "Frustrated by Glacial Improvement Process, Part Two." *Quality Digest* (February 2). www.qualitydigest.com/inside/quality-insider-column/frustrated-glacial-improvement-progress-part-two.html.
Balestracci, Davis. 2013. "Off to the Milky Way." *Quality Digest* (April 9). www.qualitydigest.com/inside/quality-insider-article/milky-way.html.
Balestracci, Davis. 2013. "What Are *You* Tolerating?" *Quality Digest* (February 14). www.qualitydigest.com/inside/quality-insider-column/what-are-you-tolerating.html.
Balestracci, Davis. 2014. "Improvement: As Simple as ABC…D?" *Quality Digest* (January 20). www.qualitydigest.com/inside/quality-insider-column/improvement-simple-abc-d.html.
Connors, Roger, Tom Smith, and Craig Hickman. 1994. *The OZ Principle: Getting Results through Individual and Organizational Accountability*. Englewood Cliffs, NJ: Prentice-Hall.
Crane, Thomas G. 1999. *The Heart of Coaching: Using Transformational Coaching to Create a High-Performance Culture*. San Diego: FTA Press.
Miller, John G. 2004. *QBQ! The Question behind the Question: What to Really Ask Yourself… Practicing Personal Accountability in Business and in Life*. New York: G.P. Putnam's Sons.

CHAPTER 4

# A Leadership Handbook: Creating the Culture to Deliver Desired New Results

*Part of the problem is that we're traveling in uncharted territory. Old maps and traditional compasses can easily lead management teams astray. Many of the routes and practices that senior managers followed for their own career success now lead to mediocre performance — or oblivion. Managers need to draw new maps for themselves, their teams, and their organizations. And since there's no certain path to higher performance or sure-fire formula for success, highly effective leaders are searching out, exploring, and blazing their own new and unique trails. — Jim Clemmer*

## KEY IDEAS

- The cultural change required for unprecedented results needs to be formally managed while avoiding eight common errors.
- Leaders need to go beyond "passionate lip service" to active involvement and integrate quality improvement into the organization's daily fabric.
- A culture that emphasizes good peer and internal customer service will be able to truly serve external customers.
- The "mood map" is a helpful organizational barometer for reading the culture.
- Creating a truly empowered workforce is difficult and requires seven elements to be in place.
- Peter Block's "Employee Manifesto" is a powerful context in which to deal with organizational victim behavior.
- Addressing demotivators formally and through daily walk-arounds will improve cultural morale and integrate accountability into a culture.
- Formally addressing poor meetings as a source of organizational waste will create the time and energy for improvement.
- When people are unclear what to do, they may need to be formally facilitated as to what they need to stop doing, start doing, and continue doing in the context of clear $R_2$ results.

- Good leaders seek feedback, they do not personalize it, and they act on it.
- Leadership must develop the skills for ongoing cultural coaching that is from the heart.
- Integrating statistical thinking into daily management will liberate the time to create the desired culture.

## EIGHT ERRORS TO AVOID

John Kotter's book *Leading Change* (see Resources) might be the single most refreshingly readable, practical, and straightforward book I have ever read on organizational change and its leadership. I highly recommend it for your leadership team development and ongoing management development.

In it, Kotter indicates that many organizations are overmanaged and underled, with tendencies toward an inwardly focused culture, paralyzing bureaucracy, parochial politics, low levels of trust, lack of teamwork, arrogant attitudes, a lack of leadership in middle management, and the general human fear of the unknown, which means, according to Kotter:[1]

- New strategies are not implemented well;
- Mergers do not achieve expected synergies;
- Reengineering takes too long and costs too much;
- Downsizing does not get costs under control; and
- Quality programs do not deliver hoped-for results.

In other words, as discussed in Chapter 3, most well-meaning improvement efforts seem to routinely fall short because they fail to alter behavior. This downside of change is inevitable because of the ever-present pain induced when human communities are forced to adjust to shifting conditions.

However, despite the inevitability, Kotter identifies what he feels are the eight most common errors that make matters worse than they could be:[1]

Error 1: Allowing too much complacency. To solve, establish a sense of urgency.

Error 2: Failing to create a sufficiently powerful guiding coalition. To solve, create one, *and get it to work like a team.*

Error 3: Underestimating the power of vision. To solve, develop a vision and strategy.

Error 4: Undercommunicating the vision by a factor of 10. To solve, use every vehicle possible to communicate it and have the guiding coalition role model the expected behaviors. Conventional wisdom seems to state that important issues should be communicated eight times in eight different ways.

Error 5: Permitting obstacles to block the new vision. To solve, empower broad-based action by changing systems or infrastructure elements that undermine the change vision. Encourage risk taking in the culture to address and break down the everyday barriers encountered.

Error 6: Failing to create short-term wins. To solve, plan for visible improvements, create them, and visibly celebrate achievements.

Error 7: Declaring victory too soon. To solve, consolidate gains to produce more change by leveraging increased credibility to change systems, structures, and policies that do not fit together. Ingrain the vision through hiring and promotion processes.

Error 8: Neglecting to anchor changes firmly in the corporate culture. Until new behaviors are rooted in social norms and shared values, they are always subject to degradation as soon as the pressures associated with a change effort are removed. To solve, develop more and better leadership with more effective management.

The first four errors result from a hardened status quo, the next three affect the introduction of new practices, and the last keeps changes from sticking. In fact, a lot of frustration with most organizational quality improvement (QI) efforts is because of a tendency to deny the power of errors 1 through 4 to keep the status quo firmly entrenched and hope that taking efforts to deal with errors 5 through 7 will get results. Unfortunately, they need to be addressed in sequence (with some overlap), and omission of a step almost guarantees failure.

In this context, the distinction between "management" and "leadership" becomes even more crucial (Kotter writes extensively on this):

- Planning and budgeting must give way to establishing direction;
- Organizing and staffing must give way to aligning people; and
- Controlling and problem solving must give way to motivating and inspiring.

Ultimately, the status quo cultural need for producing a degree of predictability and order to consistently produce short-term results must give way to producing change (often dramatic), then producing even more extremely useful change.

Organizations that outperform competitors excel at four primary management practices:

1. Devising a clearly stated and focused strategy;
2. Maintaining flawless operational management;
3. Developing a performance-oriented culture; and
4. Creating a flat and flexible structure.

In addition, they also seem to embrace any two out of the following four secondary management practices:

1. Holding onto talented staff and finding more of the same;
2. Making industry-transforming innovations;
3. Finding leaders committed to the business and its people; and
4. Seeking growth through carefully selected mergers and partnerships.

Studer's *Hardwiring Excellence* suggests a framework anchored by the nine principles displayed in Exhibit 4.1.

Here are a few more of Studer's nuggets to consider as you proceed. Early in your efforts, you must:

- Re-recruit high performers, or they will think about leaving;
- Increase the substance of communication to staff;
- Develop healthier, more mature supervision in a context of empowerment, not control;
- Spotlight and share successes and knowledge;

> **EXHIBIT 4.1** ■ Studer Group's Nine Principles®
>
> 1. Commit to excellence.
> 2. Measure the important things.
> 3. Build a culture around service.
> 4. Create and develop leaders.
> 5. Focus on employee satisfaction.
> 6. Build individual accountability.
> 7. Align behaviors with goals and values.
> 8. Communicate at all levels.
> 9. Recognize and reward success.
>
> *Always* connect results back to purpose, worthwhile work, and making a difference.
>
> **It's all about hardwiring!**
>
> Source: Adapted with permission from Studer Group. *Hardwiring Excellence: Purpose, Worthwhile Work, Making a Difference.* 2003. Pensacola, FL: Fire Starter Publishing.

- Anticipate the inevitability of "the wall," where things seem to grind to a halt, which will force leaders to confront the need to:
  – Refocus and recommit;
  – Deal with poor performers (at this point, the gap between excellent or good performers and poor performers has become intolerable, and the culture is watching);
  – Continue to re-recruit high performers;
  – Increase substance of communication to staff;
  – Promote your winners; and
  – Ensure that the right people are in the right places.[2]

## A MESSAGE FROM MY SEMINAR PARTICIPANTS

As I give seminars to healthcare improvement personnel all over the world, I receive a consistent message during the summary at the end in terms of what they perceive as organizational barriers to desired results from their viewpoint of QI. Their feelings on what it will take for any culture to overcome these barriers are summarized in Exhibit 4.2. Given these, they would feel inherently empowered and be willing to "hold themselves accountable for holding themselves accountable."

## THE NEED TO SHIFT CULTURAL $B_1$ BELIEFS

### What Behaviors Are Needed to Create Activating Events for Your Organizational Culture?

The literature is virtually unanimous: Top management cannot merely be committed to QI but must also lead the quality process.

What is your level of executive commitment? Unless you believe yourself to be at least at Level 4 (involved leadership), as detailed in the following descriptions,[3] I suggest waiting and doing some serious work on your own and the leadership team's current belief systems. If you do not, all you will end up achieving is better cultural cynics for your next perceived grand announcement.

Level 1. Permission: Let people proceed as long as their progress does not cost too much and disrupt the real business.

Level 2. Lip service:
- You read a speech written for you and write memos exhorting everyone to improve service and quality.
- Some budgets and resources are allocated to a piecemeal series of improvement programs, but no overall strategic service or QI plan is in place.
- The process is not part of operational management's responsibilities, and the leadership team is not personally involved in education or training.

Level 3. Passionate lip service:
- Leaders attend an abbreviated overview of the training being given to everyone else.
- Some elements of a deployment process are shakily in place.
- Passionate stump speeches urge everyone to "get going."

Level 4. Involved leadership:
- Leaders attend all training first in its entirety then get trained to deliver the introductory education, awareness, and skill-development sessions.
- Service and QIs related to organizational strategy are the first item on all meeting agendas and priority lists.
- Managers are held accountable and rewarded for their contributions to continuous improvement.
- The leadership group leads process management.
- A strong and comprehensive deployment process — infrastructure, planning, and reporting, and assigned responsibilities — is in place.

Level 5. Strategic service and quality leadership is displayed:
- Day-to-day operating decisions have been delegated to the myriad, increasingly autonomous improvement teams.
- The majority of the leadership team's time is spent with customers, suppliers, teams, and managers. A main part of their job is now gathering input for long-term direction and managing the organization's context by providing meaning through the vision and values.

**EXHIBIT 4.2** Davis's Past Seminar Participants' Manifesto for Leaders

- *Zero* tolerance for blame
- *Clear* organizational results ($R_2$) as a rudder for driving cultural change
- *Clear* quality improvement results
  - *Clearly* aligned with desired $R_2$
  - Quality improvement as the strategy for driving organizational policy
- Applying the Pareto principle (80/20 rule) to quality efforts
  - Ask for cultural changes *only* on important things related to mission, vision, and values
- Peer coaching in the moment on $C_1$ behaviors incongruent with organizational success and values (personal success)
- Dealing with the inherent cultural victimitis virus via "What" or "How"/"I"/ "[action]" questions

**EXHIBIT 4.3** ■ The Mood Map — From Thought to Reality

**Personal Accountability**

| | Thinking State (Beliefs and Attitudes) | Feeling State (Emotional Response) | Behaviors (Actions and Reactions) | Results, Outcomes, and Impacts |
|---|---|---|---|---|
| **Higher States** | "I'm resourceful" Up to my life Worthy Enough | Confident Inspired Eager Optimistic | Graceful Creative Purposeful Responsive | Joy Peace Bliss Resiliency |
| | "I'm grateful" Appreciative Unique Precious | Generous Empowered Abundant Positive | Contribute Give Support Thanks | Fulfillment Intimacy Safety Partnership |
| | "I'm curious" Wonderment Interested Inviting | Open Accepting Fascinated Surprised | Ask questions Attentive listening Disclosing Respectful | Learning Connection Trust Rapport |

**Victimhood**

| | | | | |
|---|---|---|---|---|
| **Lower States** | "I'm separate" You vs. Me Judgment Comparing | "Better than" (arrogant) "Less than" (resentful) | Critical/discount Judgment/blame Defend/protect stuff | Tension Distance Withdrawal Compliance |
| | "I am my role" I am identified Take it personally Win/lose | Insecure Threatened Suspicious Afraid | Attributions Resistance Attack Sabotage | Conflict Struggle Politics War |
| | "I'm powerless" I can't I'm stuck I'm helpless | Depressed Out of control Alone In despair | Frozen Wait/hope Negative Reactionary | Victim Sinking Others control you Giving up |

Source: From *The Heart of Coaching — Using Transformational Coaching to Create a High-Performance Culture*, 4th ed. by Thomas G. Crane. Crane Consulting, published by FTA Press, San Diego, CA, 1999–2015, www.craneconsulting.com.

How do you ultimately transition to Level 5? Learn the philosophy of continuous improvement (read Joiner's *Fourth Generation Management* as a start; see Resources). Use process language and data sanity (see Chapters 1 and 2) in your daily interactions. Educate, educate, educate your culture through *your* behavior. This practice goes far beyond mere training classes and short courses: *Education and awareness are never finished.*

Do not let one opportunity go by to comment on quality, organizational strategy, or desired results. Reprioritize your objectives and work style accordingly. Keep track of your ongoing progress by using the assessment checklists in the sidebars. Develop the leadership team's emotional ability to read its collective thinking state in meetings via the "mood map"[4] (Exhibit 4.3). To even have a chance of success, your team should at least be displaying genuine "I'm curious" behaviors. Remember, as emphasized in Chapter 3, the culture is a mirror reflecting the emotional climate of the leadership team.

Transition is painful. Participants want to know what's in it for them. People who perceive they are losing *will* find a way to win. Help them connect the dots to their everyday work and the future of the organization. Justify the rationale for emphasis on quality and constantly repeat it. Assure them that they will have jobs (or you will see to it that they have the skills to remain employable), even though their individual roles may change in the transformed culture.

Empathize with all involved. Acknowledge that the rules of the healthcare game are changing, but let people know: "You are smart human beings. You need to help each other do it, but you can do it." As one executive said to his staff, "I understand your pain. We empathize and will gladly carry the wounded. *But* stragglers will be shot!"

### *Develop an Almost Fanatical Obsession with Customer Needs*

Developing a fanatical obsession with customer needs means recognizing one's internal customers as well as the more obvious typical focus on external customers. Constantly be aware of your external customers' needs, but at the same time, realize that you cannot even begin to satisfactorily meet their needs until your workforce truly understands its jobs. Your workforce must understand its relationship to and the needs of its internal customers. This awareness is difficult to develop, but it is one of the most vital concepts in service QI.

And remember, the employees will treat the customers no better than the way you treat them.

### *Incorporate Statistical Thinking throughout the Organization*

The most compact summary of QI available is W. Edwards Deming's statement, "If I had to reduce my message to management to just a few words, I'd say it all has to do with reducing variation." Some key skills are given in Exhibit 2.46.

Statistical thinking means looking at everything the organization does as a series of processes that have the goal of consistently providing the results your customers desire. All processes display variation, which must be studied via data to take the appropriate improvement actions and create consistently predictable processes. Thinking in terms of processes is perhaps the deepest change needed for continuous improvement.

The data skills and customer focus of continuous improvement have profound implications on the psychology of the work culture. A helpless, powerless feeling among most employees can result from the natural tendencies to:

- Blame people;
- Use arbitrary goals;
- Judge performance in a system in which the odds are at least 85 to 15 against the employee;
- Work around poorly designed processes; and
- Use "smile or else" approaches on employees as a method to handle angry customers who are also victims of the same processes.

### *Address Demotivators*

It is believed that the fate of many companies could be altered for the better if workers were more motivated. So when things go wrong, why is the knee-jerk reaction to blame the workers for their poor attitudes and lack of work ethic? As I have been emphasizing throughout this book, one needs to look within one's business systems for the true causes of low motivation and their remedies.

EXHIBIT 4.4 ■ 21 Workplace Demotivators That Breed Fear and Anger

1. Politics*
2. Unclear expectations*
3. Unnecessary rules
4. Poorly designed work*
5. Unproductive meetings
6. Lack of follow-up
7. Constant change
8. Internal competition
9. Dishonesty, feeling "lied to"
10. Hypocrisy, not "walking the talk"*
11. Withholding information
12. Unfairness, preferential treatment
13. Discouraging responses to ideas
14. Atmosphere of criticism
15. Capacity underutilization of individuals
16. Tolerating poor performance
17. Being taken for granted*
18. Management invisibility
19. Overcontrol
20. Takeaways of past privileges
21. Being forced to do poor-quality work*

* Spitzer considers these the six most serious demotivators.

Source: Dean Spitzer. 1995. *SuperMotivation: A Blueprint for Energizing Your Organization from Top to Bottom.* New York: AMACOM, 1995, page 3. Used with permission.

*Demotivators* are performance inhibitors that have stealthily and insidiously crept into organizational processes to become part of normal daily operations. They have a profound effect on performance, yet are often ignored. A lot of the fear and anger, both expressed and repressed, rampant in organizations today is caused by these demotivators.

Exhibit 4.4 lists the 21 demotivators as identified by Dean Spitzer[5] in his book *SuperMotivation* (see Resources). He developed a helpful survey to determine the "demotivational climate" in one's organization, which is reproduced on pages 112 and 113. Its ongoing use could perhaps be analyzed via plotting the dots to monitor progress.

The ongoing presence of demotivators can result in negative behavior by employees and even affect their health. Spitzer also cites research that 84 percent of workers say they could perform better if they wanted to, and 50 percent of workers say they put forth only enough effort to hang onto their jobs.[5] He writes:

> Too many managers underestimate the importance of what they consider minor irritations, not realizing how large these irritations loom in the subjective experience of employees. To employees stuck in the middle, these demotivators are not minor at all.[5]

Spitzer claims that negative behaviors in reaction to these demotivators cost American industry $170 billion a year through intentional slowdowns, procrastination, careless repeated mistakes, inattentiveness, unsafe behavior, absenteeism, tardiness, extended

## Are You Trying to Make Your Organization or Team into Something You're Not?

To what extent are you:

- ☐ Attempting to change your organization or team without changing yourself?
- ☐ Prodding your organization to be more people (customer/partner) focused when you're a technomanager (driven by management systems and technology)?
- ☐ Driving for industry or market leadership when you're afflicted with the pessimism plague and/or victimitis virus?
- ☐ Striving to stimulate and energize others when you aren't passionate about your own role and life's work?
- ☐ Promoting organization or team vision, values, and mission when your own picture of your preferred future, principles, and purpose isn't clear and/or well aligned with where you're trying to lead others?
- ☐ Pushing for a customer-driven organization while controlling and dominating, rather than serving (servant leadership)?
- ☐ Aspiring to develop new markets and fill unmet needs while spending limited time with customers, partners, or those serving them?
- ☐ Trying to build a learning organization when your own rate of personal growth and development is low?
- ☐ Declaring the urgency of higher levels of innovation while you stick to familiar personal methods and traditional command-and-control management approaches?
- ☐ Aiming for disciplined organization or team goal and priority setting when you're not well organized, a poor personal time manager, and fuzzy about your own goals and priorities?
- ☐ Setting organization improvement plans without an improvement process of your own?
- ☐ Promoting teamwork and a team-based organization without providing a personal model of team leadership and team effectiveness in action?
- ☐ Supporting high levels of skill development — for everyone else?
- ☐ Forcing accountability, performance appraisal, and measurement on others while you defend, avoid, or halfheartedly gather personal feedback?
- ☐ Proclaiming empowerment and involvement while controlling and limiting people with a centralized structure and systems that constrain rather than support?
- ☐ Talking about the need for better communications without becoming a strong and compelling communicator?
- ☐ Establishing formal reward and recognition programs when your personal habits of giving sincere recognition and showing genuine appreciation are weak?
- ☐ Espousing support for change champions while suppressing "off the wall" behavior and pushing people to follow your plans and stay within your established system?
- ☐ Advocating reviews and assessments while doing little personal reflection and contemplation?

Source: Jim Clemmer. 1995. Pathways to Performance: A Guide to Transforming Yourself, Your Team, and Your Organization, 215–216, 290–291, 293–294. Kitchener, Ontario, Canada: TCG Press. Used with permission of Jim Clemmer, leadership and organization development author, speaker, and workshop/retreat leader (www.ClemmerGroup.com).

> **Outstanding Teams Checklist**
> 
> ☐ A high-performance balance (analytical skills and disciplined management processes, technical skills and strong capabilities to use the latest technologies, and people leadership skills)
> 
> ☐ Strong self-determination with no tolerance for the victimitis virus or pessimism plague (One team agreed, "You can visit Pity City, but you aren't allowed to move there.")
> 
> ☐ Passion and high energy for rapid and continuous learning, developing, and improving
> 
> ☐ A clear and compelling picture of the team's preferred future (including desired team type and focus)
> 
> ☐ A clearly articulated set of shared principles outlining how the team will work together
> 
> ☐ A strong sense of purpose and unity on why the team exists
> 
> ☐ Solid agreement on whom the team is serving within the customer–partner chain and organization processes
> 
> ☐ Identification of, and an aggressive plan for, improving the team's customer–partner performance gaps
> 
> ☐ Relentless exploring, searching, and creating new customers and markets (if appropriate to the team's role)
> 
> ☐ A process for innovation and team learning
> 
> ☐ A handful of performance goals and priorities directly linked to the organization's strategic imperatives
> 
> ☐ A concrete process and discipline for continuous team improvement linked to the organization's improvement effort
> 
> ☐ Process management skills, roles, and responsibilities
> 
> ☐ High levels of team leadership and team effectiveness skills
> 
> ☐ Powerful feedback loops and measurements
> 
> ☐ A culture of thanks, recognition, and celebration
> 
> Source: Jim Clemmer. 1995. Pathways to Performance: A Guide to Transforming Yourself, Your Team, and Your Organization, 215–216, 290–291, 293–294. Kitchener, Ontario, Canada: TCG Press. Used with permission of Jim Clemmer, leadership and organization development author, speaker, and workshop/retreat leader (www.ClemmerGroup.com).

breaks, violence, and stealing (petty to major). He calculates that the cost of three demotivators a day per person in an organization with 100 employees working 240 days a year would be $2.26 million a year.

The current pace of change in American business practices (including healthcare) as well as society in general has unintentionally created a fertile breeding ground for these demotivators. Addressing them in an ad hoc fashion, as in the past, will no longer work.

Peter Block wrote a monthly column for several years for the Association for Quality and Participation (now absorbed into the American Society for Quality). The column reprinted in Exhibit 4.5 contains his "Employee Manifesto," which leaders could use to create a quid pro quo: They will be accountable for addressing demotivators while making employees accountable for exhibiting Block's proposed behaviors. It is my opinion that

## Change Checkpoints and Improvement Milestones

- ☐ Clear and compelling reasons for changing and improving
- ☐ Balanced focus on people, management, and technology
- ☐ Strong ethic of self-determination
- ☐ Comprehensive and balanced improvement model
- ☐ Clear and compelling picture of your preferred future
- ☐ Three or four core values
- ☐ Definitive statement of purpose, business you're in, or why you exist
- ☐ Rich and continuous customer–partner performance gap data
- ☐ Intense exploring and searching for new markets and customers
- ☐ High levels of experimentation, pilots, and clumsy tries
- ☐ Robust process for disseminating team and organization learning
- ☐ Three to four strategic imperatives for each annual improvement cycle
- ☐ Direct links between all improvement activities and strategic imperatives
- ☐ Comprehensive and balanced improvement plan
- ☐ Improvement planning structure, process, and discipline
- ☐ Well-designed, proven approach to process management
- ☐ Clear understanding of the preferred types and focus of all teams
- ☐ Well-trained team leaders and members
- ☐ Intense levels of technical, management, and leadership skill development
- ☐ Simple customer–partner, innovation, capabilities, improvement, and financial measurements
- ☐ Active feedback loops that foster learning and improvement
- ☐ Flat, decentralized, and team-based organization structure
- ☐ Systems that serve and support customers and partners
- ☐ Extensive and continuous education programs
- ☐ Effective communication strategies, systems, and practices
- ☐ Partner-designed reward and recognition programs within a vibrant appreciation culture
- ☐ Strong development of change champions
- ☐ Support for local initiatives
- ☐ Annual progress reviews and improvement assessments
- ☐ Frequent celebrations of major breakthroughs and small wins
- ☐ Annual refocus and planning for the next year's improvement cycle

Source: Jim Clemmer. 1995. Pathways to Performance: A Guide to Transforming Yourself, Your Team, and Your Organization, 215–216, 290–291, 293–294. Kitchener, Ontario, Canada: TCG Press. Used with permission of Jim Clemmer, leadership and organization development author, speaker, and workshop/retreat leader (www.ClemmerGroup.com).

## SuperMotivation Survey

How true are the following statements *as you perceive things in your work environment?*

1 = Not true at all
2 = True to a small extent
3 = True to some extent
4 = Mostly true
5 = Completely true

1. Employees in this organization are energetic and enthusiastic. _____
2. Employees are highly productive. _____
3. Employees have positive and optimistic attitudes. _____
4. There is little or no wasted effort. _____
5. The organization is highly customer focused from top to bottom. _____
6. Unsafe conditions are identified and promptly corrected. _____
7. Employees are made to feel like true business partners. _____
8. Employees have a strong sense of organizational identity. _____
9. Employees are very careful about how they use the organization's resources. _____
10. Employees have a clear understanding of the organization's mission, vision, and values. _____
11. Employee input into organizational strategic planning is solicited and used. _____
12. Employees are encouraged to make significant choices and decisions about their work. _____
13. Employees are involved in making key frontline decisions. _____
14. Employees are empowered to improve work methods. _____
15. Employees are encouraged to work closely with their internal customers and suppliers. _____
16. There is a no-fault approach to problem solving in this organization. _____
17. A concerted effort is made to identify and use the full range of abilities employees bring to work. _____
18. Employees are challenged to strive for ambitious goals. _____
19. Obstacles to effective employee performance are promptly identified and eliminated. _____
20. Personnel decisions are perceived to be fair and consistent. _____
21. There are few, if any, unnecessary policies and rules. _____
22. Effective communication is a high organizational priority. _____
23. Employees throughout this organization are well informed. _____
24. Management explains to employees the rationale behind all important decisions. _____
25. There is frequent communication between employees and management. _____
26. Senior managers regularly visit employees' work areas. _____
27. No secrets are kept from employees. _____
28. Meetings are well led and highly productive. _____
29. Company publications are informative and helpful. _____
30. Management is highly responsive to employees' needs and concerns. _____
31. Employees feel that management has their best interests at heart. _____
32. When labor–management conflicts arise, they are promptly and constructively resolved. _____
33. Management is quick to take personal responsibility for its mistakes. _____
34. Employees are encouraged to assume leadership responsibilities. _____
35. Employees receive a great deal of encouragement and recognition. _____
36. Outstanding performance is always recognized. _____

(Continues)

(Continued)

37. Both individual performance and team performance are appropriately rewarded. _____
38. Poor performance is never rewarded. _____
39. Creativity is encouraged and rewarded. _____
40. Employees consider their pay to be fair and equitable. _____
41. Employees are willing to pay part of the cost of their benefits. _____
42. Employees feel that their ideas and suggestions are genuinely welcomed by management. _____
43. Employees' suggestions receive prompt and constructive responses. _____
44. Everyone in the organization is committed to continuous improvement. _____
45. There are no barriers between departments or units. _____
46. There is a high level of trust between workers and management. _____
47. There is excellent teamwork throughout the organization. _____
48. There is a high level of trust between workers and management. _____
49. Management views problems as opportunities for improvement, rather than as obstacles to success. _____
50. Learning is a high priority in this organization. _____
51. Employees are encouraged to learn from one another. _____
52. There is consistent follow-up after training. _____
53. Employees are involved in making training decisions. _____
54. Employees are involved in determining performance requirements, measures, and standards. _____
55. Employees view performance evaluation as a positive developmental process. _____
56. Self-evaluation and peer evaluation are integral components of performance appraisal. _____
57. Discipline is perceived to be fair. _____
58. Employees consistently give extra effort. _____
59. Tardiness, absenteeism, and turnover rates are extremely low. _____
60. Employees are excited about working in this organization. _____

**Your score** (add up all responses) _____
**Your organization's percentage score** (divide by 300) _____%

**Preliminary Survey Interpretation**

Add all your responses. This is your organization's score. A perfect score would be 300 (based on a maximum response of 5 for each of the 60 items on the survey). When you divide your organization's score by 300, you will obtain an overall percentage score. The lower an organization's score, the more urgently it needs to apply the SuperMotivation strategies presented in Spitzer's book.

Here are some preliminary guidelines for helping you interpret your organization's overall percentage score:

| | |
|---|---|
| 90–100% | Congratulations! Your organization has attained SuperMotivation status. |
| 80–89% | Your organization is well on its way to SuperMotivation. |
| 70–79% | Your organization has some aspects of SuperMotivation. |
| 60–69% | Your organization has a slightly above average* motivational climate. |
| 50–59% | Your organization has an average* motivational climate. |
| <50% | Your organization has a below average* motivational climate. |

*Based on national norms for this survey.

Source: Dean Spitzer, *Supermotivation: A Blueprint for Energizing Your Organization from Top to Bottom*, New York: AMACOM, 1995, pp. 201–204.

**EXHIBIT 4.5** ▪ Turnabout Is Fair Play

I don't quite know what is happening to me, but I am beginning to feel some empathy for managers. In our efforts to create accountable, high performing and satisfying workplaces, we most often think that if the management would change, the institution would change. So we train them, write books for them, consult to them.

I have felt for some time that the problem with our leaders is not so much their behavior but the depth and intensity of our expectations of them. We persistently want our boss to be our mentor; we want them to take responsibility for our development. We get upset when they do not act with integrity or work well together, articulate a clear vision, or serve as a powerful advocate for our unit with those even higher in the institution.

It is disturbing that we expect so much of our managers. For a shift in culture, something more is required of the employees. Perhaps workers are the cause and management is the effect. Our frequent feelings of futility and frustration may be from putting our eyes on the wrong prize. Here are some wishes of myself and other employees that would balance the equation and support the transformation many of us seek.

### Employee Manifesto

1. Care for the success and well-being of the whole institution regardless of how it is managed. Stop thinking that the organization has to earn loyalty. Commit to its purpose and its customers even if management no longer is so committed to us.

2. Mentor ourselves. Find our own teachers and support, don't expect it from the boss or from human resources. Be willing to pay for our own learning, recruit our own coaches, and plan our own continuing education. Stop thinking the organization is responsible for our development.

3. View our boss as a struggling human being, no more able to walk their talk than we are able to walk ours. Have some empathy for anyone who would have to endure the reality of having us as their subordinates. Besides, most bosses are more worried about their bosses than they are about us. Why would they be any different than us?

4. Learn how to run the business. Become economically literate. Know the budget-cost-revenue connection of everything we touch. Learn as many jobs as possible, figure out what clients and customers want and how to give it to them. And do it even if the pay system is irrational and indifferent to anything that matters.

5. Be accountable for the success of our peers. Decide to support their learning and focus on their strengths, rather than criticize their shortcomings. Be their mentor, see their weaknesses as an opportunity to learn forgiveness and tolerance. And if there is a battle with them over territory or budget, give it away.

6. Accept the unpredictability of the situation we are in. The future of the organization is a mystery and no one knows how long these conditions will exist. Outsource our fortune teller, and stop asking where we are headed. Today is where we are headed and that is enough.

7. Forget our ambition to get "ahead." Ahead of whom? Why not stop competing with those around us? Maybe we are not going to get promoted and our salary grade is essentially peaking right now. The only hope we have for more prosperity is if the institution really grows and even then we will never get our fair share of the rewards. Besides, if we do get promoted, who is to say we will be any happier? My observation is that the higher you go in the organization, the more depressed people become.

(Continues)

**EXHIBIT 4.5** (Continued)

8. View meetings and conversations as an investment in relationships. Value a human relationship over an electronic one. Assume we come together to make contact with each other and any decisions we make are simply a bonus. Agree to end one meeting this week without a list or action plan. Besides, most of our best plans get changed five minutes after we leave the room and the lists are mostly a reminder of those things we do not really want to do.

9. Deliver on our promises and stop focusing on the actions of others. The clarity and integrity of my actions will change the world. Stop thinking and talking about the behavior of others. Let go of disappointment in them and how they were too little and too late. Maybe they had something more important to do than meet our requirements. Similarly, no one else is going to change. They are good the way they are.

10. If change is going to happen, it will be us. Gandhi said that "if blood be shed, let it be ours." We need to blink first. Shift our own thinking and do it for our own sake, not as a hidden bargain designed to control the actions of others.

11. Accept that most important human problems have no permanent solution. No new policy, structure, legislation or management declaration is going to fix much. The struggle is the solution. Justice and progress will always happen locally, on our watch, in our unit, only as a result of our actions with those in the immediate vicinity.

12. Stop asking "how?" We now have all the skills, the methods, the tools, the capacity and the freedom to do whatever is required. All that is needed is the will and courage to choose to move on, and to endure the uncontrollability of events.

13. Finally, stop seeking hope in the eyes and words of people in power. Hope is for us to offer, not request. Whatever we seek from our leaders can ultimately only be found in the mirror. And that is not so bad.

### The Point

The point is to confront the passivity, isolation and complaints that flood our workplaces. Employees are powerful players in creating culture and we ignore this when we act as if managers are the primary agents of change. Managers and leaders are not off the hook for how their power makes a difference. It is just that the hook has room for many players — us included.

These guidelines could easily be translated into ways to handle the difficulties of marriage or ways for citizens to rebuild the qualities of their community. They may seem to carry a strain of cynicism, but they are more a witness of faith. I have long felt that what we seek looking up in our organizations are expectations and dependency that is better directed at God rather than at a second level supervisor.

Also, I write these with full knowledge that they are rules I fall short of fulfilling. Perhaps if I could act on what I know to be true, I could stop writing, you could stop reading and we could both seek in real literature, music and art what we now seek on bookshelves filled with answer manuals. We could stop going to consultants and therapists and force them into real work. We could turn in our degrees in engineering, technology, finance and administration for ones in philosophy and religion. And this would be the most practical thing we could do.

Source: Reprinted with permission from *News for a Change*, ©1999 ASQ, www.asq.org. No further distribution allowed without permission.

using the wisdom of this column while simultaneously addressing demotivators is an as yet untapped wildcard in organizational transformation efforts.

Quint Studer, in *Hardwiring Excellence,* explains that daily "rounding for outcomes" is an absolute must for achieving desired results. It is a chance to get *honest* feedback from the culture and become aware of these demotivators (a lot of the feedback obtained will be an indirect result of these). This type of rounding will allow you to create an $A_2$ activating event by making a small thing right, which is pure gold in terms of creating a culture that will volunteer to achieve $R_2$ results.

As uncomfortable as it will be to admit that these things happen on your watch, remember: Feedback is a perception being shared, not a truth being declared. Swallow your ego, fix it, and watch what happens in terms of cultural morale and alignment toward your $R_2$ results.

And of course, the time for this rounding comes from the use of process-oriented thinking described in Chapter 1 and the data sanity concepts of Chapter 2. As emphasized repeatedly, potential exists to reduce your time spent in meetings by 50 percent and to free up an hour a day for middle managers, which then allows you to make rounding a cultural priority.

### Transition from Unconscious to Conscious Business

Are the following patterns tolerated in your current culture? If so, and you are frustrated at lack of results, one could call these the $C_1$ consequential behaviors of "unconscious business":

- Repeating the same patterns and problems over and over again;
- People not identifying themselves as the source of those patterns and problems;
- Spending a lot of time ignoring or recycling the patterns;
- Expending considerable energy trying to prove somebody else is to blame;
- Getting defensive in situations where enlightenment could be sought;
- Not talking about feelings directly;
- Carrying secrets not yet shared with the relevant person;
- People thinking of themselves as victims, resulting in:
  - Vacillating between thinking of others as perpetrators or fellow victims;
  - Arguing from the victim position, casting others as perpetrators; and
  - Resolving arguments by often joining others in being fellow victims; and
- People not expressing full creativity and having a variety of excellent reasons why they are not doing so.

An alternative $B_2$ belief system of "conscious business" is given in the list that follows. What type of $C_2$ consequential actions might this generate?

- "If a pattern or problem repeats itself, we look for the source of the pattern in ourselves."
- "We commit to learning instead of defensiveness in toxic interactions."
- "We become skilled at thanking people and the universe for giving us feedback, instead of punishing them."
- "We make conscious commitments and hold scrupulously to those commitments."
- "We make practical magic happen."

## Empower Your Employees to Act at Moments of Truth

A "moment of truth" is any interaction with a customer, external or internal. All promises to customers must be kept. Give your employees a vision to use as a guideline in making decisions when the customer's perception of quality is at stake. At the same time, realize that it is foolish to empower helpless people, that is, to promote a culture that perceives itself as powerless through "learned helplessness."[6]

It will take a consequential effort by the leadership team to create a culture that will allow its employees to accept being empowered. This effort will require eliminating demotivators, culturally inculcating new beliefs (from Chapter 3) about accountability, and having employees succeed in their attempts. For true empowerment, the culture will need processes that allow the following seven elements to be present for every employee[7] (see also Jeffrey's "Preparing the Front Line" in Resources):

1. *Knowledge.* Long-term strategy, short-term priorities, and action plans; intermediate goals and objectives.
2. *Skills.* Technical, interpersonal, and administrative training that will meet or exceed customer expectations.
3. *Product and process information.* Clear, concise information on products, services, and other details that affect their ability to make effective decisions and provide quick, responsive feedback.
4. *Performance information.* Timely feedback on key customer satisfaction, business, financial, and group and individual performance measures for the purpose of improving service.
5. *Authority.* Broader, less restrictive parameters for decision making that will allow staff to serve the customer better.
6. *Resources.* Adequate, reliable equipment, tools, and supplies to better serve customers and reduce frustration and resentment.
7. *Support.* Understanding customer needs to understand the needs of those on the front line and meet them.

## Putting It All Together

To summarize, all improvement requires:
- Customer orientation;
- Continuous improvement;
- Elimination of waste;
- Prevention, not detection;
- Reduction of variation;
- Statistical thinking and use of data;
- Adherence to best-known methods;
- Respect for people and their knowledge; and
- Use of best available tools.

Recall the two key questions related to QI:

1. How do we create activating events ($A_2$) to motivate the beliefs ($B_2$) to drive the right consequential behaviors ($C_2$) that will achieve our desired results ($R_2$)?

2. How do we stop recreating activating events ($A_1$) that reinforce old beliefs ($B_1$) that have unwanted consequential behaviors ($C_1$) and produce undesired results ($R_1$)?

How does one transition from the current $R_1$ results to the $R_2$ results needed in today's business climate? It will involve improving (and innovating) both current work processes and the emotional climate of the work environment through relentless application of the A → B → C → R model. This model applies both to organizational results and individuals' behaviors through a transformed management belief system as previously summarized in Exhibit 3.12.

The question is not whether you should create activating events and beliefs to yield a culture. You are already doing that and will continue to do so whether you want to or not. Remember:

- Every interaction between a manager or supervisor and an employee amounts to an experience that will either foster and promote or undermine and erode the desired $B_2$ beliefs;
- People tend to recognize events that reinforce their existing $B_1$ beliefs rather than those that promote the new $B_2$ beliefs, meaning that most activating events will need to be interpreted for people for them to form the $B_2$ beliefs you want them to have;
- By not understanding the experience people are having in their daily work, especially demotivators, managers can remain unaware of gaps and leave them open; and
- Culture changes one person at a time. How are people interpreting experiences? Present key words at key times to create the right perception and connect the dots for your employees.

## THE ROLE OF THE LEADERSHIP TEAM

### Lead the Transition Process

To drive new behaviors in your organization, a new leadership process with its own unique $R_2$ results will be required. In addition to coming up with the needed $R_2$ organizational results, think about the process of managing the deconstruction of your current culture and its subsequent realignment: Take ownership of the current $R_1$ results. I see the process as taking place in three phases, the first of which is defined in Exhibit 4.6.

### *Have Your Behavior Send a Clear Message*

Revisiting the mantras summarized in Chapter 3, especially in Exhibit 3.12, and putting them in the context of mission, vision, values, and $R_2$, ask, "How do I have to change to get them to want to volunteer to change?" (Exhibit 4.7).

### *"What Should I Keep Doing, Stop Doing, and Start Doing?"*

One of Clemmer's favorite questions when people are confused is, "What should I keep doing, stop doing, and start doing?" He encourages asking it of yourself, your improvement teams, or any work team when faced with three to five clear $R_2$ results and not sure how to proceed (Exhibit 4.8). Answering that question is a helpful technique to encourage people to take a realistic view of their daily work and actions. This approach will be especially useful when "those darn humans" feign confusion (using a stated reason) as to what they should change in their work.

**EXHIBIT 4.6** ■ Creating Leadership and Organizational Accountability Toward Clear Results

1. The leadership and other leaders need to formally hold themselves accountable for current $R_1$ results by publicly admitting, "We have managed to $R_1$ and we own up to it."
2. Have everyone understand and own up to his or her current $R_1$ results to establish the $B_2$ belief that "Everyone is 100 percent responsible for current results."
3. Through the lens of your mission, vision, and values, facilitate a process of clearly defining cascading $R_2$ work results for every employee with the help of middle and lower levels of management.

It is best to initially start with no more than three to five $R_2$ at each level.

**EXHIBIT 4.7** ■ Changing Me to Change Them

1. Use Studer's concept of the daily walk-around to proactively solicit honest feedback and create an atmosphere of safety regarding feedback:
2. Use data sanity and meeting sanity to create the time to do this;
3. Try to gain insight into your culture's demotivators; and
4. *Act* on the feedback when appropriate.
5. Exhibit $C_2$ consequential behaviors to demonstrate the desired $B_2$ cultural beliefs and values in daily tasks, interactions, and meetings (see Exhibits 3.12 and 4.1).
6. Ask "What should we keep doing, stop doing, and start doing?" Perform a continue/stop/start analysis (see Exhibit 4.8) for *all* key $R_2$ results to determine needed leadership team $C_2$ actions:
    - Begin with your team's desired $R_2$ result: "Dealing successfully with cultural barriers and resistance to organizational business $R_2$"; and
    - Remember that your team's current behaviors are perfectly designed to produce $R_1$.

As will be explained in the next two sections, it is not only useful to motivate change initially but also in the future, when the culture inevitably seems to hit a wall regarding progress toward $R_2$.

## Take Control of the Culture

My good friend Faith Ralston has developed a useful technique for dealing with a work group infected with the victimitis virus.[8] I call it "The 100 Percent Responsibility Exercise" (Exhibit 4.9). It is very easy to address instances of victim behavior in an individual via a "What" or "How"/"I"/"[action]" question, but with a group such as physicians, nurses, departments, or middle managers, you have to be a bit more clever to respond to their stated reason, which may be along the lines of, "It's not us, it's them. And here's what they're going to do."

I used this exercise on a group of nurses who were "sick and tired of not being respected by physicians." I began with Step 1 and determined that they felt the physicians were 85 to 90 percent responsible for the situation, that is, the nurses were willing to accept 10 to 15 percent of the responsibility.

## EXHIBIT 4.8 ■ "What Should I Keep Doing, Stop Doing, and Start Doing?" Analysis

Given organizational values and my specific $R_2$, I need to...

STOP: What I do that doesn't make sense is...

STOP: If I were brave, I would stop doing...

STOP: I question the effectiveness of the following activities but do them anyway: ...

STOP: I could immediately stop doing...

START: I can better understand why...

START: I can improve the way we...

START: I don't do the things in the six statements above because I need to start...

KEEP: Meanwhile, I must continue to keep...

## EXHIBIT 4.9 ■ The 100 Percent Responsibility Exercise: Changing the Belief Window on a Situation

In addressing a significant organizational issue, ask each group involved:

1. What do you see as the biggest frustrations and challenges in this situation?
   - How have others contributed to this problem? What percentage is out of your control? Who are these groups, and what percentage does each contribute?
   - How have you contributed to this problem? What percentage is your fault?

2. Specifically,
   - How did others contribute to the problem? "They said/did/forgot/denied/made, etc."
   - How did you contribute to the problem? "I thought/forgot/neglected/assumed, etc."

3. Now, take a deep breath, and assume full responsibility for the entire situation and repeat the exercise. Then consider:
   - What are all the things you could have done to prevent the problems that were created by someone or something else?
     - "They said...but I could have..."
     - "They did...but I could have..."
     - "They forgot...but I could have..."

Address all items in both lists generated by answering item 2.

4. Without blaming yourselves, identify why you did not take these actions.
   - "I did not have the skill, permission, time, willingness, etc."
     - Do you see patterns that allow you to intuit cultural $B_1$?
     - What insights do you have?
     - What changes can you make?
     - What attitudes are blocking your way? What are the belief systems of both sides?
     - Could there be perceived threats to jobs, status, autonomy?
     - Do groups' windshields through which they view and filter the situation need some cleaning?

Source: Faith Ralston, professional speaker and author of *Play Your Best Hand* and *Emotions@Work*. Used with permission.

As I facilitated Step 2, the nurses gleefully generated four flip-chart pages of behaviors the physicians exhibited. When I asked what they, the nurses, did to contribute, they were able to come up with three items.

I then hit them with Step 3, assume 100 percent responsibility for the entire situation, and heard an audible collective gasp. When I revisited *each* instance of the four flip charts' worth of physician behaviors, there was indeed something the nurses could have done to prevent each one.

Now this is very important: Step 4 asks the group to *nonjudgmentally* examine why they did not do the things they could have done. The discussion exposes the current cultural handcuffs, both real and perceived. Solving these issues is not as simple as the typical patronizing response, "Well, then, just do it." It takes some deep organizational conversations. Exhibits 3.5 and 3.11 could be very useful as follow-up guides.

Four types of organizational roadblocks can come up in dealing with groups:

1. *Brick walls.* External factors inhibiting performance that are not likely to change and are well beyond individual or collective control. They are immovable and real, and one needs to act through the belief, "Get over it and deal with it."
2. *True cultural handcuffs.* These will most likely require the involvement of leadership, management, or supervision to get resolved. It will take interdepartmental effort, time, money, and/or additional personnel or resources (recall the section titled "Code 13" in Chapter 3). Your organization is currently perfectly designed to have these handcuffs, and ingrained cultural $B_1$ beliefs allow them to continue.
3. *Perceived cultural handcuffs.* The roadblock exists *in the group's mind* (group $B_1$ belief system). However, it only looks impenetrable to employees because isolated events have made them *believe* it is. Testing the perception will show it not to be true. You have to make it safe for them to be able to take a risk to test that it is indeed only an illusion and have them succeed.
4. *Victim mind-set.* Untested beliefs and perceptions, usually from fear, leading to paralysis. They believe they cannot achieve an outcome and thus make it self-fulfilling.

In their wisdom, the nurses in the preceding exercise said to me, "Davis, wouldn't it be a good idea to do this exercise with the physicians and get them to take 100 percent responsibility as well? Then we could have a nondefensive dialogue going over each of our lists." *Bravo!* But in this situation, I could never get the physicians to agree to a meeting.

This case is a great example of the new definition of accountability. The issue is not one of splitting the responsibility 50-50 between doctors and nurses; rather, each side has to take 100 percent responsibility if the situation has any hope of being resolved. And notice how the exercise forces a new belief system by changing the window on the situation and creating a visceral discomfort.

## Be Prepared for the Inevitable Cultural Red Flags of Transition

A lot of your team and individual energy will be spent working to convince the culture and get them involved in the change by connecting the change with $R_2$ results and changes in the business environment. If you have been careful and proactive, you have every right to expect results; however, transition is awkward and painful. Those darn humans will:

- Demonstrate lack of enthusiasm and ownership;
- Take inconsistent actions even when they've said they agree with you;

- Remain silent when asked how it is going;
- Continually bring up issues you thought were resolved;
- Exhibit the victimitis virus; and
- Still openly say they disagree with a direction that has been committed to.

If results are not attained, the challenge will be to examine how *your* belief system might be standing in the way while simultaneously asking people: "So, what is it going to take?" and "What will it take from me to support you in that effort?" when they tell you why they can't instead of how they can, and helping them via:

- Asking and facilitating "What should you keep doing, stop doing, and start doing?" for their needed $C_2$ behaviors on the desired result;
- Creating $A_2$ activating events to seed the $B_2$ belief that stonewalling is not an option;
- Formalizing the feedback process;
- Creating time for feedback in meetings;
- Counseling saboteurs out of the company through objective feedback on behaviors or increasing intensity of experiences until they make a choice. In the case of the saboteur being a known organizational jerk, this tactic could be leveraged as an $A_2$ to help create some positive $B_2$ beliefs in the culture about the leadership's commitment to the newly espoused cultural values; and
- Working around people considered indispensable personnel, who consistently resist change, to isolate them from the larger organization. This practice prevents them from propagating toxic $B_1$ beliefs.

## THEY'RE WATCHING YOU

Realize that leaders are watched closely in anticipation of backsliding (perceived or real) and that the victimitis virus permeates the culture via remembered negative experiences, persistent useless beliefs, and ineffective habitual actions as well as external obstacles, inexperience, and human nature (territorialism and self-protection).

Exhibit 4.10 describes some issues that will arise as you begin the initially awkward process of integrating a more proactive leadership feedback process into the culture.

Many stated reasons will emerge as the feedback process is initiated. In reacting to the feedback, especially difficult feedback, say to yourself, "This is only a belief (perception) being shared, not necessarily a truth being declared," then ask yourself:

- Is that a belief I want people to have?
- If that belief continues, will it get in the way of desired results?
- What do I have to do to change that belief?

## CREATE EDUCATIONAL MOMENTS

As a leader, here are ways to create those educational moments:

1. Create the experience that it is safe for people to point out a (perceived or real) behavioral inconsistency. Determine if it is just a stated reason. If so, what might be the real reason?
2. *Always* preface any remarks with "Thank you for that feedback," and, intuiting from the feedback, identify the belief that needs changing. Listening closely to view the experience from their perspective, ask yourself, "Is this a belief I want them to have?"

EXHIBIT 4.10 ■ How to Actively Solicit, Listen to, and Process Cultural Perceptions of Leaders

- Create the positive $A_2$ activating events to drive the $B_2$ belief, "Open dialogue and positive confrontation are desirable and can occur without negative consequences."
- Realize that strong emotions will probably be unleashed. Expect 10 percent jerk time. Foster positive confrontation, the practice of *openly* discussing differences without creating interpersonal or organizational damage. *Where there is no emotion, there is no investment.*
- A needed $B_2$ for leaders is "I *don't* necessarily expect people to coach me if I am not proactively seeking their feedback. That is, I will hold myself accountable for holding myself accountable."
- Seek feedback on, and peer coach to, alignment checkpoints: "As the culture observes our leadership team behaviors, have we created the perception, that is, would they conclude that we are aligned around:
  - The urgency of the need to shift the way we think and act?
  - Our cultural beliefs?
  - The actions we expect people to take?
  - The $A_2$ events we think we are creating as a team in leading the change?
  - The personal commitment each of us needs to make in creating new activating events for the organization?
  - How we agreed to hold ourselves accountable for the change?"

3. Restate their beliefs to their satisfaction. Plan to change the experience they are having.
4. Tell them the belief you want them to have. Communicate that you sincerely want to understand their perception. This step lets them know that their current beliefs are not the ones you want them to hold. Tell them the belief you do want them to have, if possible, in the context of the $B_2$ beliefs or values. You could say, "Based on your feedback, it seems like I got it wrong. Let me get it right next time. Here's the belief I want you to hold, and I will ask you next week for honest feedback as to whether I'm modeling that belief."
5. Describe the experiences you are going to create for them. Use the situation that just occurred and state how you will handle it differently in the future. (You are accountable for generating the appropriate $A_2$ event.) This statement will signal your commitment to change and will focus others on interpreting future behavior in terms of the needed cultural shift so that people will recognize it. In this way, you are helping them break the pattern of viewing $A_2$ through $B_1$.
6. Culture change occurs one observation, one conversation, one belief, one person at a time — intense attention to detail must be maintained. Those darn humans are looking for *any* excuse not to believe you. Do not give them one.
7. Ask them for feedback on the planned experience and also ask, "What other activating events might I need to create to form a $B_2$ belief?" People usually have some idea of the events they feel *should* be happening to support the desired belief. It is your responsibility to find out what that is.
8. Enroll others in giving you feedback on your progress. Ask for both reinforcing and constructive feedback. Tell them what to watch for in the future and make sure they know that you will be asking for feedback on your progress. As a result,

they will now be looking for reasons to *think differently* about the beliefs they hold. This shift automatically and subtly focuses the observers' attention on their own beliefs and behaviors. In this way, you are involving them in the process of change. Leaders and their subordinates are co-creators of the new culture and must show it at the day-to-day action level. Openness followed by ownership represents the only useful posture toward feedback.

## SUMMARY

Many employees in the current culture will kick, scream, and stonewall as the organization transitions through the QI process. Leaders must manage this process to ensure a successful transition. Here is a list of steps for leadership to follow to take charge of the culture and the change.

1. Map desired $R_2$ onto current $R_1$; note the gaps; and look at resulting cultural, deployment, and development issues involved for needed transitioning of each $R_1$ to $R_2$.
2. As described in Chapter 3, facilitate the performance of a cultural audit through an affinity process to (a) expose the hidden cultural $B_1$, (b) facilitate needed $B_2$, and (c) brainstorm $C_2$ that would result from $B_2$.
3. Leverage this audit to create the needed visceral conscious cultural realizations that these $B_1$ beliefs will *not* allow attainment of $R_2$ and a culture of feedback is needed that will coach to the brainstormed $C_2$.
4. Dialogue and create an environment where each person will ask himself or herself, if given the needed organizational $R_2$ results, what specifically should they keep doing, stop doing, and start doing? If they don't ask the question of themselves, *you* should ask it.
5. Through your walk-arounds, hear the hard things about what to culturally keep doing, stop doing, and start doing.
6. Create a $B_2$ belief in the culture that victim behavior will not be tolerated. Reinforce this $B_2$ through the consistent creation of a gently challenging $A_2$ for individuals (i.e., "What" or "How"/"I"/"[action]" questions. Offer to help them make that happen to support their risk.) For groups, use the 100 Percent Responsibility Exercise (see Exhibit 4.9). Promise appropriate involvement on your part to remove any barriers encountered. This will motivate a $B_2$ context to create needed healthy interdepartmental dialogue.
7. Deal with behavioral problems in alignment and transition in a context of results-oriented, nonjudgmental peer coaching and expected cultural value of personal responsibility and accountability.

Key elements to succeed in implementing change include leadership demonstrating commitment to change with leading by example, addressing demotivators, seeking solutions not blame, and not tolerating victimization. Leadership should also solicit feedback and perceptions throughout the change process. This will help ensure that behavior and beliefs consistently demonstrate commitment to the transition and that the change doesn't include any unexpected consequences

A performance-based, feedback-rich organization that is supported by coaching as a predominant cultural practice creates a sustainable competitive advantage over its competitors.[4] It reflects a culture that displays:[4]

# EXHIBIT 4.11 — Some Cultural Phrases to Keep Reinforcing New Beliefs

- I think we might need a "What" or "How"/"I"/ "[action]" question here.
- Accountability does not mean "account for." It means asking oneself, "What else can I do?"
- What is my belief window?
- If you can't talk about it, you can't fix it. Period.
- If I assumed 100 percent of the responsibility for this situation, what else could I do to get the results I need? Without judging myself, why didn't I do those things? What would it take?
- The only person I can change and speak for is myself.
- No sweat — that was your 10 percent jerk time.
- Sorry, that was my 10 percent jerk time.
- What else can I do?
- You must assume accountability for giving feedback when you've got it, not just when you're asked to provide it.
- The organization must value feedback (or you will not make time for it).
- The supervisor is no longer responsible and to blame.
- We expect individuals to demonstrate competency in team leadership and people skills before they are placed in management or supervisory positions.
- We trust employees until they show us we can't.
- If there are performance issues, we address them immediately.
- When employee tensions arise, we encourage them to speak directly to each other and work things out and, if necessary, volunteer to facilitate such a conversation.
- We create environments where it is safe for people to tell the truth.
- Instead of blaming others, we seek information.
- Becoming responsible means looking our old job in the face and seeing all the ways it didn't work and could be better. We know what needs to get done, and we take the responsibility for doing it.
    - When we need something, we ask for it.
    - When we see something wrong, we talk about it.
    - When we want something to be different, we take action. And we don't do it alone.
- The role of the manager is to coordinate the decision-making process, build effective alliances and partnerships, create high-performing teams committed to a common goal, persuade and motivate rather than control and inspect.
- Meetings will respect people's time, be well planned, and be energy creating.
- Managers need the skills to be able to motivate people who don't report to them.
- Managers will understand the potential destructiveness of demotivators and be open to feedback about them, while engaging the workforce to be proactive in reporting them and solving them.
- Don't personalize. Feedback is a perception being shared, not a truth being declared.
- Our success will demand levels of collaboration and teamwork that we never dreamed were possible. It will depend on our ability to trust each other, share our resources, and build bridges to other people and organizations.
- We must create a sense of community where employees can confront bosses, where business decisions can be questioned, where it is safe to say, "I'm unhappy here," where rocking the boat is expected, where honesty is the norm, and where deep feelings are shared.
- We will respond to the needs of the world and its customers in a brilliant and creative way.
    - We will foster and support the personal and professional growth of the individuals who serve it.
- We must learn new ways to relate to each other that include listening and caring and the ability to set limits and say "No."
- Unless we provide seamless basic services, the customer will see our efforts at "delighting them" as getting in the way of their perceived needs.

- Mutual accountability;
- Willingness to learn;
- No fear;
- No surprises;
- Truthfulness; and
- Self-responsible language.

## Some B₂ Cultural Mantras

I gave quite a few new leadership $B_2$ mantras in Chapter 3. Quint Studer's message is that key words at key times are integral to creating the right perception and connecting the dots for your employees. In addition, I share a set of phrases (Exhibit 4.11) that might be helpful for such a purpose if they were to creep into your daily cultural conversations. I have no doubt that you will come up with others as well.

## REFERENCES

1. Kotter, John P. 1996. *Leading Change*, 16. Boston: Harvard Business School Press. Used with permission of Harvard Business Publishing. All rights reserved.
2. Studer, Quint. 2003. *Hardwiring Excellence: Purpose, Worthwhile Work, Making a Difference*, 45, 61, 75, 109, 118, 139, 167, 189, 211, 231. Pensacola, FL: Fire Starter Publishing.
3. Clemmer, James. 1992. *Firing on All Cylinders: The Service/Quality System for High-Powered Corporate Performance*, 340. Homewood, IL: Business One Irwin.
4. Crane, Thomas G. 1999. *The Heart of Coaching*, 12, 141, 199. San Diego: FTA Press.
5. Spitzer, Dean. 1995. *SuperMotivation: A Blueprint for Energizing Your Organization from Top to Bottom*, 42–57. New York: AMACOM/American Management Association.
6. Clemmer, Jim. n.d. "Organization Structure Limits or Liberates High Performance." www.clemmergroup.com/organization-structure-limits-or-liberates-high-performance.php.
7. Turner, Dan. 1994. "Redesigning the Service Organization." *Journal for Quality and Participation* (July/August): 32–33.
8. Ralston, Faith. 2002. *Emotions@Work: Get Better Results by Encouraging Accountability and Resolving Conflicts*, 55–57. Bloomington, IN: 1st Books.

## RESOURCES

Autry, James A. 1992. *Love and Profit: The Art of Caring Leadership*. New York: William Morrow and Company.

Autry, James A. 1995. "Love and Profit: The Art of Caring Leadership" (video). Cambridge, MA: Enterprise Media.

Clemmer, Jim. 1992. *Firing on All Cylinders: The Service/Quality System for High-Powered Corporate Performance*. Homewood, IL: Business One Irwin.

Clemmer, Jim. 1995. *Pathways to Performance: A Guide to Transforming Yourself, Your Team, and Your Organization*. Kitchener, Ontario, Canada: TCG Press.

Clemmer, Jim. 2003. *The Leader's Digest: Timeless Principles for Team and Organization Success*. Kitchener, Ontario, Canada: TCG Press.

Clemmer, Jim. 2005. *Growing the Distance: Timeless Principles for Personal, Career, and Family Success*. Kitchener, Ontario, Canada: TCG Press.

Clemmer, Jim. 2008. *Moose on the Table: A Novel Approach to Communications @ Work*. Kitchener, Ontario, Canada: TCG Press.

Clemmer, Jim. n.d. "A Coach's Playbook for Workplace Teams." www.clemmergroup.com/a-coach-s-playbook-for-workplace-teams.php.

Clemmer, Jim. n.d. "Culture Change Starts with the Management Team." www.clemmergroup.com/culture-change-starts-with-the-management-team.php.

Clemmer, Jim. n.d. "Education and Communications Pathways and Pitfalls." www.clemmergroup.com/education-and-communications-pathways-and-pitfalls.php.

Clemmer, Jim. n.d. "Improvement Planning for Taking Charge of Change." www.clemmergroup.com/improvement-planning-for-taking-charge-of-change.php.

Clemmer, Jim. n.d. "Leaders Care for Organization Culture and Context." www.clemmergroup.com/leaders-care-for-organization-culture-and-context.php.

Clemmer, Jim. n.d. "Organization Structure Limits or Liberates High Performance." www.clemmergroup.com/organization-structure-limits-or-liberates-high-performance.php.

Clemmer, Jim. n.d. "Signs of Stagnation." www.clemmergroup.com/signs-of-stagnation.php.

Clemmer, Jim. n.d. "Stop Managing and Start Leading." www.clemmergroup.com/stop-managing-and-start-leading.php.

Clemmer, Jim. n.d. "Stop Whining and Start Leading." www.clemmergroup.com/stop-whining-and-start-leading.php.

Clemmer, Jim. n.d. "Two Keys to Adding Values." www.clemmergroup.com/two-keys-to-adding-values.php.

Connors, Roger, and Tom Smith. 1999. *Journey to the Emerald City: Achieve a Competitive Edge by Creating a Culture of Accountability.* Paramus, NJ: Prentice-Hall, 1999. Revised edition, New York: Penguin, 2004.

Connors, Roger, Tom Smith, and Craig Hickman. 1994. *The Oz Principle: Getting Results through Individual and Organizational Accountability.* Englewood Cliffs, NJ: Prentice-Hall.

Crane, Thomas G. 1999. *The Heart of Coaching.* San Diego: FTA Press. (The first three chapters can be downloaded for free at www.craneconsulting.com.)

Jeffrey, J. R. 1995. "Preparing the Front Line." *Quality Progress* (February): 79–82.

Joiner, Brian L. 1994. *Fourth Generation Management: The New Business Consciousness.* New York: McGraw-Hill.

Kemp, Jana. 1994. *Moving Meetings.* New York: McGraw-Hill.

Kotter, John P. 1992. "Leadership with John Kotter" (video). www.enterprisemedia.com.

Kotter, John P. 1993. "Corporate Culture and Performance with John Kotter" (video). www.enterprisemedia.com.

Kotter, John P. 1996. *Leading Change.* Boston: Harvard Business School Press.

Kotter, John P. 2007. "Succeeding in a Changing World with John Kotter" (video). www.enterprisemedia.com.

Murphy, Emmett C. 1996. *Leadership IQ: A Personal Development Process based on a Scientific Study of a New Generation of Leaders.* New York: John Wiley & Sons.

Ralston, Faith. 2002. *Emotions@Work: Get Great Results by Encouraging Accountability and Resolving Conflicts.* Bloomington, IN: 1st Books Library.

Scholtes, Peter R. 1998. *The Leader's Handbook.* New York: McGraw-Hill.

Scholtes, Peter R., Barbara J. Streibel, and Brain L. Joiner. 2003. *The TEAM Handbook*, 3rd ed. Madison, WI: Joiner/Oriel.

Spitzer, Dean. 1995. *SuperMotivation: A Blueprint for Energizing Your Organization from Top to Bottom.* New York: AMACOM/American Management Association.

*(Note:* Clemmer's books may be ordered through www.clemmergroup.com. Many are also available as audio books, and some have accompanying workbooks to develop good leadership behaviors through personal growth. I recommend Clemmer's articles as particularly relevant to culture.)

## HELPFUL WEBSITES

The Clemmer Group: Jim Clemmer offers more than 300 free articles on a wealth of topics related to quality improvement. www.clemmergroup.com/.

Studer Group: Website contains good information and newsletters, often on leadership. www.studergroup.com.

CHAPTER 5

# Deeper Implications of Process-Oriented Thinking: Data and Improvement Processes

**KEY IDEAS**

- Although service outputs may seem more difficult to define than manufacturing outputs, all processes in both settings have measurable outputs.
- Significant quality improvements result only when data collection and analysis are used to establish consistent work processes and to identify elements of work processes that do not provide value.
- All work is a process, including the unique interactions between clinicians and patients.
- All processes exhibit variation and have measurable values associated with them.
- Outputs are those quantifiable things, such as tests, reports, examinations, or bills, which go to internal and external customers.
- Inputs to a process include people, methods, machines, materials, measurements (including data), and environment. All inputs carry variation, the aggregate of which is reflected in the output.
- Flowcharts reduce problems created by disagreement and variation in perceptions (human variation) about how processes currently operate.
- Processes represent repeatable actions occurring over time and must be studied that way.
- Data collection is a process — actually four processes — with inputs, outputs, and variation.
- There are eight questions to answer for any data collection.
- Common errors in quality improvement that result when process-oriented thinking is not used include action based on anecdotes and the addition of unnecessary complexity to a process.
- Operational definitions can prevent inappropriate actions based on anecdotes.
- To create significant lasting improvement, appropriately collected data must be used for decision making.
- Statistics can provide a unified language to break down barriers created by varied perceptions of how a process works.

## INTRODUCTION

### Manufacturing Concepts in a Service Environment

Much of the statistical emphasis in current quality improvement (QI) training originated from quality control efforts developed in U.S. manufacturing around World War II. They achieved widespread popularity in Japan after the war through the efforts of W. Edwards Deming and Joseph Juran. Because manufacturing uses an observable, physical process to produce an actual measurable product, data and statistical analysis have been used routinely for QI for more than 60 years. The emphasis in that environment has been primarily on product improvement.

The concept of measuring a work process within a service environment may appear harder to define. Processes are perceived to be intangible and difficult to define numerically. Observed events tend to be anecdotal and reflect perceptions rather than data.

It can be difficult to see how techniques for improving machines are related to services. It may also be difficult to understand how statistics can be helpful other than for summarizing a company's financial performance and operational statistics. Derived indices and aggregated financial figures presented in tabular form are common examples of the service organization's standard approach to using statistics.

### "We're Healthcare — We're Different"

Healthcare professionals in particular feel that their field is unique from manufacturing. They often espouse concepts such as:

- Medicine is an art;
- People are not "widgets" — healthcare professionals and patients are unique individuals who cannot be consistently measured or categorized;
- Statistics' role is a narrow, rigorous one defined by clinical trial research and quality assurance;
- Individuals' statistical needs are a basic knowledge of descriptive statistics with an occasional hypothesis test or regression; and
- Individual accountability is the bottom line.

These perceptions have led people to believe that only huge, random data sets external to the process can provide the information needed for improvement. Donald Berwick points out that this is the misconception behind the traditional quality assurance (QA) process of identifying the "bad apples" in a "sort and shoot" mind-set[1] (see also the explanation of QA vs. QI in the appendix at the end of this book). The uniqueness of patient cases and provider skills can seem too individualized to measure.

However, the processes in which both patients and providers participate are quantifiable and, to a large extent, predictable. Collecting data on the processes themselves is the key to identifying and eliminating the problems that people experience. Studying the number of lost medical records tells us how many records are lost. Studying the process of creating, transporting, and filing the records may tell us where and why they were lost as well as give us information necessary to permanently reduce the number of lost records.

Despite perceptions, it makes no difference whether the improvements are being made in a manufacturing or service environment. The QI process is identical. It is only the emphasis on individual components of the process that differs greatly between them.

The primary challenge for nonmanufacturing organizations is to recognize both the existence of processes and the need to standardize those processes to eliminate tasks that do not add value for the customer.

## Everything Is a Process

As already emphasized many times in this book, thinking in terms of processes is perhaps the most profound change needed to shift to continuous QI: *All work is a process.*

Personal experience has shown that concentrating on the process inherent in any improvement situation leads to:

- An atmosphere of cooperation because of a common language, which depersonalizes problems and eliminates blame; and
- Simpler, more effective, and more robust solutions to the problems presented.

Processes are sequences of tasks aimed at accomplishing a particular outcome. Everyone involved in a process has a role of supplier, processor, or customer. A group of related processes is called a system.

Because all processes produce measurable data (outputs), it is as valid to apply statistical methods to healthcare processes as to manufacturing processes.

The interactions between an organization's processes and systems can be understood by collecting data on key business outputs. Studying patterns of variation allows more predictable processes and systems to be established.

A short list of service process outputs is shown in Exhibit 5.1. You may find some entries surprising.

All output data collected from a process exhibit the aggregated effects of the variation from six inputs: people, work methods, machines, materials, measurements (data), and environment. When brainstorming problems about a process, any theory can be categorized into at least one of those six sources.

It is worth noting that the measurements source can have two interpretations. Obviously, measurements can affect our perception of process outputs, but measurements can be inputs to the process, too. In fact, many processes have a resulting measurement as a primary output, which is in turn an input to another process. Examples include a lab test result, used by a physician to decide the course of action for a patient, and an accounting system, the numerical output of which is used by management to evaluate the state of the organization.

Many quality programs focus only on people, their attitudes, and simply "doing

**EXHIBIT 5.1** Some Service Process Outputs

- Patient length of stay
- Cost variances
- Lost time from accidents
- Percentage patient "no shows"
- Cancelled operations
- Absenteeism
- Lab tests ordered
- Complaints
- Meetings
- Telephone calls
- Days per 1,000 patients
- Patient satisfaction scores
- Medication error rate
- Time from order to shipment
- Data entry errors
- Percentage of meetings rescheduled
- Percentage of meetings missed
- Number of referrals to X specialty
- Percentage of junk mail
- Percentage waste
- Time to retype documents
- Accounts receivable by payer

it right the first time." Although well intentioned, these motivational programs address only one of six inputs to an organizational process: people. Each of the six inputs contributes variation that must be addressed. One-day "smile training" (usually "smile or else") customer service courses are not effective because they reinforce a "you're the problem" message rather than address the underlying problems in the processes. What problems in the process are causing people not to want to smile?

## VARIATION AND PROCESS ANALYSIS: IMPROVEMENT PROCESS CORNERSTONES

As stated in Chapter 1, the seven sources of problems with a process probably provide the most useful road map in educating people about process analysis and problem solving. A common initial reaction to a problem is to immediately and feverishly collect data solely on the output (Source 7). Jim Clemmer has a wonderful saying: "Weighing myself ten times a day won't reduce my weight."[2] This approach is inefficient and will be horribly contaminated by ignorance of the effects of variation caused by Sources 1 through 6.

Immediate data collection could be an initial strategy whose objective is to establish a baseline for the current extent of the problem. Although this process is important, deeper issues related to the seven sources of problems cannot be accurately exposed and separated by looking merely at outputs. Sources 1 through 6 can introduce multiple sources of variation into the process output. Each will need its own uniquely designed data collection process to address variation of the inputs as well as outputs.

Further complications arise when poorly planned output data are combined with previously collected data that have been stored in a computer "just in case." The usefulness of the just-in-case data is further diminished because the data were not collected with the process improvement objective in mind. It is easy to draw false conclusions about cause-and-effect relationships when looking at data that were not intended to study those relationships. Deeper insight into the sources of variation is needed to identify the true causes. Data collected without any clear purpose have the potential to eventually prove someone's hidden agenda. A wonderful discussion of this concept is given by Mills in "Data Torturing."[3]

Many of a typical organization's work efforts are devoted to problem containment rather than discovering a problem's root cause — the Level 1 fix (see Chapter 1). Many times, root cause problems are buried deep in procedures and processes. (Recall that it is not the problems that march into your office that are important but the problems of which no one is aware.)

One coding improvement project found that its coding problems were intertwined with larger issues of billing and claims follow-up. Several of the common errors made in improvement efforts can result from taking a problem-containment approach. For example, people often try to improve a process by adding or rearranging steps instead of learning how to prevent the problem. This can make a process more complicated without necessarily adding any value.

Another common error is to create a project that is a mere disguise for implementing an anecdotal solution, generally considered the "known" solution to a long-standing problem. This ad hoc problem solving can result in unforeseen distortion of other parts of the process and further unexpected consequences. Implementing solutions does not necessarily address root causes.

Processes become complex as extra steps are added to work around root causes. As other problems appear resulting from this distortion, more and more steps are added elsewhere to compensate. The effects of the distortions often multiply and cause problems with other processes, which in turn are solved with extra steps adding still more complexity. Studying the reasons the steps were added can often bring true root causes to the surface.

Complexity is typically the first problem identified when teams begin to study problems with a process. There are at least four kinds of complexity: mistakes and defects, breakdowns and delays, inefficiencies, and variation.

**1. Mistakes and defects.** Mistakes and defects cause repeated work, take extra steps to correct, and require damage control to repair customer relationships. Could these have been prevented by proper design of earlier process steps? The sole focus of many QI efforts is a Level 1 fix, treating each mistake or defect as a special cause. This approach is often inefficient because it addresses a symptom and not necessarily the deeper root causes. The same problems end up being solved repeatedly. Deming referred to this as "scraping burnt toast."

**2. Breakdowns and delays.** Breakdowns and delays interrupt the work flow and cause waiting time. Waiting times are sometimes designed into work processes because of the prevalence of breakdowns and delays. Good questions to ask are:

- Which input is the major cause?
- Are internal customer needs fully understood?
- How do these breakdowns and delays affect the external customer?
- Could breakdowns and delays be eliminated?
- What would the process look like if it were one continuous flow?

A danger is that these have become so accepted as a natural part of work that people are blind to them as sources of waste.

**3. Inefficiencies.** Inefficiencies are the result of either the design of work processes or limitations of the physical space. Why was the process *originally* designed this way?

**4. Variation.** A wide range of unintended, unplanned results forces workers to react with myriad Level 1 fixes. With the best of intentions, they individually add steps to compensate for unpredictability and typically document none of their changes. (Standardization and documentation are discussed extensively in Chapter 8.) Good questions to ask in this situation are:

- Why are results inconsistent?
- What scenarios caused the added steps?
- Can the process be designed more robustly?
- Are people doing the right things?
- Are people doing the right things right?

Each of these factors causes rework. Rework is:

- Handling products more often than is necessary;
- Fixing an existing product; and
- Redelivering a service.

Rework introduces unnecessary costs to the organization and compromises customer satisfaction. Although some of the procedures tied to rework are ingrained into the work culture, they must be recognized as opportunities for improvement. A much deeper understanding of the implications of waste must be developed.

So although an organization might be able to show standards auditors their "process documentation," the atmosphere of constant Level 1 fixes can render them useless: They bear no resemblance to what really goes on.

## Flowcharts: Describing the Current Process

Perhaps the most serious problems in service processes result from variation caused by a lack of agreed-on processes. Inappropriate and unnecessary variations experienced by customers stem from excessive, unintended variation in individual work processes and from variation in management's perceptions of these processes. Flowcharts provide an opportunity for those involved in a process to describe its current operation in a concise, visual way. They give everyone involved new perspectives on process complexity and variation.

> Systems are unlikely to be defined in practice unless they are both suitable and adequate for the jobs for which they are intended, *and are written down in a way comprehensible to all involved* [emphasis in original]. … One or more forms of flowchart may be helpful, or the definition may be purely textual — but the system does need to be documented in some way.
>
> Yet again, there can be big differences between what is written down — the way the system is intended, or thought, to operate — and what actually happens. Incidentally, the acquisition of this latter information can be difficult if not impossible in an unfriendly work environment. …But, even in a constructive environment, it may still turn out to be almost impossibly difficult to complete a flowchart or other description because what is going on is so *un*systematic [emphasis in original].
>
> To be blunt, if a system cannot be written down, it probably doesn't exist: that is to say it probably functions more on the basis of whim and "gut feel" rather than on any definable procedure. This surely implies that the variation being generated is some scale of magnitude higher than really necessary, with the resulting well-known effect on quality.[4]

Let's consider something as simple as a process to assemble three parts to make a product: "Assemble A, B, and C to make D and move it to the next process step." That's how it should work. But here is what really happens:

- Sometimes A is missing, so people assemble B and C, create an inventory of "waiting for A," and move it to the inventory stockroom where it is logged into a notebook.
- Sometimes B is missing, so people assemble A and C, create an inventory of "waiting for B," and move it to the inventory stockroom where it is logged into a notebook.
- Sometimes C is missing, so people assemble A and B, create an inventory of "waiting for C," and move it to the inventory stockroom where it is logged into a notebook. (*Note:* Three distinct inventories have been created that must be tracked.)

These three processes create an inventory process and a job for a supervisor:

- Receive a shipment of parts;
- Before delivering parts to the line, review notebook for inventoried assemblies needing parts;
- Retrieve partial assemblies;

- Deliver partial assemblies and parts to assembly line;
- Interrupt worker with instructions; and
- Expedite completed assembly.

I can just hear someone who is considered an "excellent" supervisor proudly declare, "It's a good thing we're organized around here, or we wouldn't know which assemblies are missing which parts." If a smooth flow of available parts were guaranteed to avoid this, this whole subindustry, which is nothing but wasted time and effort, could be avoided.

A simple data collection suggested by the description provided would be to determine whether part A, B, or C tend to be missing from the kit most often (suggesting a special cause localization of the problem) or if the missing parts are evenly distributed (a common cause, deeper issue of organizational procurement). This example demonstrates an important implication of process-oriented thinking in terms of the use of data to isolate major sources of variation, be they common or special causes.

The preliminary work of flowcharting creates a common team understanding and terminology. It exposes and helps eliminate process inconsistencies often rooted in a lack of process documentation and inadequate training and reduces the human variation in perception.

There are three basic types of flowcharts: top down, detailed, and deployment. Processes must be understood in their current, actual form if they are to be improved.

### Top-Down Flowchart

The top-down flowchart provides a macro view of the basic processes, showing their natural relationships to each other as well as supplier/customer relationships. Simple descriptions of the task describing each subprocess are listed under each basic process (usually five to seven basic processes are shown). This type of flowchart describes what work is supposed to be done but does not show how the work actually gets done. Without comment, its purpose is to expose the various work tasks and where in the process they occur.

### Detailed Flowchart

The detailed flowchart provides a more specific version of a major process identified in the top-down flowchart. It shows how the actual tasks are transformed from the inputs into outputs. Parts of this chart include:
- Beginning and ending boundaries of the process, usually designated by ovals;
- Key process steps, usually designated by rectangles (the description typically includes a verb); and
- Any decision steps containing a "Yes/No" question, usually designated by diamonds and showing the individual subprocess of each path.

### Deployment Flowchart

The deployment flowchart can be used with either the top-down or detailed flowchart, or in combination. This flowchart adds another dimension to the previous charts, showing process responsibility through a spatial sequencing.

Departments involved in the process are listed horizontally across the top of the chart. The process flow is drawn from top to bottom, indicating the passage of time. Each specific process activity is placed in the vertical column below the department responsible for it.

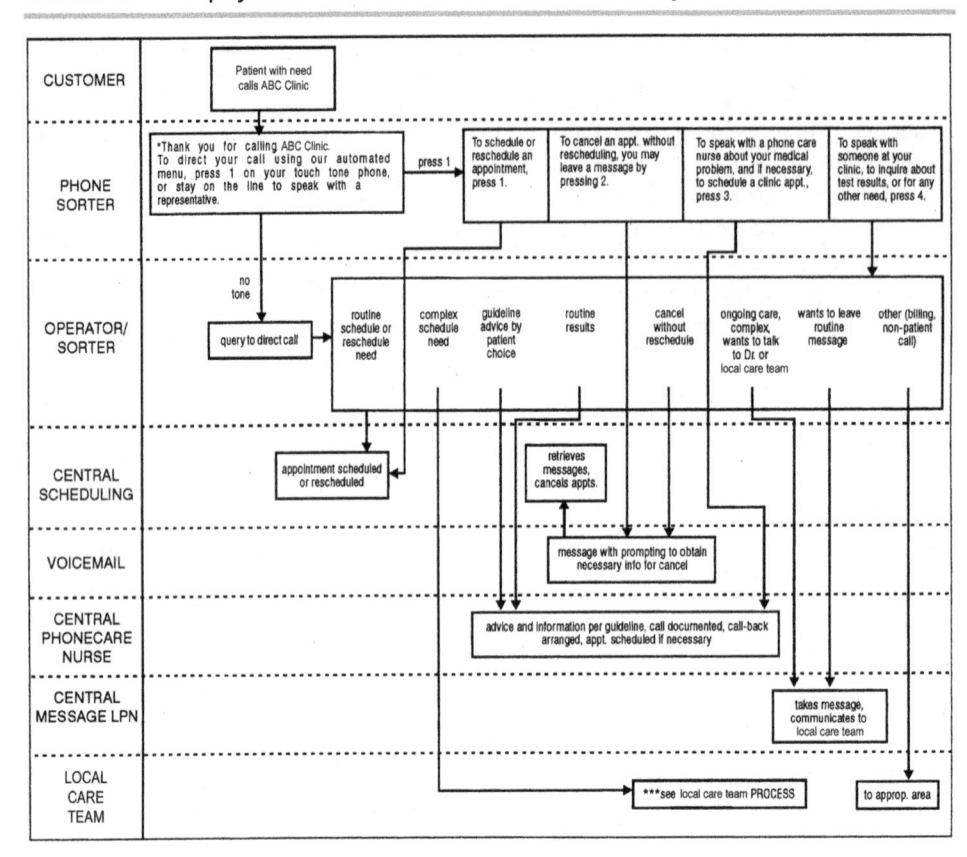

**EXHIBIT 5.2** ■ Deployment Flowchart of an Automated Phone System

| | |
|---|---|
| CUSTOMER | Patient with need calls ABC Clinic |
| PHONE SORTER | *Thank you for calling ABC Clinic. To direct your call using our automated menu, press 1 on your touch tone phone, or stay on the line to speak with a representative. → press 1 → To schedule or reschedule an appointment, press 1. / To cancel an appt. without rescheduling, you may leave a message by pressing 2. / To speak with a phone care nurse about your medical problem, and if necessary, to schedule a clinic appt., press 3. / To speak with someone at your clinic, to inquire about test results, or for any other need, press 4. |
| OPERATOR/ SORTER | no tone → query to direct call / routine schedule or reschedule need / complex schedule need / guideline advice by patient choice / routine results / cancel without reschedule / ongoing care, complex, wants to talk to Dr or local care team / wants to leave routine message / other (billing, non-patient call) |
| CENTRAL SCHEDULING | appointment scheduled or rescheduled / retrieves messages, cancels appts. |
| VOICEMAIL | message with prompting to obtain necessary info for cancel |
| CENTRAL PHONECARE NURSE | advice and information per guideline, call documented, call-back arranged, appt. scheduled if necessary |
| CENTRAL MESSAGE LPN | takes message, communicates to local care team |
| LOCAL CARE TEAM | ***see local care team PROCESS / to approp. area |

Obscure relationships requiring other departments' consultation, participation, and/or approval are indicated by horizontal lines extending from the primary department.

The deployment flowchart can be useful for indicating time bottlenecks caused by too many parallel approval steps. It can also show inefficiency created by too much back-and-forth work between departments. This is a very useful chart in medicine's multiple supplier/customer/processor environment. A deployment flowchart of an automated telephone system is shown in Exhibit 5.2.

To find a problem's true root cause, exposure of individual variations in what was thought to be a standard process is crucial. The flowcharting process helps to establish not only that people are doing the best job possible with the current process but also that the process can be further improved and standardized. Sometimes, obvious problems are exposed during flowcharting that can be fixed using minimal data. Flowcharts can establish agreement on:

- What the current process actually is;
- What the best current process might be; and
- The need to collect data.

Flowcharting provides motivation and can help identify the most effective leverage points for data collection. It also answers two crucial questions of the seven sources of problems with a process: (1) How does the process actually work? (2) How should the process work? Goals and objectives for the rest of the improvement project can be set based on the answers.

This process allows for the most efficient data collection because human variation in perception has been minimized and more specific objectives have been defined. In addition, flowcharts can be used for current process documentation and future employee training.

In the early stages of a project, it is common to concentrate too much on flowcharting the specific details of the process. Too much detailed flowcharting and lack of a good baseline estimate of the extent of the problem are the two major reasons why many improvement projects fail. It is best to narrow the scope by:

- Getting a macro view of the problem by using a top-down flowchart to document tasks;
- Discovering where data may be available;
- Collecting data to localize which process represents the major opportunity within the larger system; and
- Flowcharting the details of how that specific process gets its work done.

A lot of teams get bogged down in flowcharting minutiae. Too many resources teach flowcharting as an isolated tool and very few put it in the proper context. Many good references are available on the various flowcharts (see Resources), which provide more explanation and excellent examples.

Beware of another common error in the early stages of a project of skipping the task of flowcharting because "Everyone already knows what goes on" or "We already have the answer." Experience has shown that it always takes the team far longer to flowchart and understand the current process than anticipated. "Oh, my gosh! We do that?" is a common remark heard during flowcharting.

Flowcharts, while not numerical, meet a definition of data I like to use, which is any physical piece of information that aids in understanding variation. Flowcharts provide critical data in any improvement effort by reducing *human* variation in perceptions of the process and by improving the subsequent quality of the team process. The goal in the early stages of a project is to understand the existing process and the supplier/customer relationships it contains, not necessarily to understand all the microprocesses required to get the work done.

## Teaching Frontline Staff That Their Work Is a Process

Before any numerical data are collected, we must determine how the process currently works and how the process should work. *The TEAM Handbook* (see Scholtes and colleagues Resources) provides excellent guidance in the area of studying a process prior to collecting numerical data (some of this discussion is presented in Chapter 8).

The questions posed in Exhibit 5.3 can be used to get a frontline group to see their job as a process or at least help you to understand a situation as a process. It is very common for the hard-working front line to have no concept of process. They see their jobs as a series of tasks they proudly tailor to the uniqueness of each customer interaction.

**EXHIBIT 5.3** ■ Questions to Ask about a Process

**Instructions:** Working with your team, select several questions you think are most relevant to the project. Divide those questions among individuals or small groups, decide whether you want to use a standard reporting format, and set a (reasonable) deadline for reporting back to the team. Between meetings, gather whatever available data you can, talk to process operators, etc. Repeat this process until all relevant questions have been answered.

The process being studied is _____ .

1. Who are its external customers? What individuals, groups, or systems outside our organization rely on or could benefit from this process? Who has (or could have) expectations about this process?

2. How do we know what the external customers like or don't like about this process? What satisfies or dissatisfies them?

3. Who are its internal customers? Describe those within our organization who do (or could) rely on the successful operation of this process or the resulting product or service.

4. How do we determine what the internal customers like or don't like about this process? What satisfies or dissatisfies them?

5. What are the operational definitions of quality in this process? What specifically determines whether the process is working well or poorly?

6. What records are kept regarding quality? Who uses this information? How do they use it? Are these record formats suited to how they are used?

7. What are the most common mistakes or defects that occur? What is the operational definition for each mistake or defect? What proportion of these is commonly assumed to be a worker's fault? What proportion do we usually attribute to the system? How do people arrive at these conclusions?

8. By what process do we inspect, evaluate, and report problems regarding:
   - Planning required for this process?
   - Incoming materials, supplies, and information critical to this process?
   - The process itself?
   - The final product or service received by the external or internal customer?

9. List the critical elements of this process: materials, ingredients, components, parts, information, etc.

10. List the suppliers or vendors of each critical element.

11. Describe the company's procedures for purchasing materials or ingredients brought in from outside the facility (plant office, company, etc.). To what extent is "low bid" a governing factor in our purchasing decisions?

12. Describe the impact of the most common mistakes or defects in this process. What do they cost in time, money, customer loyalty, or worker pride?

13. Who is responsible for quality in this process? Who is responsible for detecting mistakes and defects? Who is responsible for identifying and correcting the causes of mistakes or defects?

© Joiner Associates. Used with permission.

These questions are a powerful way to teach employees the process language in a just-in-time manner. Used in conjunction with Berwick's questions from Chapter 1, it gets them thinking deeper about waste (especially wasted time). The best result would be to use a resulting simple data collection to expose a deep cause within one of their most frustrating ongoing issues, among the most typical being:

1. Do you ever waste time waiting when you should not have to? Exactly how long, how often, and under what circumstances? What accounts for the bulk of the time spent waiting? What about time wasted in meetings? Does it happen to anyone else?
2. Do you ever redo your work because something failed the first time? Which things? What accounts for the bulk of rework? How often? What percentage of your total work time does it take? Does it happen to anyone else?
3. Do the procedures you use waste steps, duplicate efforts, or frustrate you through their unpredictability? Which procedures? Are there a few procedures that cause the bulk of this rework? What caused the need for such procedures? What have you noticed as a result of these procedures? Does it happen to anyone else?
4. Is information that you need ever lost? Which information? What accounts for the bulk of it? How often? What happens as a result? Does it happen to anyone else?
5. Does communication ever fail? Exactly what does this mean? What observable events does this cause? How often are these occurring? Does it happen to anyone else?

The data suggested by the follow-up questions are not the type of data normally collected in an organization. The data needed to run a business are often quite different from the data needed to improve its everyday clinical processes. And, once they are improved, the process-specific data are no longer needed. However, data will be needed to maintain any gains and to make sure leaders do not overreact to daily common cause variation.

## Next: Focus, Focus, Focus

Recall the accident data example in Lesson 2 of Chapter 2. A simple stratification exposed three significant sources of variation that remained hidden as long as the focus was on the actual number of accidents. This example demonstrates the Pareto principle, which is described in Exhibit 5.4.

In conjunction with considering special and common causes of variation, understanding the Pareto principle is critical to improvement efforts. It motivates staff to recognize the importance of identifying and exposing the real underlying, hidden opportunity in what is many times initially an anecdotally vague situation or project definition. This occurs through using existing data or focused, simple, efficient data collection strategies. The goal is to expose and localize major improvement opportunities or, to use the Pareto principle, the "20 percent of the process causing 80 percent of the problem."

Using a series of data collections and the questions uniquely generated subsequent to each collection — implicitly the plan-do-study-act (PDSA) cycle (mentioned in the preface and discussed in several Deming resources) — demonstrates a powerful statistical technique: exposing major sources of process variation by stratification via process inputs. Special causes are isolated as a result, allowing a more specific action to focus on solving the problem.

EXHIBIT 5.4 ■ The Pareto Principle

In the 1920s, Joseph Juran noticed that when faced with an improvement opportunity, 80 percent of the observed variation was generally caused by only 20 percent of the process inputs. For example:

- 20 percent of the customers usually account for 80 percent of the sales.
- 20 percent of one's expenses probably account for 80 percent of one's monthly checking statement, either individually or by class.
- 20 percent of the types of food bought make up 80 percent of one's food bill.
- 20 percent of a company's products produce 80 percent of its sales.
- 80 percent of an organization's "quality problems" are due to 20 percent of the potential improvement opportunities.
- 20 percent of the diagnosis classes represented or 20 percent of the physician's panel of patients account for 80 percent of a physician's practice activity.

Juran called this phenomenon the *Pareto principle*, after a Renaissance Italian economist who studied the distribution of wealth.

Quality improvement (QI) uses this principle to its fullest advantage. When studying an improvement opportunity, it makes sense to isolate and attack the 20 percent of the variation causing 80 percent of the problem. This gives the greatest return on investment of precious time.

Juran called the 20 percent the "vital few" and the others the "trivial many" or, more recently, the "useful many." It should be emphasized that these problems are most assuredly not trivial to the people who must work in those situations. They are trivial only in terms of their current effect on the entire organization. As the more significant opportunities for improvement are solved, some of these trivial opportunities will either be addressed in the context of a larger problem or eventually become vital.

The vital few are generally long-standing, perennial opportunities that have never been solved despite repeated efforts. Their root causes are deeply entrenched in the culture of interconnected processes of many departments, and they will require more formal and higher-level guidance and participation to address them, including that of top management. Their solution processes will be lengthy and require patience and persistence. However, the solutions should have a significant effect on organizational culture.

The useful many are important to individuals. However, because of their sheer number, there is a common tendency for them to distract teams from their primary tasks. This is particularly true if the team's mission is not clear. The useful many take just as much time to solve as the more significant problems, but with less value to the organization. The best reminder is that "There is no such thing as improvement in general." The goal must be to expose and focus, and then further focus on a major opportunity.

### What about the Useful Many?

If all of the organization is educated in statistical thinking and awareness of processes and customers, the existing work teams can form informal task teams (generally intradepartmental) of two to three months' duration to work on these problems. In other words, "working on their work" should become a routine part of people's daily jobs. These projects are important for educational purposes. They empower people by giving them proof that they are making a difference in the organization as well as solving a frustrating work problem, thus providing people with more joy in their current job.

These task teams should be ad hoc. Forcing them to become part of an organization's "quality machinery" drains their inherent energy by bogging down a seemingly spontaneous effort in dreadful formality. Ideally, QI becomes the organization's work culture, existing parallel to the necessarily more formal higher-level improvement efforts. Managers and supervisors are part of this culture, communicating with each other through an informal network to share results with other similar groups in the organization. Juran was adamant that working on the useful many would be successful only if such a structure were in place. The miserable failure of the Quality Circle movement of the 1980s in the United States certainly bore his wisdom out.

Source: Peter R. Scholtes, Brian L. Joiner, and Barbara J. Streibel. 2003. *The TEAM Handbook*, 3rd ed., C-20. Madison, WI: Oriel. Used with permission.

## Data Aggressiveness: Four Strategies

Although data collection is very important, there is a tendency to overuse it or collect too much in the early stages of understanding an improvement opportunity. If the data collection is not carefully designed and defined, it is easy to accumulate too much data with vague objectives. This leaves people scratching their heads about what they should do with it. And, as I have found at times, any resemblance between what the team intended and what actually gets collected also can seem purely coincidental.

When data collection objectives and methods are unclear, the project team unduly inconveniences the work culture involved in the collection. Those providing data understandably become peeved when told, "We're sorry. We forgot to think about _____. Would you mind doing it again?"

Credibility for the project is now lost, as is credibility and cooperation for future collections and projects. In addition, this error feeds into some of the natural initial cultural cynicism, leading to comments such as, "This QI stuff implies I'm not doing a good job."

Do not lose sight of the fact that data collection itself is a process. People collecting the data must be educated in the objectives of the data, the forms used to collect it, and operational definitions of what they collect. Forms must also be user friendly and allow the data to virtually collect themselves. Once again, people's jobs are already perceived to take up at least 100 percent of their time; they are doing you a favor by participating in the data collection, so make it easy for them.

In the course of designing a data collection effort, project teams should also ask the following questions before one piece of data is collected:

- What is our plan for using these data?
- Suppose we had the data in hand right now. What is the potential action?
- What specifically would we do with them once we got them?
- What analysis is inherent in our collection process?
- What tools would appropriately analyze them?
- Would we know the right processes for interpreting the analysis and taking action?

Thinking once again about the seven sources of problems with a process, apply the sources of problems to the data collection process as well as the process under study. Think of examples where a data collection effort was not as effective as it could have been. Was this due to the effects of the first six sources of problems with a process or failing to consider input variation? Did the data collectors understand how the data were to be collected? Did data have to be retaken?

Each source of process problems requires its own unique data collection based on understanding its contribution to the variation in the work process. Without awareness of variation and what can cause it, people (including the data planning team) tend to overcomplicate a situation and perceive it to be full of special causes.

This discussion demonstrates one of the many that I like to call nonmathematical aspects of statistics and statistical thinking. With apologies to Yogi Berra (former Major League Baseball player and coach famous for his head-twisting quotes), who once said about baseball, "Ninety percent of this game is half mental." I suggest that "Ninety percent of statistics is half planning."

The key is to have extremely focused objectives on major opportunities. This focus encourages an inherent strategy of a series of simple, efficient data collection processes that progressively isolate significant root causes of variation.

When special causes of variation exist, exposing them allows quick localization of both the problem and solution. It also makes the problem much easier to solve. If no significant special causes are exposed, the improvement process gets more difficult and one needs to move on to different, more complex problem-solving strategies.

Four basic data collection strategies exist to allow accurate understanding of a situation and testing for potential improvements. They are discussed in ascending order of "aggressiveness," or disturbance to the daily work habits of people involved. Careful consideration of the effect of a data collection on a department or other group will go a long way toward obtaining that group's ultimate (and future) cooperation, especially if they can see there is high potential for making their lives easier. Even deeper buy-in can occur by involving key department personnel in the design of the data collection.

Strategies of low aggressiveness should be used to expose major potential sources of variation and opportunity. Low aggressiveness strategies can sometimes help screen out initial theories regarding causes of the problem.

### Data Strategy 1: Exhaust Existing In-House Data

The first data strategy is to exhaust already existing in-house and routine data. Use the current data to define any recurring problems, assess the effect of each problem, and localize each major problem. You can use the following questions to identify recurring issues[5]:

- How often does this problem occur?
- How severe is it when it occurs?
- When does or doesn't the problem occur?
- Where does it occur, or where is it first observed? Where doesn't it occur? Where is it not observed?
- Are there other problems that always or often occur together with this problem? Could these be related somehow?
- Who tends to have the problem most often?
- Does the occurrence correlate with any particular vendor's product in terms of higher or lower rates?

You can also use the current in-house data to assess the impact of human variation both in definition of data and data collection and in the reporting process. Some changes may be needed to reduce variation by redefining what and how data should be collected and reported. You will also need to identify if other data will be useful to determine the problems' impact and how the data should be obtained.

It can be dangerous to use data that originally were collected with no clear objective. However, at a project's early stage, simple stratifications, scatterplots, and time plots of existing data may shed light on possible theories for significant sources of variation and their causes. These theories can then be tested by subsequent, properly designed data collection.

In-house and routine data frequently consist only of process outputs. Because they normally cannot be traced directly to their inputs (as a participant in one of my seminars woefully discovered), outputs themselves are not necessarily helpful for improving processes. However, through run and control charts, these output data can establish a baseline for evaluating the progress of improvement strategies. They will also indeed show whether any gains made from the project have been maintained.

It is usually not advisable to institute a change or solutions based strictly on in-house data. However, they can be a rich source for suggesting significant theories to be tested. Because someone went through the trouble of collecting the data, they may as well be used for what they are worth. This exercise also creates an opportunity to assess the value of continuing to collect the data.

### Data Strategy 2: Study the Current Process

The second data strategy is to study the current process. This allows work processes to proceed normally while recording data that are virtually available for the asking. It is almost like taking a time-lapse video of the work as it occurs.

If no in-house data are available, sometimes the solution can be just as simple as observing the process over time and plotting the dots to get a process baseline. The dialogue in planning this process will also be helpful for subsequent action. This aspect of studying the current process is discussed extensively in Appendix 8A at the end of Chapter 8 through three very simple, eye-opening examples.

For high-level projects, usually in-house data are available. This stage typically involves stratification of an important output, which is tracing it to its input sources. Through minimal additional documentation of normal work, stratification and subsequent Pareto analysis can expose potentially significant sources of variation.

These first two levels of aggressiveness, looking at routine data and studying the current process, expose many sources of special causes and allow localized efforts to fix these obvious but previously hidden problems. They are also useful in dealing with:

- The fourth source of problems with a process, errors and mistakes in executing the procedures; and
- The possible need to address the fifth source of problems with a process, current practices that fail to recognize the need for preventive measures.

Solutions to these problems frequently involve redesigning the process to include an error-proofing element.

When data show a problem to be common cause, it means that, given the current process, occurrences of the problem are inevitable; they are not under the control of people working in the system. Many times the cause is due to the limitations of human attention, sometimes placed under the umbrella of "multiple simultaneous responsibilities."

The root cause in this case may be inadequate knowledge of how a process should work, current practices that fail to recognize the need for preventive measures, or even a poor overall organizational training process. Some examples of preventive measures and error proofing include a written script for receptionists or a computerized billing system that does not accept incomplete forms. A robust process redesign that inherently forces use of the desired behavior or technique is often a good strategy and a major component of Lean enterprise thinking.

Identifying deep causes of variation can also expose some elements of the sixth type of problem in a process, unnecessary steps, rework, and wasteful data collection. Examples include extra paperwork (especially inspections and pseudo-inspections) and time buffers, which merely condone an inefficient process.

Many times, additional steps are unnecessarily added to the process because of one-time events that created chaos for workers in the past. They were added as a knee-jerk reaction to a special cause (happened only once) that was treated as a common cause (perceived potential to happen often in the future). I recently had an example in one of my seminars for the Department of Veterans Affairs: A suicide in one state prompted a whole new paperwork industry for reporting suicides in all states, treating each suicide as a special cause.

Also seen is a tendency for processes to grow over the years with many steps losing whatever value they once had. Elimination of this slack strengthens and improves the process by addressing root causes of variation and reducing opportunities to add further variation to a process.

At this point, many of the ongoing underlying special causes of variation have been addressed and eliminated. One can now assess the value of each step of the process by review and revision of the original flowchart: Has process redesign eliminated the need for some of the nonvalue work?

### *Data Strategy 3: Cut New Windows*

Juran called the third data strategy "cut new windows." This approach takes studying the current process (stratification) one step further by gathering data that are, once again, not routinely collected. However, for this strategy, much more disturbance in the daily work flow is required to get at these data. And many times it is a major disturbance because of the level of detail needed; hence, it is more aggressive.

A possible improvement opportunity has been identified through Pareto analysis via the first two strategies. For further knowledge, however, the process now has to be deeply dissected beyond any routine requirements or easily obtainable data. The good news is that it only has to be done for 20 percent of the process causing 80 percent of the problem (Pareto principle) — a very high probability of being productive.

Using lab test turnaround time as an example, data strategy 1 can help get an approximate baseline of problem extent. Strategy 2 (possibly even some in-house data as well) can then help stratify data to isolate and identify the lab test procedures, departments, or times of day accounting for the majority of excessive times.

These initial studies of the current process would be based on an agreed-on global definition of "overall lab test turnaround time." One possibility might be the elapsed time from the test being ordered to the time the result is available to the patient; another is time from order to result delivered to the physician. Make sure agreement is achieved on just such definitions.

For deeper issues regarding the measurement process input, it would also be interesting to stratify these results by recording any words on the order such as "STAT," "Rush," "Priority," and so forth. Do they result in lower turnaround times?

If a major opportunity is isolated, this overall lab test turnaround time would now have to be broken down into its various components or disaggregated. Such component times might include "transportation to the laboratory," "waiting in the work queue," "performing the test," "communicating the result to the physician (or hall nurse)," "time to get the result to the patient," and so on. Further, the definitions of each individual component will need to be very clearly defined for everyone involved.

As you can see, the overall process has now been dissected into its subprocesses. There might even be an additional factor for consideration regarding potential collection, for example, the previous analyses may have exposed that it is only necessary to collect these data for one or several specifically isolated time periods during the day. But it might also have shown that Mondays or weekends had unique specific problems vs. a more "typical" day.

Breaking apart the total time is, in effect, cutting a new window into the process, dissecting it to look at different perspectives and smaller pieces. And note that this level of detail is done only on the tests that have been identified as a major problem, from Pareto analysis of the data in data strategies 1 and 2, the 20 percent of the test types causing 80 percent of the excessive test times.

With such a focused data collection, gathering the required information will involve no more personnel than necessary: Data collection in other areas would add little value for the effort expended. A further benefit is that this study of the process for lab test procedures with the most problematic turnaround times might also ultimately provide some benefit for all procedures.

For planning purposes, the previous work on an appropriate detailed flowchart would expose the best leverage points for data collection. It would also allow creation of an effective data collection sheet (see Exhibit 5.12 and the "Eight Questions for Effective Data Collection" section later in this chapter).

Use process dissection only after a significant source of variation has been exposed and isolated. Realize that it is a very common error for teams initially to jump directly to this step. This results in too much data and, more importantly, inconveniencing people who did not need to be inconvenienced. The data collection has no ultimate benefit for them, and your credibility as an improvement leader is now suspect.

As you know, this strategy is a major upset to daily routine. Make sure that its use has been preceded by the only mildly inconveniencing data strategies 1 and 2 to isolate a major opportunity on which to focus. Make sure any perceived additional work by staff members has ultimate value for them. This will enhance your reputation as well as create better members organizational beliefs about QI.

### Accident Data in the Context of Data Strategies 1 through 3

Let us revisit the accident data example from Chapter 2; it is such an elegantly simple and insightful example of using this data sequence to review in this context. As the run chart of the monthly performance shows (Exhibit 5.5a), the variation is common cause. As emphasized, this does not mean that one must passively accept this current situation. It does mean, however, that the current special cause approach to reducing accidents (a Level 1 fix analyzing each accident individually) has been ineffective and a common cause strategy is needed. So in-house data were used to get a baseline.

Now consider the Pareto matrix stratification shown in Exhibit 5.5b. With a little research, data became available on the nature of each accident and in which department it occurred. If this information was not available, it could easily be recorded (along with other information that was easily available) on subsequent accidents if the data continued the common cause pattern.

Employing stratification by process input, the Pareto principle applies:
- Two departments account for most of the accidents; and
- Two accident types account for most of the accidents.

This is what is desired from this type of analysis — the ability to localize and focus in on true causes, which then allows more focused solutions.

However, the matrix form shows even further insight. Summarizing the matrix:
- The "people" input was one source of variation in that process.

EXHIBIT 5.5 ■ Run Chart and Pareto Matrix of Accident Data

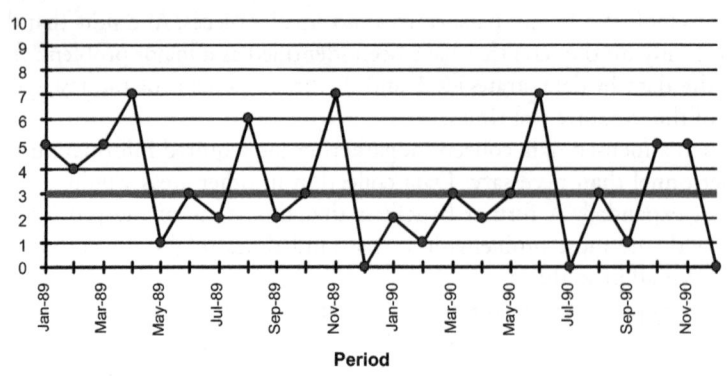

**a. Run Chart of Accident Performance**

**b. Matrix of Adverse Events**

| Event Type | Unit | | | | | | Total |
|---|---|---|---|---|---|---|---|
| | A | B | C | D | E | F | |
| 1 | 0 | 0 | 1 | 0 | 2 | 1 | 4 |
| 2 | 1 | 0 | 0 | 0 | 1 | 0 | 2 |
| 3 | 0 | 16 | 1 | 0 | 2 | 0 | 19 |
| 4 | 0 | 0 | 0 | 0 | 1 | 0 | 1 |
| 5 | 2 | 1 | 3 | 1 | 4 | 2 | 13 |
| 6 | 0 | 0 | 0 | 0 | 3 | 0 | 3 |
| 27 | | | | | | | |
| 28 | | | | (less than 6 each) | | | |
| 29 | | | | | | | |
| Totals | 6 | 19 | 7 | 3 | 35 | 7 | 77 |

- Departments B and E were special causes inside the people input;
- There was a further special cause (accident type 3) within Department B; and
- Department E showed no further potential localization.

■ The "measurement" input, by operationally defining individual accident types, showed:
- Accident types 3 and 5 were prevalent;
- Accident type 5 was an issue in the entire plant (common cause); and
- Accident type 3 was localized to a specific department (special cause).

■ It is now time to answer the workers' natural question, "Well, then, what should I do differently from what I'm doing now?" Otherwise:
- Department B would continue to have problems with accident type 3;
- Department E would continue to have a terrible safety process;
- The plant would continue to see accident type 5 as a problem everywhere; and
- These predictable performances would continue to aggregate predictably and demonstrate a predictable (common cause) output.

During the two years that performance data were collected, the safety process was a monthly meeting analyzing every single accident from the previous month, which is a Level 1 fix and special cause strategy.

The run chart has shown this process to be ineffective at accident reduction. The organization was treating common cause as special cause, and the underlying aggregate of all these perfectly designed processes continued to be predictable. Further, unless a common cause strategy — in this case, stratification — was employed instead, more future new policies, safety seminars, safety posters, and new reporting forms would be implemented and no change would occur.

Statistics on the number of accidents do not prevent accidents. All these special causes were combined and aggregated with normal day-to-day variation. This procedure produced the predictable monthly output seen by management. Understanding variation and prediction is rarely as easy as acting on the numbers seen in a summary table.

Strategy 3 now needs to be employed to further dissect Department E's accidents and accident type 5, which will probably be a lot of work. But it is only being applied to localized areas where the probability of further insight is high.

A plant manager, after seeing the run chart showing no change, might well say, "We need to go from a two-page reporting form to a five-page reporting form." That change, in and of itself, might guarantee fewer accidents, because no one would bother to report them. In the short term, however, temporarily doing deeper analysis on Department E's accidents and accident type 5 occurrences might find a solution. Leadership could then go back to the normal reporting form until a special cause is indicated on the run chart monitoring subsequent performance.

Now, if some potential solutions are found, it is time for data strategy 4.

### Data Strategy 4: Designed Experimentation

The final strategy is designed experimentation. This involves making a major fundamental structural change in the way a process is performed, then measuring whether it is indeed an improvement. It also involves even more disturbance to the daily work culture than the process dissection described in the previous section. This strategy should be used only sparingly.

The first three strategies help to expose all existing underlying special causes of variation. They also provide necessary insight into how the current process came to be and allow construction of a baseline for assessing the effects of a designed experiment.

The current process has now been optimized to its fullest capable extent. If the process remains incapable of meeting customer needs and some root causes still have not been addressed, a designed experiment is appropriate to evaluate a fundamental redesign of the process.

### The Same Tempting and Common Error

Again, initially, it is common for teams to jump right to this step to implement a "known" solution based on anecdotes. When this occurs, there is usually lack of a clear problem definition, which will even further compound this error because of:
- Poor understanding of how the process really works;
- Lack of good baseline data;
- The presence of unexposed special causes; and
- Reliance on poorly planned data collection.

These factors have serious potential ramifications in the subsequent evaluation and prediction from its results: It will be no better than looking into a crystal ball.

This approach naively begins the challenging problem-solving journey with the most aggressive data strategy. Such changes will result in major disturbance to a work culture that thrives on predictability. Especially if the strategy is unannounced and perceived as being forced on a work culture, it will also inhibit cooperation and understanding from the department involved in the experiment (see "Juran's Rules of the Road" in Chapter 8).

*Think Again about Your Credibility*

To summarize, flowcharts and data collections allow people to focus on the significant improvement opportunities. It also ensures that the right solution is applied to the right process. The team will gain substantial political credibility if it:

- Considers the staff's feelings;
- Respects the use of people's time during the project or experiment;
- Demonstrates its competency in the improvement process; and
- Involves members of the workforce at the appropriate times.

*Other Things to Consider in Designing an Experiment*

Candidates for solutions should be generated, prioritized, and initially tested *on a small scale*. As stated in the preface, rapid-cycle PDSA has emerged as the favored methodology to do this. One should always pilot any proposed solution on a focused, small scale first. It is not desirable to put a large work environment through a major disturbance. It will create unintended variation, add to confusion, and cloud the results (see Chapter 10). A pilot will expose the lurking unexpected problems that compromise the experimentation process itself, as well as lurking cultural "sabotage."

"How will we know if things are better?" is the question that must be answered in the planning of the experiment and then tested with appropriate data collection (which might initially include a test of the data collection process).

If you have proceeded to this stage via strategies 1 through 3, you should have some baseline data — hopefully at least a run chart — describing the problem. If there is a good baseline, the run chart can continue and the statistical rules given so far can be used to determine whether the desired special cause was created. Additional rules for determining the effectiveness of an intervention are discussed in Chapter 6.

*Summary of the Four Data Strategies*

Data aggressiveness is summarized in Exhibit 5.6. Each level of aggressiveness is listed along with its purpose, common approaches, and the amount of what I like to call cultural disturbance — disruption to routine work processes.

## INFORMATION GATHERING AS A PROCESS

As John Tukey said, "The more you know what is wrong with a figure, the more useful it becomes."[4] Good data collection is so important to process improvement, yet it is rarely taught as a skill. The teaching of passive analysis through applying traditional tools to any data set is no substitute. Precious time can be saved by knowing and leveraging the skills of simple, efficient data collection. In addition to collection, the skills also include awareness

EXHIBIT 5.6 ■ Data Aggressiveness

1. Exhaust in-house data (minimal disturbance):
   - Establish baselines to assess current process.
   - Isolate process problems through stratification if possible.
   - Expose variations in perceptions of data definitions.
   - Suggest theories needing further consideration for possible testing.
2. Study current process (tolerable disturbance):
   - Establish extent of problem(s).
   - Establish baseline for measuring improvement efforts.
   - Develop operational definitions suited to data collection objectives.
   - Reduce data contamination due to human variation.
   - Further localize problems.
     – Use current data collection methods to establish traceability to process inputs.
     – Capture and record available data that, while currently uncollected, are virtually there for the taking.
     – Conduct Pareto analyses and stratified histograms to localize problems.
3. Cut new windows — process dissection or disaggregation (uncomfortable disturbance):
   - Place intense focus on a major isolated source of localized variation.
   - Split process into subprocesses for further study.
     – Collect data not needed for routine process operation — the data collection process may be awkward and disruptive to routine operation.
4. Designed experimentation (major disturbance):
   - Test a process redesign suggested by one of the previous three levels.
   - Use a run or control chart to assess success.

of human factors lurking to add unintended, contaminating variation, which masks the actual process variation and renders useless any collected data.

Data-based decisions and statistical skills should not be reserved exclusively for the formal teams that develop during the course of the improvement process. As Chapter 2 demonstrated, it is important for all staff to have the skills to collect, manage, understand, analyze, and interpret data in the simplest, most efficient manner possible.

Chapter 2 also showed that part of management's transformation should be a serious reevaluation of the way data are used throughout the organization. A data inventory process is suggested later in this chapter (see "A New Perspective for Statistics"), and also provided is a survey to evaluate the robustness of your current organizational data collection process (see Exhibit 5.12); you may even consider taking that survey now.

The use of data is four processes: measurement definition, collection, analysis, and interpretation. Each of these processes has the universal six sources of inputs: people, methods, machines, materials, measurements (data), and environment. Think of a process needing improvement and these six inputs. If it is desired to quantify the output, a measurement process is used to produce an actual piece of data. These individual measurements undergo a collection (or formal accumulation) process. After collection, the data are input into an analysis process whose output then goes through an interpretation process (interpreting the variation). The interpretations usually result in a management action (reacting to the variation). This action then feeds back as an input into the process being studied. This cycle is summarized in Exhibit 5.7.

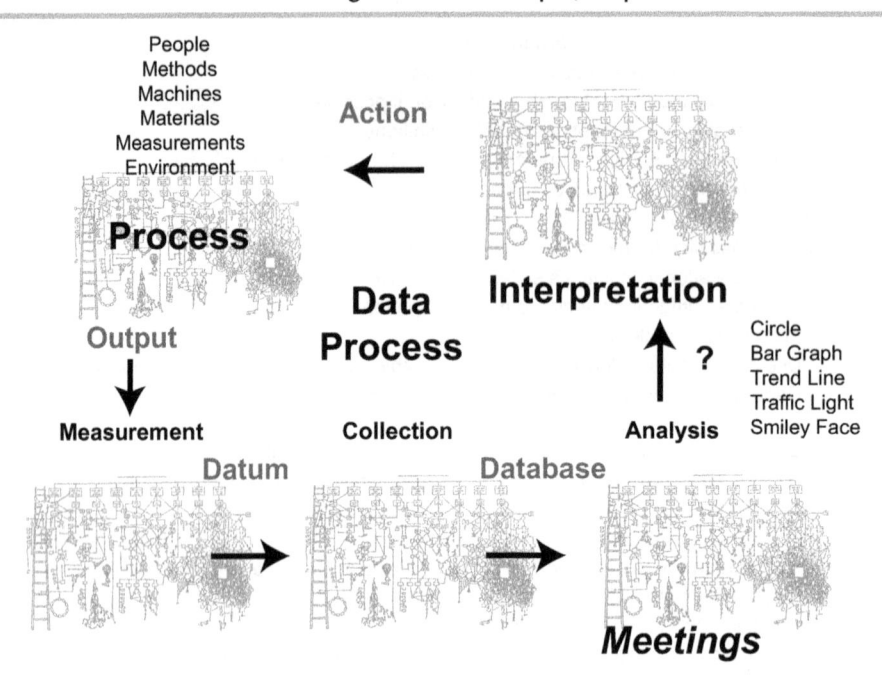

**EXHIBIT 5.7** ■ Information Gathering as a Process — Input/Output Flowchart

```
        People
        Methods
        Machines
        Materials        Action
        Measurements       ←
        Environment

        Process              Interpretation
                     Data                       Circle
         Output      Process           ↑ ?      Bar Graph
           ↓                           |        Trend Line
                                       |        Traffic Light
        Measurement    Collection    Analysis   Smiley Face
            Datum       →  Database  →

                                              Meetings
```

Any of these four data processes can be improved by using the now familiar seven sources of problems with a process. As with any other improvement opportunity, any one of the six inputs can be a source of variation for any one of these four processes. This variation, usually caused by human factors, lurks to contaminate your data process, which could ultimately mislead you as to what is going on in the actual process you are trying to improve.

Unless the variation in these processes is minimized, there is a danger of reacting to the variation *in the data process* and not the process one is trying to understand and improve.

Do you remember the seventh source of problems with a process, which is variation in inputs and outputs? Not only is it applicable to any project, but it is also applicable to data from any process, for example, clinical, operational, financial, administrative. Look at it from a routine managerial perspective, dealing with any typical variation of any process:

- Daily managerial reaction based on anecdotal incidents or poorly collected data (e.g., crisis-of-the-moment meetings, emergency budget revision meetings, extremely dissatisfied customers);
- Scheduled quarterly or annual review meetings accounting for current results;
- Meetings based on arbitrary numerical goals, including budgeting; and
- Routine scheduled meetings that unknowingly treat common cause as special cause.

Human variation is the enemy of quality in this process. This includes differences in perceiving the variation being studied (objective), in the process of defining a literal number to collect (measurement), and in actually executing the methods of measurement, collection, analysis and display, and interpretation.

Measurement and collection are very important. The critical thinking needed to address them can be motivated by looking at any data's routine current use, and most of this use takes place during scheduled meetings involving data.

How could you look at the current use of data and apply your improvement expertise? Look at a sample of any routine meeting's raw data and objectively ask:

1. What could these data tell you?
2. What is actually being done with these data?
3. What graphical displays are being used?
4. What other displays are being used (e.g., traffic lights, rolling averages)?
5. What is the reliance on using tables of raw numbers?
6. Is any difference between two numbers being treated as a special cause (e.g., smiley faces, thumbs up or down, month-to-month comparison, variance to goal)?
7. What actions result from these data? Do they consider whether the variation being acted on is common or special cause?
8. And especially, does a plot of these data over time exist? *How could you construct one?*

## The Four Data Processes

### Measurement Definition

Any process produces outputs that are potentially measurable. If one chooses, one can obtain a number (a piece of data) characterizing the situation through a process of measurement, called an *operational definition*. If the objectives are not explicitly clear or people have varying perceptions of what is being measured, the six sources of input variation will compromise the quality of this measurement definition process.

For QI purposes, crude measures of the right things are better than precise measures of the wrong things: As long as the measure is "consistently inconsistent" and defined in a way to ensure that anyone put in the situation will get the same number, you will benefit from the elegant simplicity of the statistical techniques inherent in QI.

### Collection

These individual measurements must then be accumulated into some type of data set, so they next pass to a collection process.

If the objectives are clear, the designed collection process should be relatively well defined because the analysis is known ahead of time; the appropriateness of an analysis depends on how the data were collected. If the objectives are not clear, the six sources of input variation will once again act to compromise the process. (From my experience, it is guaranteed that the six sources will compromise the collection process anyway.) Many organizational data sets comprising "operations" performance are collected with no clear purpose in mind.

The cultural implementation of QI and data sanity as strategies will result in an intense process focus. This will demand one particularly challenging change regarding organizational data collections: the need for smaller, more frequent samples collected in "real time." It will also be important to retain the samples' individuality (for potential future stratifications) and to plot them. Contrast this approach to most common practice and experience: Most organizational data are routinely aggregated into a large, pristine random summary sample — a table of numbers that begs people to "draw little circles," as discussed in Chapter 2.

Part of overcoming this seemingly overwhelming task will be to pilot collecting the data in this manner on the 20 percent of the organizational data that causes 80 percent of the organizational "perspiration."

### Analysis

Your analysis should be known before one piece of data has been collected. If the objectives are passive and reactive, eventually someone seems to retrieve the data and use a computer to "get the stats." This, of course, is an analysis process (albeit not necessarily a good one) that also has the six sources of process inputs as potential sources of variation. Or maybe more commonly, someone extracts the data and hands out tables of raw data presented as computer-generated summary analyses at a meeting. As described in Chapter 2, the meeting then becomes the analysis process, which is affected by the human variation in perceptions and abilities of people at the meeting.

Further, data not collected specifically for the current objective can generally be "tortured" to "confess" to someone else's hidden agenda. When people analyze data whose sole purpose is a quantitative summary to make causal inferences, they are usually asking for trouble.

I once saw an article summarizing some published academic research that used Nielsen television ratings. The only purpose of these ratings was counting answers to the question "How many?" and estimating how many people watched a show. Two researchers inappropriately took it further to imply causation. Analyses like these allow stereotypes about statistics to continue:

> [An] associate professor…and Chicago-based economist…reviewed Nielsen television ratings; 259 locally televised NBA games were analyzed. …They attempted to factor out all other variables — such as the win-loss records of teams and the times games were aired [torturing the data].
>
> The economists concluded that every additional 10 minutes of playing time by a white player increases a team's local ratings by, on average, 5,800 homes.[6]

I have a term for this type of analysis, which will be discussed in a later section of this chapter, "A New Perspective for Statistics."

### Interpretation

Statistics is not a set of techniques to "massage" data. The purpose is to appropriately interpret the variation with which you are faced in a situation. The variation can occur as one of two types, common cause or special cause, and treating one as the other makes things worse.

Ultimately, all analysis boils down to interpreting the variation with which one is faced. So the interpretation process (with the same six sources of process inputs) results in an *action* that is then fed back in to the original process.

Think of the many meetings you attend — in essence, analysis and interpretation processes — with tabular data, bar graphs, and trend lines being compared with arbitrary goals, resulting in interventions (usually special cause strategies). Could human variation in perception also manifest through the six input sources to affect the quality of each of the four data processes and subsequent decisions? How many meetings are reacting to variation in the data processes and not necessarily the process attempting to be improved?

When data are looked at as a process in the role of QI, statistics is not the science of analyzing data but becomes the art and science of collecting and analyzing data, simply and efficiently. As I like to say to my clients, "I'm the statistician, I know nothing. You're the healthcare workers, you know too much. That makes us a good team. My job is to keep you out of the data swamp. Your job is to come up with theories to test by simple data collection that I help you design."

## Eight Questions for Effective Data Collection

There are eight questions that need to be asked to result in an effective data process (see also Exhibit 5.12 for an implementation process):

1. *Why collect the data?* What is the objective? Data should not be collected for "museum" purposes and should be an immediate basis for action.
2. *What method(s) will be used for the analysis?* (This question must be answered before one piece of data is collected.)
3. *What data will be collected?* What concept or process output are we trying to capture?
4. *How will the data be measured?* How will we obtain either a number to characterize the situation or a decision point determining whether an event did ($x = 1$) or did not ($x = 0$) occur? This approach will never be perfect, and, for QI purposes, crude measures of the right things are better than precise measures of the wrong things. In other words, as long as a measurement is consistently inconsistent and allows one to successfully take the desired action, one can deal with it.

These first four questions help to reduce human variation in the design of the data collection. The ensuing problems of consistency and stability remain. The unintended ingenuity of human psychology that lurks to sabotage even the best of designs is a most formidable force to overcome. It is only when the human variation in the collection process and its logistics are also minimized that data can be trusted enough so that you can take appropriate action on the process being improved. These are addressed by the next four questions.

5. *How often will the data be collected?* Given the nature of process-oriented thinking, one of the biggest changes in thinking will be to realize the benefit of studying a process by collecting *more frequent samples over time*. This will cause the need to redefine many current pristine operational definitions to become "good enough." Because your processes are perfectly designed to get the results they are already getting, taking more frequent samples is like taking a time-lapse movie of your process rather than one snapshot (which contains no context of variation within which to interpret).
6. *Where will the data be collected?* Where will disruption be minimized to allow the opportunity for the highest quality data to be captured?
7. *Who will collect the data?*
8. *What training is needed for the data collectors?* Do the people collecting the data understand why they are collecting the data, how to get the number, where to collect it, and how often to collect it? In other words, is the variation in the collection process itself minimized?

Questions 7 and 8 need serious consideration and are usually neglected. If people do not know why they are collecting the data and/or how to obtain the number and/or how

EXHIBIT 5.8 ■ Initial Envelope Thickness Measurements

| | |
|---|---|
| 0.25" (top corner) | 1.02 mm |
| 0.019" (bottom corner) | 0.0125" |
| 0.017" (bottom corner) | 0.0106 |
| 12.600 mils | 0.0106 |
| 0.01875" | 0.015625 (blue) |
| 1.02 mm | 0.01219 (green) |
| 0.018" | 0.02 |
| 0.01875" | 0.01 |
| | 0.017" |

to record it, any data obtained are worthless. It is best to do an initial short pilot study of any proposed data collection to make sure this data process is stable. Otherwise, human variation will ultimately cause a poor-quality data set.

### Are You Measuring Envelopes?

As an example of the hidden dangers of data collection, Exhibit 5.8 shows an actual data set I obtained while teaching a class. Quantities of envelopes and various types of rulers were distributed. I gave the class an (intentionally vague) assignment: Find the thickness of an envelope and record it on a flip chart. Some were curious as to how much pressure to apply, to which I responded (with a straight face), "a moderate amount." There were no other instructions. Very few clarifying questions were usually asked by the class, or I would put up an intimidating demeanor if they did and demand, "Just get me the thickness of an envelope. *What's your problem?*"

The numbers that the class arrived at were all different. The class was asked to brainstorm why so much variation was present, which usually resulted in at least 30 reasons. Significant differences in measurement techniques, calculation of the number, and location of the measurements became evident. The lack of an objective for the data collection resulted in a variety of perceptions regarding what problem was being addressed and, therefore, how to measure it. Some people had perceived the exercise as a total waste of time (this scenario may seem familiar to some of your routine processes) and gave it a half-hearted effort. All these factors resulted in a poor-quality data set.

Think of this exercise as a process and ask yourself why the numbers might be different. Can you classify the reasons for variation into people, methods, machines, materials, measurements, or environment?

What should be done with these data? Often, the response is, "Put them in the computer." Seriously, do these data have any use? In fact, they are quite useful because they show there is neither an agreed-on objective nor measurement process. However, if this same collection process were followed with data taken in a similar manner day after day, month after month, it would immediately cease to be useful. Consistent, repeated collection would just institutionalize the lack of objective and process.

In effect, variation in human perceptions became nonquantifiable variation that could not be understood through a formal statistical analysis. Suppose the data had been sent to a computer center to be keyed into the database just as it was — a list of numbers. Any formal statistical analysis would have been ludicrous.

EXHIBIT 5.9 ■ Conflicting Mental Models about Data

- Research
- Inspection (comparison/finger pointing)
- Micromanagement (from "on high")
- Results (compared to arbitrary goals)
- Outcomes (for bragging)
- Improvement

The numbers would have been different even if there was agreement on the objective and measurement process. However, they would have exhibited less variation, and an initial attempt could be made to statistically analyze them. Less variation translates into a higher quality data set. Recall Tukey's comment: "The more you know what is wrong with a figure, the more useful it becomes."

A seemingly trivial exercise became quite complicated, generating much confusion and chaos. Are not daily work processes more complicated than measuring envelopes?

Two major points can be made with this exercise:

1. A good statistical analysis of a bad set of data is worthless; and
2. If we can agree on what to measure but cannot agree on how to measure it, any data generated will essentially be worthless.

In my experience, one can never overestimate how the ingenuity of human psychology can add variation to a data collection. When instructions go through someone's personal filter (or underlying hidden agenda, especially if motivated by fear), they are often unintentionally altered, thus adding variation to the process.

Conflicting mental models about data (Exhibit 5.9) also contribute significant human variation. A measured result could change depending on someone's belief about the objective of the data (including fear of the consequences of the result; generally, frightened humans will find a way to meet a goal). Even more likely, the presentation, analysis, and interpretation of the data will differ from one mental model to another. Indeed, the first and last models in Exhibit 5.9 are the only two of value.

The others are statistically dysfunctional manifestations of the improvement mode (and a sincere desire to improve). They are contaminated by human psychology and rely heavily on faulty assumptions in their data processes as designed (collection, analysis and display, interpretation). They result in much inappropriate, though well-meaning, action. Nonquantifiable human variation in a data set will render statistical analysis virtually meaningless.

Improvement of data quality occurs as both quantifiable and nonquantifiable sources of variation are reduced. That is, prediction capability is enhanced by understanding, controlling, and reducing variation through study of the measurement process that produced these numbers. Confidence is thereby built into the system, and the data can be used for their true objective.

## A Key Emphasis in a Service Culture: Operational Definitions

Words have no meaning unless they are translated into action, agreed upon by everyone. An operational definition puts communicable meaning into a concept. "There is no true value of anything."[4]

The concept of operational definitions is so important that it is worth more formal discussion. Quality problems often persist because of different perceptions of the meaning of words. All meaning begins with concepts — thoughts, notions, images in the mind. These perceptions bring the element of human, nonquantifiable variation into data processes. Human variation complicates the interpretation of a process's true variation by (unknowingly) invalidating the statistical analysis. Several people assessing the same situation can come up with conflicting sets of data if operational definitions are not clarified up front. Operational definitions of all key process terms are critical for data to be comparable across individuals, departments, or organizations.

An operational definition is not open to interpretation, but instead quantitatively interprets a concept by describing what something is and how it is measured, that is, how to get a number out of a situation. It defines a procedure that yields consistent results regardless of who measures the process.

Although people may not fully agree on an operational definition, the definition provides at least some consensus. Regardless of who measures a given situation, the desire is to obtain virtually the same number. If an operationally defined measurement procedure is replaced with a different operationally defined procedure, the same situation will likely yield a different number. Neither procedure would be right or wrong, but the effects of changing the procedure would be clear. However, if the procedure is not operationally defined, latitude taken by individuals practically guarantees different numbers even with supposedly the same procedure.

This was demonstrated at a meeting I once attended where three health centers presented mammography rates data to a customer. After viewing the presentation, the customer had two comments: "The way you've each defined your data, I can't compare you," and, smiling, added, "You've also each defined your data in a way that was self-serving." Thus the definitions were appropriate for each organization's internal objective, but not for a customer's objective of comparing the health centers' results.

As an exercise in identifying terms that require operational definitions, consider what is meant by the following vague terms: grossly contaminated, late, clean, careful, satisfactory, attached, correct, level, secure, fresh, user-friendly, too many, complete, uniform, significant improvement, on time, majority, large majority, rush, RUSH!, STAT, unemployed, accident, error. Now, for a hospital you work with, define:

- How many beds does it have?
- How many patient deaths occurred there last year?

How these are counted will depend on what the objective is. For those of you who work in hospitals, state and national databases contain your hospital's name and numbers for these categories and each database probably has a different number for the same item.

The sheer magnitude of human variation in the contamination of data sets because of lack of clear operational definitions is astounding. Consider the following examples.

Does a hospital's length-of-stay definition use midnight census in its definition? This definition may have been appropriate when I had my appendix out in 1966 and stayed in the same bed for four days. Today's processes of practicing medicine are radically different. One can still get a length-of-stay number using midnight census, but does it allow one to take meaningful, desired action?

How can you tell whether you have cut the smoking rate from 26 percent to 21 percent? Before you answer, think about these qualifications: (1) Define *stopped smoking* and (2) define *smoking rate*. (Do you include pipes, cigars, or smokeless tobacco? Make sure agreement is reached.)

Who won the 2000 U.S. presidential election? It all boiled down to counting the votes in Florida the day after the election. Definitions were attempted depending on whether the paper ballot chads were not completely punched out, on how far it was hanging, and so forth. But what if more than one hole seemed to be punched? What if one was clearly punched out, but another contained a hanging chad? There were also issues of what constituted a "legal ballot." However, even if all of these issues could have somehow been made consistent, recounting the ballots on two different days would most likely still yield different numbers.

And then there's poor Pluto, who a few years ago was no longer considered a planet. When protests persisted, an astronomer arrived at a revised definition of "planet" that would reinstate Pluto and create the necessity to declare 100 other heavenly bodies as planets.

When creating an operational definition, the team should not view any procedure as right or wrong, but should instead question if the measurement satisfies the current objectives of the data collection and analysis. Is it consistent and good enough, and does it result in the desired action?

In the absence of operational definitions, people often resort to anecdotal data, that is, stories about the seriousness of a problem and the solution to it, which are influenced by the perspective of the person telling them. To prevent inappropriate action based on anecdotal information, the following process is recommended (the process described in Exhibit 5.3 may also be used):

1. Ask further questions about the anecdote to clarify exactly what is meant by the terms it includes. Try to develop operational definitions of key terms that are consistent and good enough. Then collect data on the number and types of occurrences; or
2. Recognize the anecdote as a breakdown of a process. Ask whether there is adequate knowledge of how the process works or how it should work. Clarify this human variation in perception by facilitating a session to develop a map, that is, a flowchart, of the situation. Talk to customers to determine their needs and then operationally define them.

## How Are You Using Data?

What data are routinely collected in your organization? Is there an objective? Organizations can have a tendency to routinely amass numerical data on various perceived key process outputs and business indicators and produce monthly reports at incredible rates. One could say (with apologies to Samuel Coleridge and the Ancient Mariner), "Data, data everywhere, and not a thought to think."

An interesting clinical perspective comes from Heero Hacquebord, who notes in an article about his hospital stay during back surgery (a wonderful example of healthcare as a process):

> While the health care professionals that I came in contact with collected and recorded a great deal of data about me during my stay, it is not clear to me that this information was fully utilized to improve my care, or the care of future patients. Vital signs on a patient's condition should not be just simply recorded; it is necessary to interpret such data effectively so that correct remedies and actions are taken. I believe this problem of data overload comes about in health care because there is often no explicit theory that one is

testing that could then be used to drive data collection and the identification of key information.[7]

Unless a process has been analyzed using the seven sources of problems with a process sequentially, the danger exists that any data collection will be significantly contaminated with excessive variation. Data with excessive variation that are used for business or clinical decisions could have a serious negative impact.

### A Process to Evaluate Your Organization's Overall Measurement System

Think about how your organization measures itself. Mark Graham Brown developed an insightful survey that is given in Exhibit 5.10.[8] Brown's philosophy and design are based on the seven Malcolm Baldrige National Quality Award criteria:

1. Customer satisfaction;
2. Employee satisfaction;
3. Financial performance;
4. Operational performance (e.g., cycle time, productivity);
5. Product/service quality;
6. Supplier performance; and
7. Safety/environmental/public responsibility.

This particular survey allows an organization to assess its own measurement system. The 50 questions are divided into three categories and address the overall approach to measurement, specific types of measures, and how to analyze and use the data to improve the organization.

Following an assessment with Brown's survey, a process can be developed to define goals and critical success factors, after which one redefines the measures.

This process must start from the top and cascade down to all levels in the organization with the net result being that each employee has a balanced set of no more than 10 measures covering the seven categories.

Are your data collections truly adding value to your organization? As mentioned earlier, data collected without any clear purpose can eventually be used to prove virtually any hidden agenda. Does today's constantly changing business environment have time for such nonsense?

What implications does the process of data collection have if you are collecting process outputs in the absence of clear objectives communicated to the people involved in the measurement definition, collection, analysis, and interpretation processes? Consider a new perspective.

## A NEW PERSPECTIVE FOR STATISTICS

"Statistical theory is helpful for understanding differences between people and interactions between people; interactions between people and the system that they work in, or learn in."[9] Because all work is a process that exhibits variation, and quality aims for consistently excellent results, QI can be defined as using the context of process-oriented thinking to:

1. Understand observed variation;
2. Reduce inappropriate and unintended existing variation; and
3. Control the influence of detrimental outside variation, including uncontrolled variation in human behavior.

## EXHIBIT 5.10 ■ Survey for Evaluating Your Current Organizational Data Collection Process

**Questionnaire directions** — The questionnaire is divided into three sections, each addressing an aspect of your measurement system.

- Part I (questions 1-5) is about your overall approach to measurement.
- Part II (questions 6-40) questions ask specific types of measures.
- Part III (questions 41-50) is about how you analyze and use the data to improve your organization.

Read each statement and check the appropriate box, depending on the extent to which you strongly agree (5) or strongly disagree (1) with the statement. Answer every question even if you have to guess.

The scope of the questionnaire should pertain to your entire organization, or at least a large enough portion of the company or organization that could be a stand-alone business/organization. For example, you could do a business unit rather than the whole company, or one hospital in a chain of hospitals. You could and should not use the questionnaire to apply to a single department such as radiology, or human resources.

### Part I: Overall approach to measurement

1. Our organization has developed a specific set of criteria for screening out extraneous measures from our data base.
   ___ ⑤ Strongly agree ④ Agree ③ Somewhat ② Disagree ① Strongly disagree

2. Our data base was built with a plan, rather than something that just evolved over time.
   ___ ⑤ Strongly agree ④ Agree ③ Somewhat ② Disagree ① Strongly disagree

3. Our CEO or President looks at no more than 20 measures every month to evaluate the overall organization's performance.
   ___ ⑤ Strongly agree ④ Agree ③ Somewhat ② Disagree ① Strongly disagree

4. Measures of performance are mostly consistent across our business units/locations.
   ___ ⑤ Strongly agree ④ Agree ③ Somewhat ② Disagree ① Strongly disagree

5. We have a well balanced set of measures, with about equal amounts of measures/data in each of the following categories: financial performance, operational performance, customer satisfaction, employee satisfaction, product/service quality, supplier performance, and safety/environmental performance.
   ___ ⑤ Strongly agree ④ Agree ③ Somewhat ② Disagree ① Strongly disagree

### Part II: Specific types of measures on your scorecard

*Customer related measures*

6. Our data base includes good hard measures of customer satisfaction such as repeat/lost business, returns, etc.
   ___ ⑤ Strongly agree ④ Agree ③ Somewhat ② Disagree ① Strongly disagree

7. Our organization collects data on customer feelings/satisfaction levels using a variety of techniques such as telephone surveys, mail surveys, and focus groups.
   ___ ⑤ Strongly agree ④ Agree ③ Somewhat ② Disagree ① Strongly disagree

8. Our scales for measuring customer satisfaction focus on delighting customers rather than just satisfying them.
   ___ ⑤ Strongly agree ④ Agree ③ Somewhat ② Disagree ① Strongly disagree

9. What we ask customers in our satisfaction surveys or discussions is based upon thorough research to identify customers' most important requirements.
   ___ ⑤ Strongly agree ④ Agree ③ Somewhat ② Disagree ① Strongly disagree

10. We combine various hard and soft measures of customer satisfaction into an overall Customer Satisfaction index.
    ___ ⑤ Strongly agree ④ Agree ③ Somewhat ② Disagree ① Strongly disagree

*Employee related measures*

11. We survey our employees at least once a year to determine their satisfaction levels with various aspects of how the organization is run.
    ___ ⑤ Strongly agree ④ Agree ③ Somewhat ② Disagree ① Strongly disagree

12. Employee surveys are anonymous and more than 75 percent are returned each year.
    ___ ⑤ Strongly agree ④ Agree ③ Somewhat ② Disagree ① Strongly disagree

13. Research is done to determine what is important to employees before putting together or buying a survey with standard questions.
    ___ ⑤ Strongly agree ④ Agree ③ Somewhat ② Disagree ① Strongly disagree

14. Our organization collects data on other metrics that relate to employee satisfaction such as voluntary turnover, absenteeism hours worked per week, requests for transfers, et cetera.
    ___ ⑤ Strongly agree ④ Agree ③ Somewhat ② Disagree ① Strongly disagree

15. Individual measures of employee satisfaction are aggregated into an overall employee satisfaction index, similar to the customer satisfaction index.
    ___ ⑤ Strongly agree ④ Agree ③ Somewhat ② Disagree ① Strongly disagree

*Financial measures*

16. We have identified a few (e.g. 4-6) key measures of our overall financial performance.
    ___ ⑤ Strongly agree ④ Agree ③ Somewhat ② Disagree ① Strongly disagree

17. Financial measures are a good mix of short and long-term measures of financial success
    ___ ⑤ Strongly agree ④ Agree ③ Somewhat ② Disagree ① Strongly disagree

18. Financial measures are consistent across different units/locations.
    ___ ⑤ Strongly agree ④ Agree ③ Somewhat ② Disagree ① Strongly disagree

19. We collect financial data on our major competitors to use in evaluating our own performance and in setting goals.
    ___ ⑤ Strongly agree ④ Agree ③ Somewhat ② Disagree ① Strongly disagree

(Continues)

## EXHIBIT 5.10 (Continued)

20. The organization aggregates financial data into one or two summary statistics that reflect overall performance, such as economic value added (EVA) or return on assets (ROA).
___ ⑤ Strongly agree ④ Agree ③ Somewhat ② Disagree ① Strongly disagree

### Operational measures

21. The organization has developed a set of 4–6 common operational measures such as value-added per employee that are used in all locations/functions.
___ ⑤ Strongly agree ④ Agree ③ Somewhat ② Disagree ① Strongly disagree

22. Any process measures that are collected are directly related to key product/service characteristics that customers care about.
___ ⑤ Strongly agree ④ Agree ③ Somewhat ② Disagree ① Strongly disagree

23. Cycle time is used as a key operational measure throughout the organization.
___ ⑤ Strongly agree ④ Agree ③ Somewhat ② Disagree ① Strongly disagree

24. Operational measures allow you to prevent problems rather than just identify them.
___ ⑤ Strongly agree ④ Agree ③ Somewhat ② Disagree ① Strongly disagree

25. The organization has established measurable standards for all key process measures.
___ ⑤ Strongly agree ④ Agree ③ Somewhat ② Disagree ① Strongly disagree

### Supplier measures

26. The organization has a rating system for evaluating supplier performance.
___ ⑤ Strongly agree ④ Agree ③ Somewhat ② Disagree ① Strongly disagree

27. Our supplier rating system is a mix of hard data such as products returned/shipments rejected, and soft measures such as our satisfaction levels with suppliers' responsiveness.
___ ⑤ Strongly agree ④ Agree ③ Somewhat ② Disagree ① Strongly disagree

28. The quality of goods and services purchased from suppliers is measured on a regular basis.
___ ⑤ Strongly agree ④ Agree ③ Somewhat ② Disagree ① Strongly disagree

29. Our organization asks suppliers for process data and encourages self-inspection.
___ ⑤ Strongly agree ④ Agree ③ Somewhat ② Disagree ① Strongly disagree

30. Staying within our price guidelines is only one of many measures used to evaluate and select suppliers.
___ ⑤ Strongly agree ④ Agree ③ Somewhat ② Disagree ① Strongly disagree

### Product/service quality measures

31. Characteristics of products/services that are measured are those that are most important to customers.
___ ⑤ Strongly agree ④ Agree ③ Somewhat ② Disagree ① Strongly disagree

32. If 100 percent of products/services are not checked, then large enough sample sizes are used to ensure that all products/services meet standards.
___ ⑤ Strongly agree ④ Agree ③ Somewhat ② Disagree ① Strongly disagree

33. Automated measurement devices are used wherever possible to avoid errors caused by poor human judgement.
___ ⑤ Strongly agree ④ Agree ③ Somewhat ② Disagree ① Strongly disagree

34. Measures for services are related to accomplishments rather than behaviors (e.g. percent of correct orders filled, or percent of flights that take off on-time versus smiling when greeting customer).
___ ⑤ Strongly agree ④ Agree ③ Somewhat ② Disagree ① Strongly disagree

35. Measures of product/service quality are expressed as actual number rather than percentages of defect-free products/services.
___ ⑤ Strongly agree ④ Agree ③ Somewhat ② Disagree ① Strongly disagree

### Safety/environmental/public responsibility measures

36. The organization collects data on safety and environmental performance at least once a month, using several different metrics.
___ ⑤ Strongly agree ④ Agree ③ Somewhat ② Disagree ① Strongly disagree

37. Measures of safety are more behavioral and preventative in nature rather than the typical lost time accidents.
___ ⑤ Strongly agree ④ Agree ③ Somewhat ② Disagree ① Strongly disagree

38. Environmental measures go beyond those mandated by the EPA and other regulatory agencies.
___ ⑤ Strongly agree ④ Agree ③ Somewhat ② Disagree ① Strongly disagree

39. The organization collects data on measures of public responsibility such as hours of community service or awards received from community/civic groups.
___ ⑤ Strongly agree ④ Agree ③ Somewhat ② Disagree ① Strongly disagree

40. The organization has developed a public responsibility index that is an aggregation of safety, environmental, and community service measures.
___ ⑤ Strongly agree ④ Agree ③ Somewhat ② Disagree ① Strongly disagree

### Part III: Reporting and analyzing data

41. The organization reports data from all sections of its scorecard in a single report to all key managers.
___ ⑤ Strongly agree ④ Agree ③ Somewhat ② Disagree ① Strongly disagree

42. Data are presented graphically in an easy to read format that requires minimal analysis to identify trends and levels of performance.
___ ⑤ Strongly agree ④ Agree ③ Somewhat ② Disagree ① Strongly disagree

43. Data on customer satisfaction, employee satisfaction, and public responsibility are reviewed as often and by the same executives as data of financial, operational, product/service, and supplier performance.
___ ⑤ Strongly agree ④ Agree ③ Somewhat ② Disagree ① Strongly disagree

44. The organization has done research to identify correlations between customer satisfaction levels and financial performance.
___ ⑤ Strongly agree ④ Agree ③ Somewhat ② Disagree ① Strongly disagree

(Continues)

## EXHIBIT 5.10 (Continued)

45. The organization understands the relationship between all the key measures in its overall scorecard.
    ___ ⑤ Strongly agree  ④ Agree  ③ Somewhat  ② Disagree  ① Strongly disagree

46. Performance data are analyzed and used to make key decisions about the organization's business.
    ___ ⑤ Strongly agree  ④ Agree  ③ Somewhat  ② Disagree  ① Strongly disagree

47. The key measures are consistent with the organization's missions, values, and long-term goals and strategies.
    ___ ⑤ Strongly agree  ④ Agree  ③ Somewhat  ② Disagree  ① Strongly disagree

48. The organization continuously evaluates and improves its measures and the methods used to collect and report performance data.
    ___ ⑤ Strongly agree  ④ Agree  ③ Somewhat  ② Disagree  ① Strongly disagree

49. Automated and human (e.g. surveys/checklists) measurement devices are calibrated on a regular basis to assure accuracy and reliability.
    ___ ⑤ Strongly agree  ④ Agree  ③ Somewhat  ② Disagree  ① Strongly disagree

50. The measures in the organization's scorecard are the same ones on which annual and longer-term goals are set during the planning process.
    ___ ⑤ Strongly agree  ④ Agree  ③ Somewhat  ② Disagree  ① Strongly disagree

**Calculating your score** — Questions 1-5 relate to your entire measurement system, so they are worth more than the rest of the questions. Add up the total for questions 1-5. A perfect score would be 25, if you answered Strongly Agree for all five questions. Write the total for questions 1-5 in the space below.

Proceed by adding up the total for questions 6-40. Next add up the total points for questions 41-50, and multiply this number by 2.

Add the three sub-totals to give yourself a grand total score. A perfect score on this assessment is 330, so if you ended up with more than that, go back and check your math.

Total questions 1-5 _____ X2 = _____
Total questions 6-40 _____ = _____
Total questions 41-50 _____ X2 = _____
Grand total = _____

*Interpreting your score*

*Scores of 276-330* — If your score on this survey ended up in this top band, you truly have a worldclass approach to measuring your organization's performance. You have narrowed down your database to a few key metrics and must have a well-balanced set of metrics. It also is evident that you actually use the data you collect to make decisions about improving organizational performance. Yours should be an organization that others benchmark for measurement.

*Scores of 226-275* — If your score ended up in this second band you have a systematic approach to measurement that approaches being well-balanced. Chances are you are weak in measure of customer satisfaction and employee satisfaction, and may not do a good job of aggregating individual metrics into summary statistics, and analyzing the data to improve organizational performance. You have made a great deal of progress in improving your organization's approach to measurement. However, additional refinement is needed over time, and more research needs to be done to identify correlations between long-term measures such as customer satisfaction/employee satisfaction and shorter-term measures such as financial performance. Being in this band probably means that your measurement system is better than 75-80 percent of organizations in North America.

*Scores of 176-225* — A score in this range puts you in about the middle, which says that you are off to a good start in re-engineering your approach to measurement. You probably have a good set of measures for some of the seven boxes on an organization's score card. You also probably have some major weaknesses in some types of measures. You are probably strong in financial, operational, and product/service quality data, and weak in the other four areas. Chances are you still have too many measures, and have inconsistencies across the different units/locations in your organization. A score in this range says that you are making some refinements in your approach to measurement, but still need to do quite a bit of work to put together a good solid measurement approach.

*Scores of 175 or less* — This puts you at the 50 percent o below level, which means that you are a long way from having a balanced score card. You're in good company at this level, however. In my experience, this is where most businesses are, and where almost all government and healthcare organizations are. Most business organizations are only just starting to measure customer satisfaction and employee satisfaction. Government and healthcare organizations are weak in these two areas, and also tend t be weak in product/service quality data and measures of supplier performance. Organizations that score at less than 50 percent on this survey probably still have not convinced upper management that strategic longer-term measures are just as important as the traditional financial and operational metrics.

Source: This survey originally appeared in *Keeping Score: Using the Right Metrics to Drive World Class Performance* (New York: Productivity Press, 1996) by Mark Graham Brown and is reprinted with permission.

**EXHIBIT 5.11** ■ Data Inventory Considerations

1. What is the objective of these data?
2. Is there an unambiguous operational definition to obtain a consistent numerical value for the process being measured?
    - Is it appropriate for the objective?
3. How are these data accumulated or collected?
    - Is the collection appropriate for the objective?
    - Is the data process producing consistent data?
4. How are the data being analyzed or displayed?
    - Is the analysis or display appropriate, given the way the data were collected?
5. What action, if any, is currently being taken with these data?

**Given the objective and action, is anything "wrong" with the current number?**

Statistics is the only sound theoretical basis for interpreting variation and coming to objective conclusions. However, it could be terribly misleading to use statistics on any data set unless one can answer these questions:

1. What is the objective of these data?
2. How were these data collected?
3. Was the process, including the data process that produced these data, stable?

Analyses must be appropriate for the way the data were collected.

Also implicit in proper statistical applications of QI is a proactive data strategy that considers data to be a basis for action. Unless the objective of data is clear, data collection can merely add cost without adding value, and statistical analysis can be inappropriate and misleading.

As previously stated, statistics is the art and science of collecting and analyzing data. Whether or not people understand statistics, they are already using statistics to interpret observed variation. Every day, many decisions are made based on data, whether planned or unplanned, real or anecdotal, statistically analyzed or not. When people use data, they perceive, interpret, and react to observed variation to make a prediction. As repeatedly emphasized, the variation in a given situation is generally one of two types — common cause and special cause. It is a common error to mistake one for the other, and action based on this error actually makes things worse.

These concepts are summarized in Exhibit 5.11. Look at the data you work with every day. Can you answer the five questions posed in the exhibit? They can be the basis for discussion about your current key organizational measurements.

Unfortunately, the framework within which statistics is often taught in academia incorrectly treats statistics as sets of techniques to perform on existing data sets. An acronym I use for this type of analysis is PARC. Given how I see statistics practiced, the letters in the acronym have a variety of meanings. Some examples are practical accumulated records compilation, passive analysis by regressions and correlations (including trend lines), profound analysis by relying on computers, and planning after research completed.

Of course, such acronyms exist for a reason. Service industries and medicine are flooded with data. Databases and computers with user-friendly statistical packages are easily available and allow the generation of literally thousands of reports that give people the illusion of knowledge and control of their processes. Analysis in this context generally gives a PARC analysis in reverse (the proof is left to the reader; recall the TV ratings analysis to determine racism described in the "Analysis" section earlier in this chapter).

Now, consider two other manifestations of PARC:

1. A typical organizational amalgam of *continuously recorded administrative procedures*, collected with no clear purpose in mind; and
2. What seems to be a specialty of individuals particularly resistant to change: the *constant repetition of anecdotal perceptions.*

One need not be a statistician to use statistics effectively in QI. The statistical thinking mind-set involves five skills. Given any improvement situation (including daily work), one must be able to:

1. Choose and define the problem in a process and systems context;
2. Design and manage *a series of* simple, efficient data collections to expose undesirable variation (Pareto principle: expose the 20 percent of the process causing 80 percent of the problem);
3. Use comprehensible methods presentable and understandable across *all* layers of the organization; they will all be graphical yet avoid raw data or bar graphs (with the specific exception of a Pareto analysis), trend lines, or exclusive traffic light interpretations;
4. Numerically assess the current state of an undesirable situation, further expose inappropriate and unintended variation through deeper dissection, and assess the effects of interventions; and
5. Hold the gains of any improvements made, which generally requires a much simpler data collection.

Significant improvement can occur only when statistics are used in a framework of both appreciating a system and understanding its variation. Only such understanding can result in effective decisions based on planned data collection. Neither a focus solely on results nor arbitrarily imposed numerical goals or standards will improve a process.

## SUMMARY

Statistical thinking through process focus is the key to continuous improvement. The role of statistics is to enhance prediction by:

- Understanding existing variation;
- Reducing inappropriate and unintended variation in a context of systems thinking; and
- Controlling the detrimental influence of outside variation.

Whether or not people understand statistics, they are already using statistics. It is not necessary for everyone to become a statistician to participate in an organizational QI effort. However, everyone must become aware of the continuous presence of variation and how to deal with it.

Any application of statistics to a QI opportunity must be preceded by:

- A process and systems understanding of the observed problem;
- An assessment of critical inputs and outputs from an internal supplier/customer perspective of the system; and
- Agreement on numerical (not anecdotal) measures of these indicators through clear operational definitions.

Even though it is sometimes not perceived as formal statistics, there is a statistical perspective inherent in process-oriented thinking. It creates essential readiness for subsequent efficient, more appropriate use of statistical methods.

- Although service outputs may seem more difficult to define than manufacturing outputs, all processes in both settings have measurable outputs.
- Significant quality improvements result only when data collection and analysis are used to establish consistent work processes and to identify elements of work processes that do not provide value.
- Flowcharts reduce problems created by disagreement and variation in perceptions about how processes currently operate.
- Processes represent repeatable actions occurring over time and must be studied that way.
- Data collection is itself four processes, each with inputs, outputs, and variation.
- There are eight questions to answer for any data collection.
- Common errors in QI include action based on anecdotes and the addition of unnecessary complexity to a process. These result from lack of a process-oriented thinking perspective.
- Operational definitions can prevent inappropriate actions based on anecdotes.
- To create significant lasting improvement, data collection that is appropriate for the situational objectives and subsequent analysis must be used for decision making.
- Statistics can provide a unified language to break down barriers created by varied perceptions of how a process works.

## An Everyday Strategy for Using Data

Effective action requires a fast response to problems that arise, so chart the freshest data you can get, even if they are not precise measurements. Charting an estimate of a day's production on that same day is much better than waiting a week for a more accurate figure to be released from your accounting department. You can always revise the estimate later on.

If you like to use a computer to store and manipulate your data, do not let the lack of a sophisticated graphics program keep you from making charts. Most spreadsheet programs that people already use can do a good job.

Keep your data close to the source. The people who actually are doing the work should take the measurements, if possible, and chart the results. That way, they retain ownership of the data. And people who work on a process will often notice things that others would miss.

Of course, just keeping charts is no guarantee that you will learn anything. The critical decisions are what you chart and how you measure it. You will learn more if you chart data linked to something important in your work and measure it the right way.

There is no need to chart every process; that just creates extra work and ultimately leads to frustration.

Three questions to ask yourself before you decide which data are worth charting are:

1. What component or characteristic of your work is most important to your next internal customer, or to the final customer?
2. When you get daily, weekly, or monthly figures, which number do you look at first?

3. What is the one thing your boss asks about when he or she wants to know, "How's it going today?"

In administrative areas, it is particularly important for data gatherers to agree on the operational definition of the measurement. For example, does medical information nurse cycle time start from the moment a patient places a call (and perhaps gets placed on hold) or from the entry of the patient's situation into the computer?

The greatest leverage comes from emphasizing data displays that all employees can use. Simple time-ordered, coded plots let everyone use their eyes, intuition, and experience, and common theory to identify opportunities for improvement.

A final summary of data planning and collection is given in Exhibit 5.12.

EXHIBIT 5.12  Summary of Data Collection

1. Questions should relate to *specific* information needs of the project. For the best, most simple, efficient collection, objectives should be as narrow and focused as possible and relate to a potential major source of observed variation.
   - People involved in the actual data collection should have confidence that the team knows *exactly* what it is asking and looking for as well as that it is going to *do* something with the information.
   - The level of data aggressiveness should be appropriate for the stage of the project.
2. Imagine you have the data already in hand. Have the necessary data been collected to truly answer your question? What data tools will be used? Is the proposed analysis *appropriate* for the way the data are collected?
3. Where is the best leverage point in the process to collect the data? Where will the job flow suffer minimum interruption?
4. Who should be the collector? Is this person unbiased, and does he or she have easy and immediate access to the relevant facts?
5. *Understand the data collectors and their environment.*
   - What effect will their normal job have on the proposed data collection? Will data be complete? Do the forms allow efficient recording of data with minimum interruption to their normal jobs?
6. Design of a data collection form (check sheet) is not trivial. When possible, involve some of the collectors in the design.
   - Reduce opportunities for error; design traceability to collector and environment; make the form virtually self-explanatory; make their appearance professional.
   - *Keep it simple.*
7. Prepare simple instructions and possibly a flowchart for using the data collection forms.
8. Train the people who will be involved. Have a properly completed form available.
   - Answer the following natural questions of the collectors: What is the purpose of the study? What are the data going to be used for? Will the results be communicated to them?
   - Reduce fear by discussing the importance of complete and unbiased information.
9. *Pilot the forms and instructions on a small scale.* Revise them if necessary using input from the collectors.
   - Do they work as expected? Are they filled out properly? Do people have differing perceptions of operational definitions? Are they as easy to use as originally perceived?
   - When possible, sit with and observe the people collecting the data.
10. Audit the collection process and validate the results.
    - Randomly check completed forms and occasionally observe data collection during the process: Are data missing? Any unusual values? Is bias being reflected in the data collection process?

## REFERENCES

1. Berwick, Donald M. 1989. "Sounding Board: Continuous Improvement as an Ideal in Health Care." *New England Journal of Medicine* 320 (1): 52–56.
2. Clemmer, Jim. n.d. "Organizational Measurement and Feedback Pathways and Pitfalls (Part One)." www.clemmergroup.com/organizational-measurement-and-feedback-pathways-and-pitfalls-part-one.php.
3. Mills, J.L. 1993. "Data Torturing." *New England Journal of Medicine* 329 (16): 1196–99.
4. Neave, Henry R. 1990. *The Deming Dimension*, 113, 125–26, 151. Knoxville, TN: SPC Press. © 1990. Used by permission of SPC Press. All rights reserved.
5. Balestracci Jr., Davis. 2012. "Wasting Time with Vague Solutions, Part 2: Some Wisdom from Joseph Juran." *Quality Digest*. www.qualitydigest.com/inside/quality-insider-column/wasting-time-vague-solutions-part-2.html.
6. Wiener, Jay. 1998. "Study: Whites May Sway TV Ratings." *Star Tribune* (April 19). www.highbeam.com/doc/1G1-62577964.html.
7. Hacquebord, Heero. 1994. "Health Care from the Perspective of a Patient: Theories for Improvement." *Quality Management in Health Care* 2 (2): 70.
8. Brown, Mark Graham. 1996. *Keeping Score: Using the Right Metrics to Drive World-Class Performance*, 29–37. New York: Quality Resources.
9. Deming, W. Edwards. 1989. "Theory of Variation." Lecture transcript. Institute for Management Sciences, Osaka, Japan (July 24; revised May 1, 1990). www.yumpu.com/en/document/view/22048146/w-edwards-deming-gotas-de-conocimiento/7.

## RESOURCES

Executive Learning. 2002. *Handbook for Improvement: A Reference Guide for Tools and Concepts*, 3rd ed. Brentwood, TN: Healthcare Management Directions.
Joiner, Brian L. 1994. *Fourth Generation Management*. New York: McGraw-Hill.
Scholtes, Peter R., Brian L. Joiner, and Barbara J. Streibel. 2003. *The TEAM Handbook*, 3rd ed. Madison, WI: Joiner/Oriel.

I have written many columns for *Quality Digest* that go into more depth and with some clarifications on the topics in this chapter. For those who are interested in a deeper understanding, the following resources are suggested.

## IMPROVEMENT APPROACH

Balestracci Jr., Davis. 2014. "Can We Please Stop the Guru Wars? The Universal Road Map for Improvement." *Quality Digest* (February 11). www.qualitydigest.com/inside/quality-insider-column/can-we-please-stop-guru-wars.html.
Balestracci Jr., Davis. 2014. "The 'Actual' vs. 'Should' Variation Gap: Nonquantifiable Human Variation Plays a Large Role in This Gap." *Quality Digest* (March 10). www.qualitydigest.com/inside/quality-insider-column/actual-vs-should-variation-gap.html.
Balestracci Jr., Davis. 2014. "Finding Unnecessary and Everyday Variation: The Last Two Sources of Problems." *Quality Digest* (March 19). www.qualitydigest.com/inside/quality-insider-column/finding-unnecessary-and-everyday-variation.html.

### Data Issues

Balestracci Jr., Davis. 2012. "Four Data Processes, Eight Questions, Part 1: Variations on a Theme of Process Inputs." *Quality Digest* (October 11). www.qualitydigest.com/inside/quality-insider-article/four-data-processes-eight-questions-part-1.html.

Balestracci Jr., Davis. 2012. "Four Data Processes, Eight Questions, Part 2: Minimizing Human Variation in Quality Data." *Quality Digest* (October 12). www.qualitydigest.com/inside/quality-insider-article/four-data-processes-eight-questions-part-2.html.

Balestracci Jr., Davis. 2014. "The Universal Process Flowchart × 4: This Tends to Get a Whole Lot of Emotional Interpretation Flowing." *Quality Digest* (April 7). www.qualitydigest.com/inside/quality-insider-column/universal-process-flowchart-4.html.

## Issues of Using Data during Projects and Common Cause Strategies

Balestracci Jr., Davis. 2012. "The Sobering Reality of 'Beginner's Mind': 'It Only Has to Average 100%.'" *Quality Digest* (June 28). www.qualitydigest.com/inside/quality-insider-column/sobering-reality-beginner-s-mind.html.

Balestracci Jr., Davis. 2012. "Wasting Time with Vague Solutions, Part 1: Helping Management Deal with Common Cause." *Quality Digest* (September 14). www.qualitydigest.com/inside/quality-insider-article/wasting-time-vague-solutions-part-1.html.

Balestracci Jr., Davis. 2012. "Wasting Time with Vague Solutions, Part 2: Some Wisdom from Joseph Juran." *Quality Digest* (September 18). www.qualitydigest.com/inside/quality-insider-column/wasting-time-vague-solutions-part-2.html.

Balestracci Jr., Davis. 2012. "Wasting Time with Vague Solutions, Part 3: You've Exhausted In-House Data. Now What?" *Quality Digest* (September 19). www.qualitydigest.com/inside/quality-insider-article/wasting-time-vague-solutions-part-3.html.

Balestracci Jr., Davis. 2012. "Another Strategy for Determining Common Cause: Cut New Windows but Try Not to Upset the Daily Routine." *Quality Digest* (November 5). www.qualitydigest.com/inside/quality-insider-column/another-strategy-determining-common-cause.html.

Balestracci Jr., Davis. 2012. "The Final Common Cause Strategy: 'Statistical Control' (Common Cause Only) is a Major Achievement." *Quality Digest* (December 14). www.qualitydigest.com/inside/quality-insider-column/final-common-cause-strategy.html.

CHAPTER 6

# Process-Oriented Statistics: Studying a Process in Time Sequence

### KEY IDEAS

- Most basic academic statistics requirements are based in a context of *estimation* and teach methods appropriate for research. These, unfortunately, have limited applicability in everyday work, whose need is *prediction*.
- The element of time is a key process input and generally neglected in most academic courses. This affects process data collection, use of statistical tools, and validity of analyses.
- Run charts and control charts must become routine analysis tools.
- Special causes merely indicate different processes at work. Many times the differences are unintended; sometimes they are appropriate and even desirable.
- Knowing how the data were collected is crucial to performing a good analysis.
- The stability and capability of any process being improved must be initially assessed — its actual inherent performance vs. its desired performance. Any goals must be evaluated in the context of this capability, and an appropriate strategy must be developed to deal with gaps and/or lack of stability.
- Decreasing tolerance by patients and families to medical error means that "rare events" will have to be dealt with. The tendency is to use special cause strategies such as root cause, sentinel event, and near-miss analyses. An alternative view and analysis are suggested.

### OLD HABITS DIE HARD

Many people still cannot let go of the myth that statistics can be used to massage data and prove anything. I hope that Chapter 2 began to debunk this myth by demonstrating the counterintuitive simplicity and power of merely plotting the dots — simple time plots of process outputs. These plots usually yield far more profound and productive questions than most complicated alleged statistical analyses. Here is an example that might create déjà vu.

Suppose you have been getting an increasing number of vague anecdotes that cardiac surgery mortality seems to be increasing of late. Not only that, but the organization is not making progress toward attaining a published national benchmark of 3.5 percent. There

EXHIBIT 6.1 ■ Comparison of Three Hospitals' Cardiac Mortality Performance

```
            N   Mean   SE Mean  StDev  Minimum   Q1     Median   Q3      Maximum
Hospital 1  30  5.937  0.514    2.815  0.1       3.600  5.50     8.725   10.7
Hospital 2  30  5.527  0.524    2.870  0.7       4.000  5.60     6.700   12.1
Hospital 3  30  5.853  0.571    3.125  0.0       3.625  5.05     8.725   11.9
```

EXHIBIT 6.2 ■ Comparative Histogram of Three Hospitals' Cardiac Mortality Performance

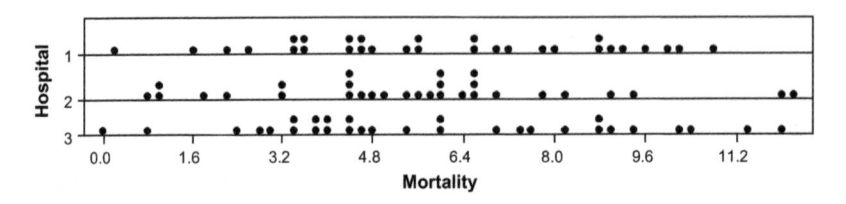

are three hospitals in your system doing this type of surgery and the tabular summary performance data for the last 30 months is shown in Exhibit 6.1.

Luckily, your local statistical guru (LSG) (every organization seems to have one) has come to your rescue, analyzed the data, and written a report, which states:

1. "Pictures are very important. A comparative histogram (Exhibit 6.2) was done to compare the distributions of the mortality rates. At a first glance, there seem to be no differences."

2. "The three data sets were then statistically tested for the assumption of normality. The results (not shown) were that we can assume each to be normally distributed ($p$-values of 0.502, 0.372, and 0.234, respectively, all of which are >0.05); however, we have to be cautious; just because the data pass the test for normality does not necessarily mean that the data are normally distributed. Rather it only means that, under the null hypothesis, the data cannot be proven to be non-normal."

3. "Since the data can be assumed to be normally distributed, I proceeded with the analysis of variance (ANOVA) and generated the 95 percent confidence intervals" (Exhibit 6.3).

4. "The $p$-value of 0.850 is greater than 0.05. Therefore, we can reasonably conclude that there are no statistically significant differences among these hospitals' cardiac mortality rates as further confirmed by the overlapping 95 percent confidence intervals."

5. "Regarding comparison to the national benchmark of 3.5 percent, none of the hospitals are close to meeting it. There will need to be a systemwide intervention at all three hospitals. I recommend that we benchmark an established hospital and copy their best practices systemwide."

## Has All the Potential Jargon Been Used?

Mean, median, standard deviation, normal distribution, histogram, $p$-value, ANOVA, 95 percent confidence interval, null hypothesis, statistical significance, standard error of

## EXHIBIT 6.3 ■ Analysis of Variance and 95 Percent Confidence Intervals

```
One-way Analysis of Variance (ANOVA)
Source  DF      SS     MS     F      P
Hosp     2    2.82   1.41  0.16  0.850
Error   87  751.90   8.64
Total   89  754.72

S = 2.940

                         Individual 95% CIs For Mean Based on Pooled StDev
Hospital  N   Mean  StDev  ------+---------+---------+---------+---
   1     30  5.937  2.815              (--------------*--------------)
   2     30  5.527  2.870  (--------------*--------------)
   3     30  5.853  3.125        (--------------*--------------)
                           ------+---------+---------+---------+---
                              4.90      5.60      6.30      7.00

Pooled StDev = 2.940
```

the mean, F-test, degrees of freedom, and benchmark: This LSG's analysis is totally worthless. Like my mother said to me after hearing me give a seminar, "Oh! You certainly *sound* like you know what you are talking about."

Three questions should become a part of every quality professional's vocabulary whenever faced with a set of data for the first time:

1. How were these data defined and collected and were they collected specifically for the current purpose?
2. Were the processes that produced these data *stable*?
3. Were the analyses *appropriate* given the way the data were collected and the stability state of the processes?

*How were these data collected?* The table was a descriptive statistical summary of the 30 previous months of cardiac mortality rates for three hospitals. These hospitals all subscribed and fed into the same computerized data collection process, so at least the definitions are consistent. From Chapter 5's discussion about operational definitions, it would still be nice to know how this mortality number is calculated, especially if being compared to other benchmarks whose definitions could differ.

*Were the systems that produced these data stable?* This might be a new question for you. As previously mentioned, *everything* is a process. All processes occur over time. Hence, *all data* have an implicit "time order" element to them that allows assessment of the stability of the system producing the data.

Therefore it is always a good idea as an initial analysis to *plot the data in its naturally occurring time order* to formally assess the process stability; the LSG did not do this. Otherwise, as you will see, many common statistical techniques could be rendered invalid. This puts one at risk for taking inappropriate actions.

*Were the analyses appropriate, given the way the data were collected and the stability state of the processes?* "But," you say, "the data passed the normal distribution test. Isn't that all you need to know to proceed with the standard statistical analysis?" And your LSG also concluded that there were no statistically significant differences among the hospitals' mortality rates.

## No Difference?

Exhibit 6.4 shows the three simple time plots for the individual hospitals. The individual median of each hospital's 30 data points has been added as a reference line. As discussed in Chapter 2, these are known as *run charts*.

Note that just by plotting the dots, you have far more insight. This insight will result in the ability to ask more incisive questions, whose answers will lead to more productive system improvements.

Compare this to analysis outputs typically encountered, such as bar graphs, pages of summary tables, and the sophisticated statistical analyses full of jargon. From your experience, what questions do people ask from those? Are they generally even helpful?

Unfortunately, healthcare workers are very smart people. They will, *with the best of intentions*, come up with theories and actions that could unwittingly *harm* a system. Or, worse yet, they might do nothing because they see no statistical differences among the systems. Or they might decide that they need more data. There will be variation in how a roomful of people perceives and wants to act on variation.

Regarding common computer-generated statistics, what do the averages of Hospital 1 and Hospital 2 in Exhibit 6.4 mean? "If I stick my right foot in a bucket of boiling water and my left foot in a bucket of ice water, on the average, I'm pretty comfortable." That is, it is inappropriate to calculate averages, standard deviations, and so forth on unstable processes such as these.

The appropriate answer to the question, "What is the average of Hospital 2?" is "When?" Over the time period of the data collection, Hospital 2 had three distinct averages. What can you *predict* about future performance?

If prediction of future mortality were the objective presented to prospective payers, the time order of the data becomes important. Looking at these plots, would you reach the same conclusion as the LSG's analysis — no difference among the three mortality rates? Hospital 1 increases during the entire time period and Hospital 2 is subject to abrupt shifts. Hospital 3, while highly variable, appears to be stable over time.

Typical summary stats, for example, average or standard deviation, are inappropriate for the processes from Hospitals 1 and 2. The process from Hospital 3 is stable and can be summarized in its current form. That does not mean it is necessarily the most desirable process, only that its current performance can be somewhat accurately assessed.

Suppose these were presented in a table as three numbers — one-point summaries — along with other such summaries of other key performance indicators? Would you prefer to make a decision with the one-point summaries or the plots of monthly results? Which type of summary allows the most appropriate follow-up actions?

It is a much higher yield strategy, after observing the time plots, to *ask questions*, especially about Hospitals 1 and 2. The nature of the plots would even result in different types of questions:

- What changes occurred during this time?
- Have any beneficial gains been made and held?
- Is Hospital 3 even capable of achieving desired goals consistently?
- What is different about their individual processes and practice environments?
- What is different about their results?

Additional data will be needed to answer these questions.

Rather than relying on single-number summaries of huge, aggregated, random samples, the goal in this type of analysis is to ensure predictive stability by using smaller

# EXHIBIT 6.4  Run Charts of Three Hospitals' Cardiac Mortality Data

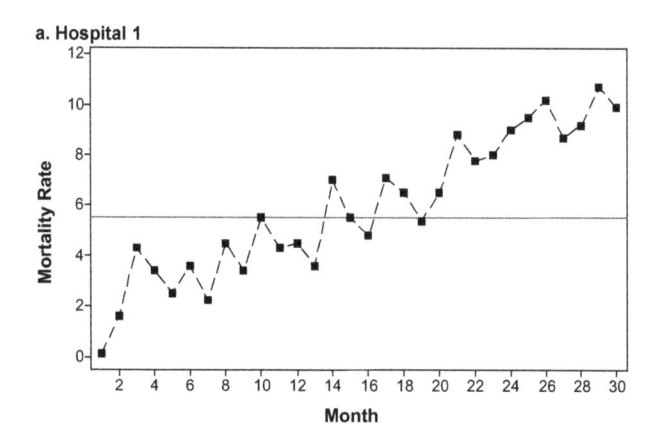

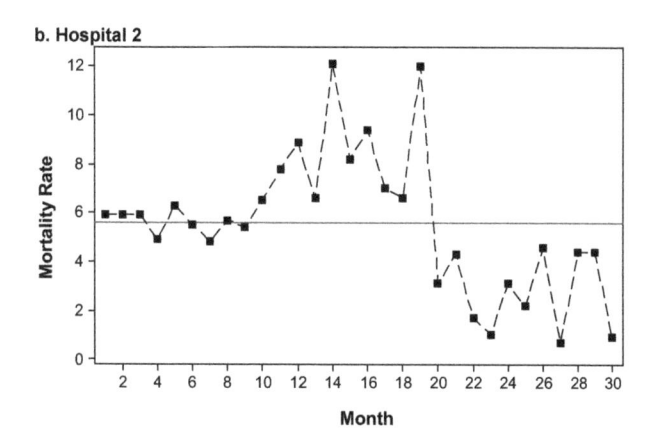

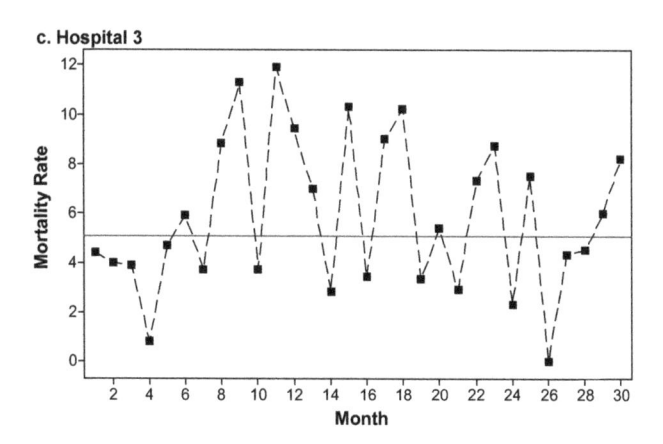

### a. Hospital 1

### b. Hospital 2

### c. Hospital 3

*Note:* If you see no difference, then plot the dots.

samples taken more frequently over time. Ignoring the time element implicit in every data set can lead to incorrect statistical conclusions. Applications of the usual descriptive summary statistics (e.g., averages, standard deviations) to an unstable process are invalid.

This introduces the concept of *analytic statistics* (process oriented, with the goal of prediction of future process results) vs. *enumerative statistics* (summary oriented, with the goal of accurate estimation of current state). The latter are generally taught in most basic statistical requirements, yet they have limited applicability in a quality improvement context where unstable processes are the rule and not the exception. And it is only analytic statistics that can expose and deal appropriately with the variation causing the process "instability"; the enumerative framework virtually ignores its presence. This will be discussed extensively in the "Statistics and Reality: The Inference Gap" section.

Note that the ultimate conclusion reached by the LSG was that one would need to "benchmark" a "cutting edge" hospital's result and copy the "best practices" discovered. However, in looking at Hospital 2, one sees two distinct shifts in the data and a current performance averaging around 2.3 percent.

There might be no need to benchmark an outside organization, which is always fraught with asking appropriate questions then encountering "not invented here" upon your return. What if one could study aspects of Hospital 2's process, determine the reasons for the shifts, and implement appropriate process changes made more recently systemwide?

Or are differences because Hospital 1 acquired some state-of-the-art cardiac technology and was now where the other two hospitals sent more complicated cases? In which case, maybe that might appropriately explain Hospital 2's recent drop in mortality.

But wait a minute, if Hospital 3 was doing that as well, why did we not observe a corresponding drop in its mortality?

- Could Hospital 3 learn some things from Hospital 2?
- Or is it that they are not appropriately referring difficult cases to Hospital 1?

Asking questions like these is a more rational, appropriate solution than implementing a systemwide redesign based on copying best practices from somewhere else. That is, assuming that the benchmarking process deciding whom to copy was even carried out appropriately.

Again, plot the dots.

The statistics needed for improvement are far easier than ever imagined. However, this philosophy in which to use them — statistical thinking — will initially be quite counterintuitive to most of you and even more counterintuitive to the people you work with.

If nothing else, it will at least make your jobs easier by freeing up a lot of time recognizing when to walk out of time-wasting meetings. It will also help you gain the cultural respect you deserve as quality professionals because your data collections and analyses will be simpler, more efficient, and ultimately more effective. The respect will also be magnified because of your ability to recognize and stop inappropriate responses to variation, that is, well-meaning current responses that make people's jobs more complicated and time-consuming without adding any value to the organization.

## More on Plotting the Dots: Common and Special Causes

Almost all quality experts agree that merely plotting a process's output over time is one of the most simple, elegant, and awesome tools for gaining deep understanding of any situation. Before plotting, one must ask questions, clarify objectives, contemplate action, and review current use of the data. Questioning from this statistical thinking perspective leads immediately to unexpected deeper understanding of the process. The end results will be valuable baselines for key processes and honest dialogue to determine meaningful goals and action.

Contrast this approach to the more typical one of imposing arbitrary numerical goals of desired performance. These are then retrofitted onto the process and enforced by exhortation that treats *any* deviation of process performance from the goal as unique and needing explanation, which is known as a *special cause* strategy.

To paraphrase the question previously used for individual undesirable events, in the context of observing a process over time, is this an isolated excessive deviation (special cause), or, when compared to the previous measurement of the same situation, does it merely reflect the effects of ongoing actions of process inputs that have *always* been present and cannot be predicted ahead of time (common cause)? Would I necessarily expect the same number the next time I measure? If not, then how much difference from the current or previous number is "too much"?

It is very important to realize that just because one can explain an occurrence after the fact does not mean that it was a unique special cause. Thinking in terms of process, there are inputs causing variation that are *always* present and conspire in *random* ways to affect a process's output. The result will not always necessarily be the same number. As will be shown, these random variations will always yield a result within a predictable *range* of possible outputs.

Many explanations merely point out things that have been *waiting* to happen, and then they happened. And they no doubt will happen again at some random time in the future. But your process tends to "prefer" some of these "bogeys" to others. So how can you collect data to discover these and minimize or even eliminate their hidden, ongoing influence (common cause strategy, which was demonstrated beautifully by the accident data summaries in Chapters 2 and 5)?

- If a process fluctuates within a relatively fixed range of variation, it is said to display *common cause variation* — stable and predictable — although one may not necessarily like the results (in the hospital example, Hospital 3's output showed common cause).
- If there is evidence of variation *over and above* what seems to be inherent, the process is said to exhibit *special cause variation* (in the hospital example, Hospital 1 showed a trend and, as discussed, Hospital 2 had two distinct shifts in its process). This usually occurs in one of two ways, either:
  - As isolated single data points that are totally out of character in the context of the other data points, indicating that another process temporarily intervened in normal operation; or
  - As a distinct shift (or shifts) in the process level caused by outside interventions (intentional or unintentional) that have now become part of the everyday process inputs.

As already discussed, the most common error in improvement efforts is to treat common cause (inherent) variation as if it were special cause (unique) variation, which W. Edwards Deming defined as *tampering*. Tampering will generally add more complexity to a process without any value. In other words, *despite the best of intentions*, the improvement effort has actually added complexity and made things worse, certainly no better.

And note that the summary statistics have serious potential to treat special cause as if it were common cause. For example, after looking at their plots, the only way to summarize the data of Hospitals 1 and 2 is by asking questions.

## STATISTICS AND REALITY: THE INFERENCE GAP

As stated earlier, there are two types of statistical study — enumerative and analytic. Enumerative study asks the question: What can I say about this *specific group's* results? Analytic study asks: What can I say about the *process* that produced *both* this specific group itself in addition to this specific group's results? Analytic study provides you with the opportunity to acquire judgment or knowledge of the subject, to look beyond the calculations. The actions taken to obtain more information increase your understanding of the sources of uncertainty and how to reduce it. Analytic statistics should also incorporate the realization that processes, events, and people are not static and can vary over time.

Think of it this way: Enumerative study envisions your organization as a stagnant pond. If you take enough data, you will eventually understand it.

Analytic study envisions your organization as a whitewater rapids, never stagnant. How do you even begin to understand it? How and where do you sample it? And even if you sample in the same place, how does your current sample compare to previous samples?

With analytic studies, there are two distinct sources of uncertainty:

1. Uncertainty due to sampling, just as in an enumerative study. This can be expressed numerically by standard statistical theory.
2. Uncertainty because we're predicting what will happen at some time in the future to some group that's different from our original sample. This uncertainty is "unknown and unknowable." We rarely know how the results we produce will be used, so all we can do is to warn the potential user of the range of uncertainties that will affect different actions.

Unfortunately, the latter uncertainty will often be much greater than the uncertainty due to sampling and may leave us with an uncomfortable feeling rather than the tidy solution for which we had hoped.

These are concepts that are crucial to understand before continuing: It is not just a matter of generating statistics and charts, but using the charts to ask intelligent questions and, something else not taught in academic courses, bridging the "inference gap."

### Objectives and Methods: Five Scenarios

As repeatedly emphasized, "What is your objective?" should always be the first question regarding any data. This will help determine which statistical and analytical methods are needed.

- **Objective 1:** Describe accurately the state of things at one point in time and place.
  *Method*: Define precisely the population to be studied and use very exact random sampling (inherent emphasis of most academic statistics courses).
- **Objective 2:** Discover problems and possibilities to form a new theory.
  *Method*: Look for interesting groups, where new ideas will be obvious. These may be focus groups, rather than random samples. The accuracy and rigor required in the first case is wasted. But this assumes that the possibilities discovered will be tested by other means, before making any prediction.

- **Objective 3:** Predict the future to test a general theory.
  *Method*: Study extreme and atypical samples with great rigor and accuracy.
- **Objective 4:** Predict the future to help management.
  *Method*: Get samples as close as possible to the foreseeable range of circumstances in which the prediction will be used in practice.
- **Objective 5:** Change the future to make it more predictable.
  *Method*: Use statistical process control to remove special causes and experiment using the plan-do-study-act cycle to reduce common cause variation.

Objective 1 is enumerative; all the rest are analytic. Have any of your past statistics textbooks or courses made these obviously necessary distinctions? If not, despite all classic textbook rigor, statistical studies can be virtually useless. Many studies are not well fitted to any one aim, which is a real-world issue. See my 2009 articles called "The Wisdom of David Kerridge" parts 1 and 2 in Resources for a deeper evaluation of enumerative vs. analytic statistical studies.

## DEEPER ISSUES OF COLLECTING DATA OVER TIME

The processes we are trying to improve function continuously. The factor of time becomes a major consideration in the data planning and collection. Therefore we use process-oriented statistics (analytic statistics) to assess the ongoing, continuous processes that produce any summary snapshots. The process-oriented framework asks:

- Because these data reflect the process frozen at one moment in time, is it a typical snapshot?
- How does this snapshot relate to previous summaries? Is the process that produced the current data set the same as the process that produced previous data sets?
- What are the significant sources of variation?
- Do people agree on how these numbers should be measured?
- What can be predicted from these data?
- What would we like to predict with these data?

The primary initial objective is assessment of the stability of the process producing the data. The obsessive accuracy of the number (estimation) is not an issue; variation is considered only a nuisance clouding whether an intervention is necessary. If the process is statistically stable, one can assess its current performance and take action either to predict future performance or to measure the effects of an improvement intervention.

The typical (erroneous) assumption made in most academic courses is that any data are frozen random samples with no time identity from an underlying stable population. Testing of process stability is, in fact, not an objective and a foreign concept. The order in which the data are collected is typically ignored and not a consideration (as demonstrated by the inappropriate analysis of the cardiac mortality data).

Think of the U.S. Census: Ideally, one would like to fix the population at one moment in time and count it. However, because of ongoing births, deaths, immigration, and so forth, the number changes minute to minute. The process one uses to decide on the actual final number (enumerative) is a much different process from analyzing how the number is changing to predict it in the future (analytic).

Whenever presented with a data summary, one should ask:

- What was the objective of these data?
- How were these data defined and collected?

EXHIBIT 6.5 ■ Run Chart of Coin Flip Data

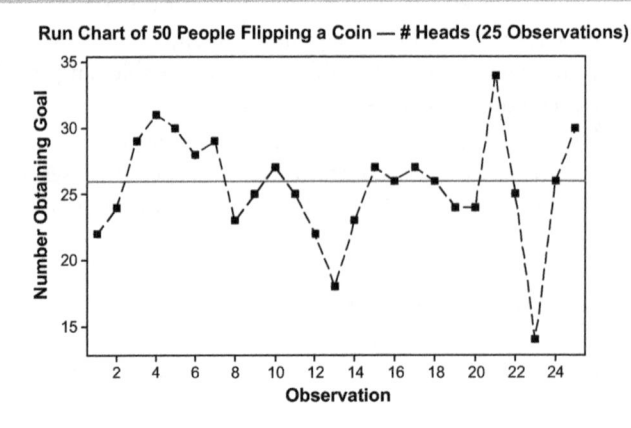

*Run Chart of 50 People Flipping a Coin — # Heads (25 Observations)*

- Is the process that produced this data stable?
- What action is being contemplated?

A good rule of thumb is to ask whether the decision being made from a statistical summary is the same as the one that would be made by looking at a time plot of the data.

## More on Common and Special Causes

### All Processes Vary

There is an inherent common cause variation present to some degree in all processes. If common causes are exclusively present, the numerical outputs will differ for multiple reasons. Looking at a run chart will discern no pattern in the data and the variation will appear to be random.

For example, consider the process of flipping coins and counting the number of heads. Suppose 50 people in a room each have a coin. At a signal, they simultaneously flip them and the resulting number of people getting heads is recorded. Twenty-five randomly generated possibilities for this process are plotted in Exhibit 6.5.

Instinctively, one feels that the number should be 25. However, when the process is repeated, successive flips do not yield exactly 25 every time. It can be shown statistically that the number of heads would usually be between 18 and 32 and occasionally could even extend as far as either 14 or 36.

### Sometimes There Is a Reason for the Variation

Another type of variation comes from outside the process, resulting in noticeable shifts or even occasional outliers. This type of variation is called *special cause*. For example, in the cardiac mortality data, a special cause is acting on Hospital 1 and causing its output to steadily increase. Special causes entered Hospital 2's process after observations 11 and 20, causing the output to shift. Hospital 3 showed no signs of special causes.

Returning to the coin flipping example, suppose a special cause enters via a process change. People are now told to flip their coins *twice* and only those obtaining heads on

EXHIBIT 6.6 ■ Plot of Coin Flip Data before and after Process Change

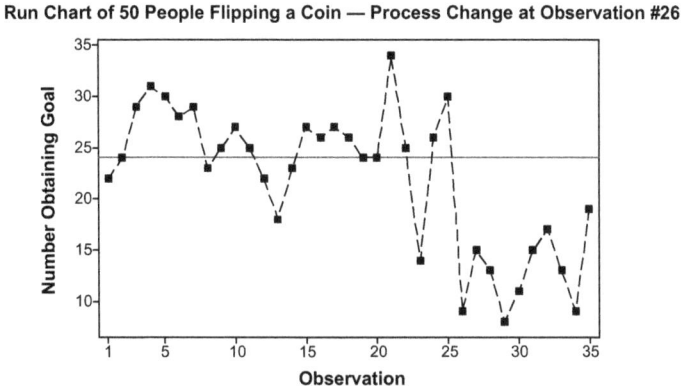

**Run Chart of 50 People Flipping a Coin — Process Change at Observation #26**

*both flips* will be tallied. Ten observations for this process have been appended onto the previous 25 observations and plotted in Exhibit 6.6.

A system of 50 people flipping a coin twice will experience "double heads" in the range of approximately 4 to 21. How long would it take for an observer of the data to detect the change? Note that this range (4–21) overlaps the range of the previous process (14–36), but, despite that, the change in the process "needle" is quite obvious in the run chart. It is further confirmed by the fact that the last 10 observations in a row are below the median, violating the special cause rule previously shown in Exhibit 2.6.

The application of simple statistical theory allows identification, interpretation, and utilization of appropriate strategies for handling each variation type. It also showed how the presence of only common causes makes the process predictable within well-defined limits. That said, it is impossible to predict where any specific individual result will lie within those limits. In addition, the limits may or may not be acceptable to one's preconceived desires.

Special causes may occur randomly in a process to make a process virtually unpredictable at any future time period. In addition, one can design studies whose purpose is to create beneficial special causes to improve a process, that is, the intention is to "move the needle."

Understanding the difference between common and special causes is crucial to statistical thinking. The strategy for improvement is very different for processes with special causes than it is for processes with only common causes of variation.

## More Déjà Vu?

In addition to the six types of process inputs (people, machines, methods, materials, measurements, and environment), there is one other major consideration when characterizing a process: time. Its presence affects process analysis, data collection, and the use of statistical methods. Every process occurs over time.

It is a common practice and seemingly part of human nature to treat the difference between two consecutive numbers as a two-point trend or a special cause. The implication is that two different processes produced the different numbers.

A partial list of two-point trends in my experience includes:
- Monthly sales;
- Unit costs;
- Quarterly reports;
- Weekly production reports;
- Annual financial reports; and
- Monthly absenteeism.

This practice is evident in questions such as:
- Utilization is up 8 percent from last month. What are you doing about it?
- Enrollment is down 4 percent from last year. What are you doing about it?

Managers demand explanations as to why current results differ from previous results. "Bad" results are punished. Attempts are made to motivate workers with rewards for achieving good results. Sometimes goals are stretched even further after good results are received.

As I have discussed, bar graphs, trend lines, reports in rows-and-columns format, and traffic light presentations are common, but they are usually deceptive ways to display data. There is also the tendency to look for trends by comparing the current result to the previous one, then comparing it to the result during the same time period of the previous year.

As shown in Chapter 2, a sequence of three different numbers can manifest in six different ways, with each having a special cause term to explain it: *upward trend, downward trend, setback, rebound, downturn,* and *turnaround*. And many times the discussion is further supplemented by aggregated year-to-date summaries with the variances from previous reports and corporate goals.

Consecutive numbers will almost always differ from each other. If the variation is due to common causes, it is of little value to attempt to explain the individual differences from point to point. Yes, the numbers are different, but what if they were all produced by the same process? What are the consequences of attributing a special cause to the observed variation? How would the action differ if it were considered common cause? With only three data points and no context of variation, it is actually quite difficult to analyze a situation.

Three questions people should consider about such data presentations are:
1. In a "this month/last month/12-months ago" display, why are the 10 in-between months ignored? (A common explanation is "seasonality.")
2. Why is January (or first month of a fiscal year) used as an essentially arbitrary cutoff point for previous data? This approach makes the previous year virtually cease to exist except for year-to-date summaries vis-à-vis the current month.
3. Why does multiple-year data presentation seem to be exclusively via bar graphs with all the Januaries together, all the Februaries together, and so forth? It implies no continuity between December of one year and January of the next year.

It is also a common practice to display only the last 12 months, at most, of either the actual data or an ongoing 12-month rolling average. Why?

On what theory are these analyses based? Right or wrong, any display and analysis of data has an inherent theory. The theory usually reflects the displayer's bias toward a particular special cause interpretation or "mental model," that is, belief system, about a situation. Unfortunately, many are arbitrary and based on intuition.

My mentor, Dr. Rodney Dueck, told me about a financial person who expressed concern to him, "We can't use Davis's methods. There's too much variation in our data, so they're not useful," to which Rodney replied, "And that is precisely the reason we should use Davis's methods." The argument fell on deaf ears. Pretending that the variation is not there does not make it go away, and many people have made a career interpreting such variation.

## A Perspective of Statistical Theory

Variation in time is unique and different from aggregated variation. The difference results from both the lack of recognition of the time factor and the implicit mixture of the six process inputs (people, methods, machines, materials, measurements, environment). Further confusion results when one realizes that each input stream also occurs (and varies) in time.

Studying variation over time is like using time-lapse photography on a process. All processes have common cause variation, but any process also has the potential to be affected by special causes. Processes exhibiting no special causes can for the moment be considered statistically stable.

Stability in time of process inputs and outputs is essential if you want to predict the process outputs. Using a time-lapse outdoor photography analogy, in the short term, some small details of each sequential picture will vary. These are analogous to common cause variation. However, as the photos continue, in some climates, one will definitely see a seasonal effect, especially winter, indicating predictable special cause. Then, unpredictably, other special causes will occasionally manifest as new road construction (as opposed to predictable post-winter road repair), a building knocked down, a shopping mall built, a new housing development on former farmland, and so forth, most definitely changing the process.

Studying any process in time is crucial to:
- Assess current process performance;
- Establish a baseline for improvement efforts;
- Assess improvement efforts;
- Predict future performance; and
- Ensure that improvement gains are held.

The following cannot be overemphasized: Ignoring the inherent time element in any process data can lead to incorrect statistical conclusions, treating common cause as if it was special cause and vice versa.

Suppose the envelope thickness exercise described in Chapter 5 was repeated, with either the same audience or a different audience. Would the numbers be different from Exhibit 5.8? Of course they would. Would the outcomes depend on whether objectives and a measurement process were discussed? Not necessarily. What could be said about the process that produced these new measurements? Is it the same? Has it improved? How would you know? How would you compare the different audiences' performances?

As repeatedly emphasized, statistical analysis of a process should always begin, whenever possible, with a plot of the data in the time order in which it was produced. By analyzing patterns in the plot, two important questions can be answered:

1. Did these data come from a stable process?
2. If the process is stable, how much variation is naturally inherent in it?

Again, the cornerstone concept in quality improvement, which is understanding the distinction between common and special causes of variation in a process, aids in formulating an appropriate response to a given situation.

Instead of asking the obvious question, "Is the current data point different than the previous data point?" when comparing two points in time, ask the key question: "Is the *process* that produced this current data point the same as the *process* that produced the previous data point?"

This is a deeper, more fundamental question that radically affects one's approach toward process improvement. Using statistical theory to interpret a situation correctly and answer this question minimizes the probability of inappropriate action.

### Common vs. Special Cause in a Time Perspective

The output over time from a common cause process represents the aggregated effect of a consistently present set of forces. These forces are inherent in the process and act on it in a seemingly random manner. Think of the individual differences of one's consecutive bowling scores, golf scores, car gas mileage, amounts spent at the supermarket, times to get to work. They are not exactly the same. One's natural obvious reply is, "Of course, they are not."

People sometimes feel that because they can explain the specific reasons for individual ups and downs of common cause processes after they occur, these are indeed special causes. However, the ability to explain a change after the fact does not make it a special cause.

### Something to Which We Can All Relate

I think back to living in Minnesota and its infamous winters. If I had plotted my winter commute times, I have no doubt that I could look at a particularly long time and say "snowstorm." Is a snowstorm necessarily a special cause in the winter? Using a common cause strategy (for winter times), I am sure it would be one random result in a consistent pattern of high commute times, that is, *every* high value corresponds to a snowstorm. To a certain extent, this helps me predict. Perhaps I cannot predict *when* a snowstorm will occur, but if we have one, I can predict that my commute time will most definitely increase by a certain amount unless I change the process by leaving work early and avoiding rush hour.

In addition, I am also willing to bet that my overall process needle predictably rose during the winter (seasonality) and, since snowstorms were not predictable, the *overall variation* in my commute times probably also increased as well.

To continue the commute analogy, an accident on a heavily traveled Twin Cities highway guaranteed a long commute and, after which, was very easy to explain. In the mid-1970s that was a special cause. As traffic flow increased over the 20 years I lived there, however, an accident during rush hour was no longer a special cause. Because of their increasing frequency, accidents are no longer a special cause, but have become common cause and are part of the process. Their unpredictability would increase my average commute time, as would its variation. There was always a consequential probability that there will indeed be an accident during rush hour.

### It's Always Something

There are many sources of common cause variation. No one can predict in advance which particular sources will affect the process at any given time. It is only certain that *some* will.

Because common causes are consistently present in a process, it is reasonable to ask, "What range of variation do they naturally impose on the process output?" Each source of common cause contributes a random, small amount of variation, and all of these sources aggregate into the output. The individual data points are not and never will be totally predictable.

When studied over time, however, the *range* of the resulting process outputs can be predicted. As in the coin flip example, one can determine maximum and minimum values that the stable process outputs will almost never exceed.

Most of the time, when the output stays within this range, it is indicative that the common cause forces have not changed. In fact, this inherent common cause is the standard measurement that determines when any observed variation is excessive, indicating a possible special cause at work.

As will be shown later in this chapter in the section "Some Other Helpful Special Cause Rules," data patterns can also be interpreted in this common cause context to postulate the presence of special causes even when all of the data stay within the limits.

When variation is excessive and attributable to forces that are not typically part of the process, it is special cause variation.

### Hidden Special Causes

There is a common misconception that a process whose plotted output exhibits only common cause variation can be improved only through radical redesign. This is inaccurate and several examples are shown to demonstrate hidden opportunity to improve a process.

*Common cause just means that the data points cannot be treated and reacted to individually.* There may still be hidden special causes present, and they are special because their effects only seem random. They actually have an underlying pattern of predictability which, if discovered, are opportunities that can be dealt with.

The set of observations can now be considered *in their aggregate* because they were all produced by the same process. The power of aggregation and the clever utilization of the strategies of stratification and disaggregation discussed in Chapter 5 will force the process to expose the hidden, underlying, consistent patterns that on a first glance only seem random. This was discussed in the accident data, medication error data, and percent conformance data examples in Chapter 2 and the commute scenarios discussed earlier in this chapter.

### A Service Culture Analogy

A service culture environment such as healthcare presents a challenge and additional opportunity. The discussion in the previous section most definitely applies to the daily data encountered by the culture. The deeper challenge in a service environment for thinking about process is to look at *every* interaction creating a service as an opportunity for something to go either "right" ($x = 1$) or "wrong" ($x = 0$). Restaurant experiences are good examples as well, both in terms of quality of the food and the service.

The random sources of variation, in addition to those in the underlying work process, are the specific endpoints of *every* human interaction involved. Was the end result appropriately delivered to the next internal customer (or patient) or not? It is the aggregated effect of this series of complicated interactions, each of which went either right or wrong, which produce the ultimate end result. And some of these interactions are more problematic than others.

Think about Berwick's questions from Chapter 1 (p. 4): What range of undesirable experiences do these experiences create for workers or customers? How come one time things go smoothly (for workers and/or customers), yet other times it's the "visit from hell" (everything that can go wrong does go wrong)?

Many workers' and customers' experiences are not, and never will be, totally predictable. However, to achieve the goal of creating a culture where the perfect experience is achieved as close to 100 percent as possible one could:

- Tally occurrences of breakdowns;
- Ask, "What is the current percent performance level?";
- Look at the gap from 100 percent as variation;
- Study the patterns of variation in occurrence patterns; and
- Reduce the potential inappropriate and unintended variation in the gap through the appropriate special cause and common cause strategies.

In a service environment, in addition to everyday numerical data, there are data potentially available to be recorded as counts of events that interacted to produce occurrences of process breakdowns. And these counts can be plotted over time to observe the process variation.

### Daily Incoming Medical Information Calls

This example describes one practice's experience with data intended to monitor incoming medical information (MI) calls. Many medical centers have purchased expensive telephone and software systems to try to manage phone usage and staffing. It is not unusual for data from these systems to be presented in a table format with averages, summaries, and other statistics aggregated in a typical rows-and-columns format and compared to performance goals. When common and special causes are not understood, management frequently circles high and low numbers and demands explanations about apparent changes in productivity. These numbers are frequently used to change staffing levels. Incorrect data collection or analysis could result in overstaffing, understaffing, or an inappropriate staffing mix.

For this example, five months of phone data were aggregated and statistically summarized (Exhibit 6.7). The objective was to gain insights into the number of MI calls received. Because the data were collected daily, one obvious potential theory was that phone calls varied by day of the week, which was a possible underlying special cause. A stratification, shown in Exhibit 6.8 using the daily average and shown as a deviation from the five-day average, reveals this to be a viable theory.

Exhibit 6.9 shows a special kind of time plot, known as a *control chart*, for Tuesday's call pattern. This particular type of control chart is also known as a *control chart for individuals* or an *I-chart* or *X-MR chart*. (Because of bad connotations associated with the word "control," Dr. Donald Wheeler coined the term *process behavior chart*.) An I-chart shows data plotted in their natural time order with three horizontal lines superimposed. As explained in Chapter 2, these lines show the average and expected natural limits of the common cause variation inherent in the process performance. These limits are easily calculated entirely *from the data*: They have nothing to do with either a desired range of values or arbitrary numerical goals that would be considered respectable to achieve. An example of this calculation is shown in Appendix 2A, but the calculation and interpretation of the limits will be discussed in more detail later in this chapter.

EXHIBIT 6.7 ■ Medical Information Telephone Data

| Hourly Calculations Box for ABC Shift 9:00 - 19:00 | | | | | | | | | |
|---|---|---|---|---|---|---|---|---|---|
| HOUR | AGENTS WORKING | TOTAL RECEIVED | TOTAL ANSWERED | TOTAL ABANDONED | PERCENT ANSWERED | AVG TIME BEFORE ANSWER | PERCENT ANSWERED IN 60 SECS | # OF CALLS ANSWERED IN 60 SECS | ADJUSTED % ANSWERED IN 60 SECS |
| 9:00-10:00 | 5 | 68 | 60 | 8 | 88% | 20 | 95% | 57 | 83% |
| Month Ave | 6.3 | 85.9 | 80.1 | 5.9 | 93.1% | 20.7 | 93.3% | 74.7 | 86.9% |
| 10:00-11:00 | 4 | 65 | 60 | 5 | 92% | 30 | 90% | 54 | 83% |
| Month Ave | 6.3 | 82.9 | 75.5 | 7.4 | 91.1% | 26.1 | 88.2% | 66.6 | 80.3% |
| 11:00-12:00 | 4 | 57 | 56 | 1 | 98% | 14 | 98% | 54 | 94% |
| Month Ave | 5.4 | 68.7 | 64.7 | 4.09 | 4.2% | 18.6 | 94.7% | 61.3 | 89.2% |
| 12:00-13:00 | 2 | 38 | 33 | 5 | 86% | 16 | 97% | 32 | 84% |
| Month Ave | 3.8 | 61.9 | 55.9 | 6.0 | 90.3% | 19.9 | 93.6% | 52.3 | 84.5% |
| 13:00-14:00 | 4 | 55 | 52 | 3 | 94% | 25 | 90% | 46 | 83% |
| Month Ave | 4.9 | 62.6 | 55.7 | 6.9 | 89.0% | 25.6 | 90.6% | 50.5 | 80.6% |
| 14:00-15:00 | 4 | 40 | 39 | 1 | 97% | 10 | 100% | 39 | 97% |
| Month Ave | 5.2 | 58.4 | 51.7 | 6.7 | 88.5% | 24.8 | 88.2% | 45.6 | 78.1% |
| 15:00-16:00 | 3 | 39 | 34 | 5 | 87% | 27 | 82% | 27 | 69% |
| Month Ave | 3.7 | 42.5 | 37.2 | 5.3 | 87.5% | 22.3 | 88.8% | 33.0 | 77.7% |
| 16:00-17:00 | 3 | 15 | 11 | 4 | 73% | 15 | 91% | 10 | 66% |
| Month Ave | 3.3 | 24.8 | 19.6 | 5.2 | 79.2 | 20.7 | 90.3% | 17.7 | 71.5% |
| 17:00-18:00 | 1 | 8 | 8 | 0 | 100% | 28 | 88% | 7 | 87% |
| Month Ave | 0.8 | 10.4 | 7.1 | 3.3 | 68.3% | 30.0 | 80.3% | 5.7 | 54.8% |
| 18:00-19:00 | 1 | 3 | 3 | 0 | 100% | 25 | 67% | 2 | 66% |
| Month Ave | 0.8 | 5.3 | 3.9 | 1.4 | 74.3% | 24.1 | 85.9% | 3.4 | 63.8% |
| DAY TOTAL | 31 | 388 | 356 | 32 | | | | 328 | |
| HOUR AVG | 3.1 | 38.8 | 35.6 | 3.2 | 91.8% | 20.7 | 92.1% | 32.8 | 84.5% |
| FM DAY AVG | 40 | 503 | 451 | 51 | | | | 410 | |
| FM HOUR AVG | 4.0 | 50.3 | 45.1 | 5.2 | 89.7% | 22.6 | 91.9% | 41.1 | 81.6% |

*When presented in a tabular format, the data and "stats" provide little insight into the process. Even labels can be confusing!*

EXHIBIT 6.8 ■ Stratification of Medical Information Data by Day of the Week

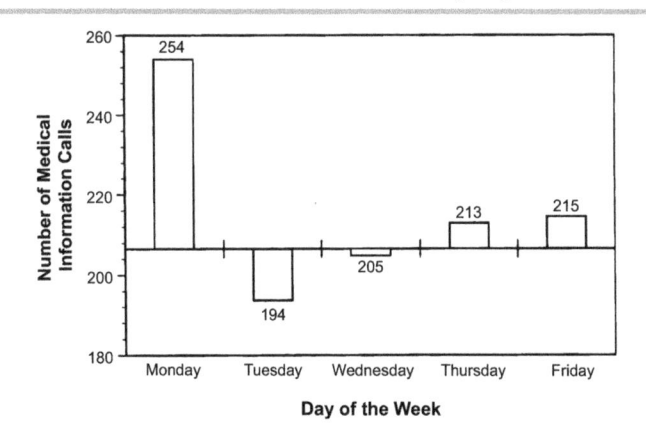

Number of Medical Information Calls by Day of the Week:
- Monday: 254
- Tuesday: 194
- Wednesday: 205
- Thursday: 213
- Friday: 215

*Note:* Three systems exist in the medical information phone call process. A stratification and further statistical analysis (discussed in Chapter 10) shows that (1) Wednesdays through Fridays represent one system; (2) due to its higher average, Mondays are in another system; and (3) due to its lower average, Tuesdays are in yet a third system.

**EXHIBIT 6.9** ■ Control Chart for Tuesday Medical Information Phone Data

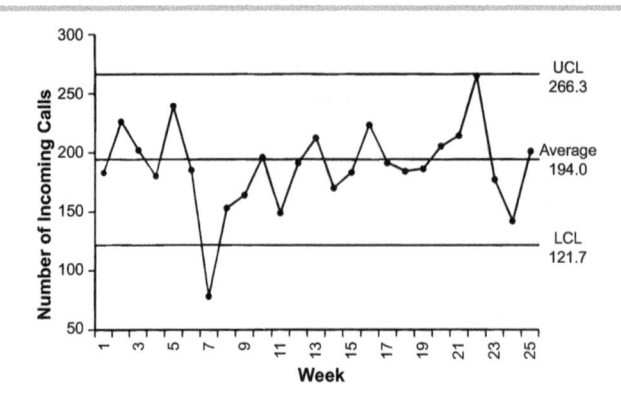

*Note:* The average for the Tuesday medical information process is 194 calls with common cause variation of ±72 calls. This means that while the Tuesday average is 194 calls, on any given Tuesday, the clinic could expect between 122 and 266 calls.

Note that the seventh point in Exhibit 6.9 lies below the lower horizontal limit. This signifies a special cause unique to that point only. Given the normal course of events, a value this low would not be expected. Investigation showed this to be December 24, Christmas Eve day. Is this a reasonable explanation? One would think so. Then does it also seem reasonable that this date should be excluded from the calculation of the average for a typical Tuesday?

Yet, overall daily averages for months are routinely reported. With all the special causes in this process (day of the week, Christmas Eve day), what does that average mean? Can that average help people determine staffing requirements? If the average is taken at face value, it is similar to the example given earlier in this chapter where a person should allegedly be comfortable though standing with one foot in boiling water and the other in ice water. Also note the common cause variation of plus or minus 72 calls for any one day. This was a much wider range than anyone expected.

Without this simple, statistical, graphical summary, is it any wonder that the temptation to tamper cannot be avoided by merely reacting to a table of numbers? *Without knowledge of the range of common cause variation, it is easy to mistake routine day-to-day variation for special causes and justify why they happened.*

Note that data point 22 lies extremely close to, but does not exceed, the upper horizontal limit. Subsequent investigations revealed nothing unusual about that particular Tuesday. It was just an extremely busy day. A day this busy will happen *occasionally* and cannot be predicted ahead of time.

Or consider this hypothetical scenario: Was this large volume because of the news story on that day's health alert? Although this is a special cause, for the future, can the increase in phone calls be predicted when there is a similar news story on a significant health issue so that one can staff accordingly?

Notice how during the subsequent week, calls returned to well within range of the average. Suppose staffing had been adjusted as a result of that demand? The result would have been tampering. Extra costs would have been caused for no reason. Natural variation (common cause) would have been treated as if action were needed (special cause).

This process is stable and predictable. It is the inherent result of the aggregation of all the inputs of the process. Assessment of its current performance can be used to ask questions as to whether that level of performance is acceptable and what implications there are for staffing. The common cause of plus or minus 72 calls is also inherent in the process as reflected in this data collection.

What is the objective of these data? Suppose they are used for staffing. Does one staff for the average, or does one staff for slightly higher than the average? Staffing for slightly above the average will result in better customer service, even though the phone system will be overstaffed on some days. One rule of thumb says to consider staffing for the 80 percent point, which, statistically, is approximately halfway between the average and upper limit.

Could these data be stratified even further? Should there be a breakdown by time of day to see whether there are special causes at certain times of the day? This could result in better predictability because variability from any time-of-day special cause is currently included in the common cause range. When any special cause such as this is removed from the data, the common cause range will be smaller than plus or minus 72 calls. Follow-up action could involve staffing higher only at certain times of the day, perhaps decreasing the phone staff at other times, or maybe even considering how to smooth out demand.

Note how the questions needed to answer a common cause situation are not as simple as taking action based on a single data point. In understanding common cause, fundamental questions that require further data collection must be asked about the underlying process. The hope is to eventually expose a hidden special cause, thus allowing a focus on both a significant source of variation and appropriate solution.

The key issue is not whether one data point is different from another data point. Variation virtually guarantees that. The more fundamental issue is whether the process that produced this particular data point is the same as the process that produced the other data point. The concept of work as a process, especially an administrative one, having a center (or average) with observed, inherent, predictable, common cause variation can be extremely difficult to grasp.

This concept is especially hard to understand when a corporate goal lies between the common cause limit (this would occur if, for example, the medical center had a goal of receiving a minimum of 225 calls per day). The result is that the goal will be achieved in some but not all of the time periods. As stated in Exhibit 6.9, numbers as high as 266 could randomly be produced by common cause variation from this process, even though it is centered at 194.

Processes do not understand goals. A process can only perform at the level that its inputs will allow. If this level does not allow the goal to be consistently achieved, fundamental changes will have to be made to the process.

The following examples once again illustrate the elegant simplicity of analysis using run charts and I-charts. These tools are essential to assess and quantify variation inherent in any data set collected over time.

### *A Review and Extension: Revisiting the Accident Data from Chapter 2*

Recall the analysis done on two years of monthly accident data (Exhibit 6.10). Every month, a safety report similar to Exhibit 6.11 was posted. One can see that it is a thinly disguised variation of the two-point trend. Does this information help people improve, especially if the variation is common cause?

Exhibit 6.12 shows a typical display of such data: the year-over-year plot. (I like to call these "copulating earthworm plots." They can have so many unique lines to the point

EXHIBIT 6.10 ■ Industrial Accident Data

|  | Accidents | |
| --- | --- | --- |
| Month | 1989 | 1990 |
| January | 5 | 2 |
| February | 4 | 1 |
| March | 5 | 3 |
| April | 7 | 2 |
| May | 1 | 3 |
| June | 3 | 7 |
| July | 2 | 0 |
| August | 6 | 3 |
| September | 2 | 1 |
| October | 3 | 5 |
| November | 7 | 5 |
| December | 0 | 0 |
| Total | 45 | 32 |

EXHIBIT 6.11 ■ Accident Data Safety Recap

**SAFETY RECAP**
September 1988

Number of doctor cases ___1___
Year-to-date doctor cases ___14___
Number of lost-time injuries ___0___
Year-to-date lost-time injuries ___0___

**THIS MONTH WAS**
same as ☐  better than ☒  worse than ☐
last month.

where one needs a Ouija board to interpret them.) One could conclude that 1990 was better because eight of its months were lower when compared to the same months in 1989. Intuitively, this seems to make sense, but what does statistical theory say? Purely random data could generate this result 23 percent of the time.

Why 23 percent? It is the odds of flipping a coin 11 times and getting at least eight heads or tails, which is the law of probability. Here, we compare 11 months (December had the same number of accidents both years and does not count in the comparison) and find 8 of them to be lower.

Thus, if one were to conclude that 1990 was truly better — the result of a special cause — there is a 23 percent chance of treating common cause variation as if it were special. When considering the risk of tampering, a statistical rule of thumb is to make this risk *5 percent or less*. This is the analog to the "95 percent confidence" mind-set taught in every basic statistics course and which has no meaning in the world of analytic statistics. These data were also previously plotted with a trend line and discussed in that context (see Chapter 2, Lesson 2).

The data needs to be considered as 24 measurements from a process output. Let the data themselves determine whether they should be plotted year-over-year or whatever. The concepts *year* and *January* are human inventions of convenience. The process does not know when a new year begins. Plotting the data in time order removes the biases created by assuming the presence of special causes. What do the data say? Exhibit 6.13 shows the run chart for these data.

Let's talk more about the construction of this run chart. To review, a run chart is a time-ordered plot with a horizontal line drawn at the median value. The median of the data set divides the data into two equal portions: Half of the data values are larger than the median, and the other half have values smaller than the median.

Let's review the concept of median.

- The median of an odd number of numbers will always be one of the actual numbers. As you will see in a later example with 19 observations ("Computer Information

**EXHIBIT 6.12** Year-over-Year Plot of Accident Data

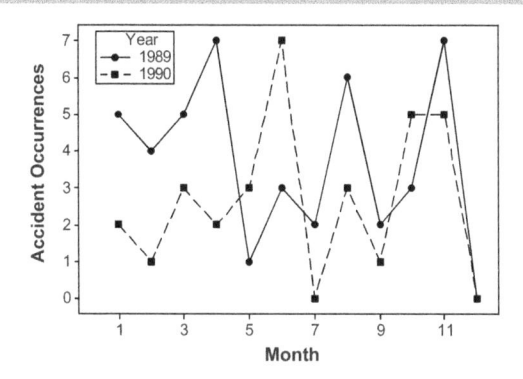

*Note:* When data are plotted in this format, it implies that special causes may be associated with the same months in each year.

**EXHIBIT 6.13** Run Chart of Accident Data

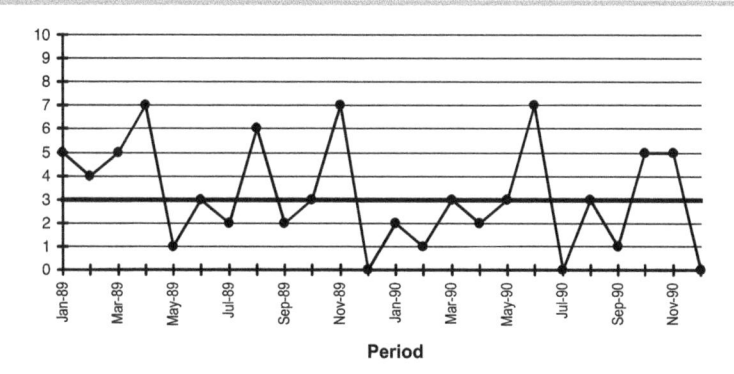

*Note:* A run chart is a time plot with a line drawn at the median.

System Percentage Uptime Example" section), the 10th in the *sorted* sequence is the median because 9 values are smaller and 9 values are larger.

- For an even amount of numbers, one must create an artificial midpoint by averaging the middle two values in the *sorted* sequence. In the case of Exhibit 6.14, which shows the accident data sorted into ascending order with 24 observations, it averages the 12th from the top of the *sorted* data with the 12th from the bottom of the *sorted* data. Counting the numbers in Exhibit 6.14, the 12th value from the top is 3 and the 12th value from the bottom is 3. The actual median is the average of these two values (12th and 13th in the sorted sequence), which equals 3.

To create the run chart then, we simply take the times-ordered plot of the data and draw horizontal lines at the median, in this case, 3.

In this or any time plot, what does "special cause" actually mean? Look again at the fundamental question to be asked: Was the process that produced the 1990 data the same process that produced the 1989 data? If a special cause was present, it would mean that

EXHIBIT 6.14 ■ Sorted Accident Data

| Month | Accidents | | |
|---|---|---|---|
| December 1989 | 0 | 1st | (Smallest) |
| July 1990 | 0 | 2nd | |
| December 1990 | 0 | 3rd | |
| May 1989 | 1 | 4th | |
| February 1990 | 1 | 5th | |
| September 1990 | 1 | 6th | |
| July 1989 | 2 | 7th | |
| September 1989 | 2 | 8th | |
| January 1990 | 2 | 9th | |
| April 1990 | 2 | 10th | |
| June 1989 | 3 | 11th | |
| October 1989 | 3 | 12th | Median is average |
| March 1990 | 3 | 13th | of 12th and 13th |
| May 1990 | 3 | 14th | |
| August 1990 | 3 | 15th | |
| February 1989 | 4 | 16th | |
| January 1989 | 5 | 17th | |
| March 1989 | 5 | 18th | |
| October 1990 | 5 | 19th | |
| November 1990 | 5 | 20th | |
| August 1989 | 6 | 21st | |
| April 1989 | 7 | 22nd | |
| November 1989 | 7 | 23rd | |
| June 1990 | 7 | 24th | (Largest) |

at least two different processes were at work during this time sequence. For an improvement in safety, we would hope to see evidence of a different process with a lower level of accident occurrences in 1990.

*Reviewing the Trend Special Cause Test*

Initially, the trend test (see Exhibit 2.5) gives no indication of such a special cause: There is no sequence of seven consecutive decreasing points (six successive decreases). The longest sequence of increases or decreases is three months, and this occurred three times: February through April 1989, September through November 1989, and April through June 1990. What additional tests based in statistical theory can be used?

## RUN CHART ANALYSIS

### Counting the Length of Runs

A *run* is defined as a consecutive sequence of data points all on the same side of the median. If the data points are connected to each other with a line, a run ends when the

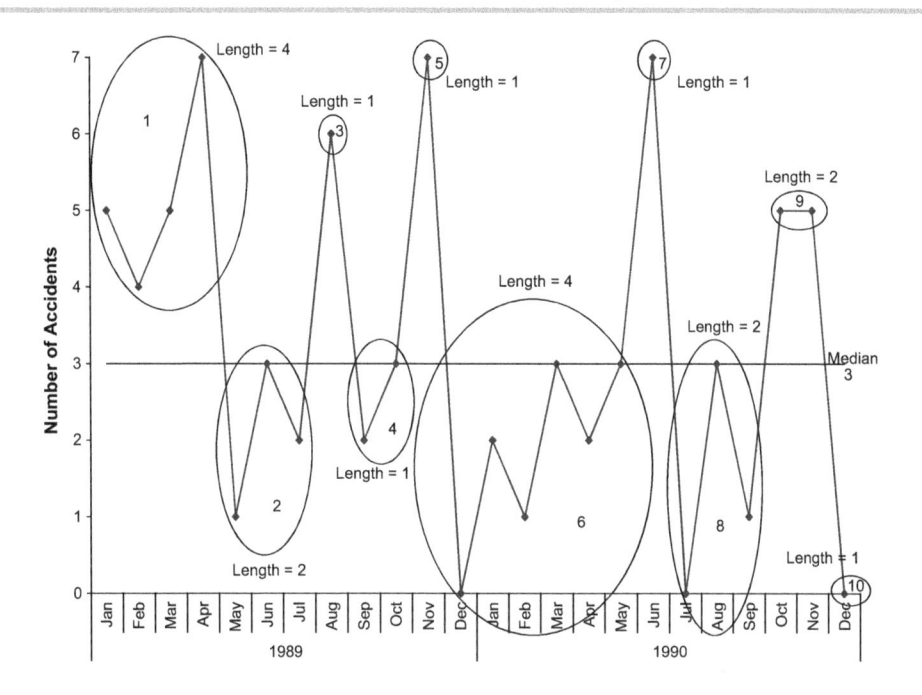

EXHIBIT 6.15 ■ Run Chart of Accident Data Showing the Length of Each Run

*Note:* Points on the median are not counted when determining the length of a run.

line actually crosses the median. A new run then starts with the next point. Points on the median are ignored in runs analysis. They neither add to nor break any run.

Exhibit 6.15 shows the run chart of Exhibit 6.14 with each run circled and numbered. The runs can be interpreted as follows. The first four data points, January through April of 1989, are called "a run of length 4 above the median." The run is broken when the line going from April to May crosses the median.

As the line continues from May, it reaches the median in June, but does not cross it, and stays below the median in July. The data point from August, however, brings the line across the median, thus the second run goes from May to July. Although three months are included in this run, one of them (June) is on the median. For the purpose of determining the length of the run, the June data point should be ignored. Thus the second run is "a run of length 2 below the median."

This analysis continues until all the plotted points are assigned to a run. Note that runs 2, 4, 6, and 8 all include points on the median, which makes their run lengths less than their actual number of months.

How long must a run be to indicate a special cause? We can make an analogy to flipping coins. When flipping a (fair) coin, there is a 50 percent chance of getting heads and a 50 percent chance of the coin landing tails. Similarly, if all variation in the accident data were due to common causes, each point would have a 50 percent chance of falling above the median as well as a 50 percent chance of falling below the median. Special cause patterns can be determined quite easily from this underlying statistical theory.

### EXHIBIT 6.16 ■ Why Eight in a Row?

There is only a 0.8 percent chance of eight consecutive points in a row appearing above the median due to common causes alone, which is less than the statistical rule of thumb of 5 percent.

Why is it 0.8 percent? Because, if this were to happen *truly* randomly, it means that it could happen either randomly all above the median or all below the median — two possibilities, the probability of which is [$2 \times 0.5^8$]. So, if eight points in a row are on the same side of the median, there is almost surely a special cause present in the process.

But isn't six in a row ($0.5^6$) less than the statistical rule of thumb for less than 5 percent risk? Yes, but to allow six in a row to occur randomly, I have to allow for the fact that it could once again occur either all above the median or all below the median, which would mean that the risk is doubled, and one would need to use at least seven rather than six.

So why use eight? Roughly 24 data points have multiple opportunities to have eight points in a row display this behavior at least once randomly: It could happen for observations 1–8, 2–9, or 3–10, all the way up to 17–24.

A table from a well-respected classic statistics text by Duncan[1] has worked out reasonable probabilities that, given 30 data points, the overall probability of observing at least one run of eight consecutive points either above or below the median is 5 percent. By the time you get to 40 data points, you might even have to use 9 in a row, and with 50 data points, 10 in a row. So let's say that eight in a row is good enough to balance reasonable risks.

---

This concept was summarized in Chapter 2, Exhibit 2.6. To minimize the risk of tampering, a run length of eight is used to signal a special cause. In other words, a special cause has occurred if eight or more *consecutive* points fall on the same side of the median. This test determines whether there were one or more process shifts over the time period of this data (Exhibit 6.16).

Returning to the accident data, if 1990 were truly lower in accidents, there might be a run of length 8 below the median to signify it and/or a similar run of length 8 above the median in 1989. Only one of these signals would be sufficient to indicate the theorized special cause of improvement. As Exhibit 6.15 shows, this did not happen.

In spite of the fact that 1990 saw fewer accidents than 1989, there is no evidence that it was necessarily a safer place to work in 1990. As far as we can tell, the process that produced 32 accidents in 1990 was the same process that produced 45 accidents in 1989. The variation in the numbers was most likely due to common causes. The fact that 1990 met the aggressive 25 percent reduction goal is probably purely coincidental. Given two numbers, one happened to have a smaller value than the other one.

The subsequent actions using common cause strategies were discussed in Chapter 5. For an additional run chart test that can be occasionally useful to test for special causes, see my 2008 article called "An Underrated Test for Run Charts" in Resources.

### Using Run Charts to Assess an Intervention and Hold Gains: The Menopause QI Team

Here is one of my first applications of a run chart in my very early days in healthcare. To say I was naive is a gross understatement. I use this example because it is a wonderful model of simplicity.

A 1991 continuous quality improvement (QI) team was trying to develop a guideline to deal with menopause. One of its objectives was reducing the inappropriate ordering of a particular diagnostic test, the level of follicle stimulating hormone (FSH). My very first week on the job, the team literally handed me 20 slips of paper from the laboratory showing how many of these tests were ordered each month for women ages 40 to 44. They wanted to know how the team was doing. All I could think of doing was plotting the dots. Exhibit 6.17 shows the resulting run chart.

A special cause is signaled by the run of the last eight data points below the median, beginning with November 1991. Thus, during this time period, the process showed some type of shift in its needle. The question became, "What special cause happened in November 1991?"

In asking the doctor who headed the team, he scratched his head a bit, his eyes lit up, and he said, "Oh, November 1991 is when we distributed our guideline recommendation regarding the appropriate use of FSH testing to diagnose menopause." It seems their intervention lowered the inappropriate use of the test, creating the desired effect. Now, how do they hold their gains?

Exhibit 6.18 shows the run chart of the intervention and subsequent data. A runs analysis of Exhibit 6.18 shows it to be stable, indicating no trends and no runs of length 8 or greater.

Exhibit 6.19 is a more comprehensive summary of the entire data set showing the overall dramatic shift in performance, taking into account that the intervention was indeed effective. It is a control chart, and not only demonstrates the step change, but the additional shifting of the common cause as well.

As I hope you are now aware, interventions cause processes to display more of a "step change" pattern rather than a "trend" (although there might be some semblance of a trend as the process *transitions* to its new needle). Because the system changed, it must be subsequently monitored by *its most current stable behavior*.

### What Range of Performance Is Expected?

The control chart (see Exhibit 6.19) shows that the process is centered at 14, and, in any one month, common cause variation leads one to expect between 2 and 27 FSH tests to be ordered. Observe that one month, August 1992, is right at the upper common cause limit of tests, 26.8. Remember the fundamental question about data: How were these data collected? It turned out that the tabulated FSH value not only includes menopausal women (inappropriate ordering) but also FSH tests given to check for infertility (appropriate ordering).

A process input phenomenon increasingly occurring during this time was that a growing number of women ages 40 to 44 were trying to get pregnant and having trouble doing so. It turns out that an exceptionally high number of FSH testing happened to be performed for infertility in August 1992. (Note a somewhat similar pattern the previous year in September through October. Is this a summer-month predictable special cause phenomenon, perhaps due to teachers?)

### Diagnosis vs. Holding the Gains: Use Medical Chart Reviews Sparingly

The issue of holding the gains brings up an interesting issue that I see bog down so many clinical projects, which is getting a "clean" number. For this menopause team, it would mean plotting only the number of tests ordered to diagnose menopause. The resulting data process then becomes doing chart reviews every month to get the number.

In my experience, one can sense the increasing tension in a room when the words *chart review* are used. They can be useful in early stages of projects, but only with clear

**EXHIBIT 6.17** ■ Run Chart of Follicle-Stimulating Hormone Test Ordering Frequency

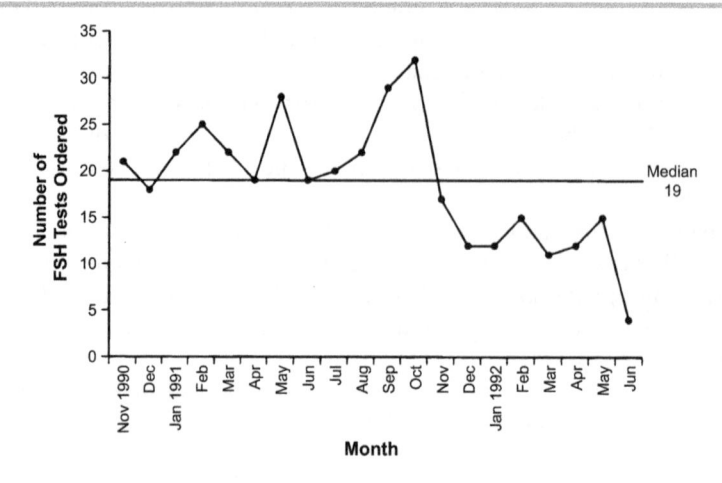

*Note:* Eight consecutive months are below the median at the end, signaling a special cause.

**EXHIBIT 6.18** ■ Run Chart of Post-Intervention Data

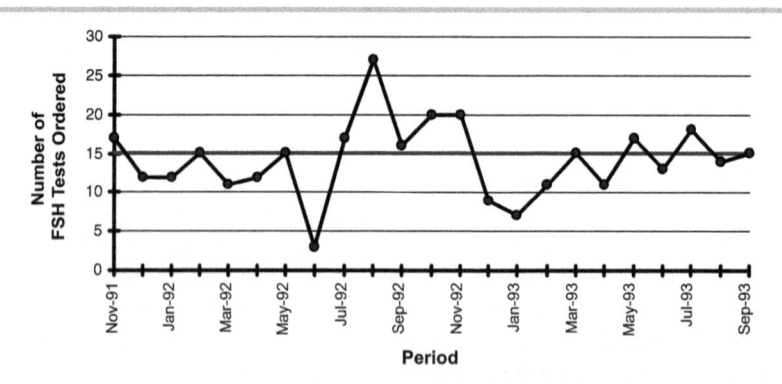

*Note:* For monitoring to hold any gains, the new process median is used for subsequent analysis.

objectives: (1) trying to quickly find the 20 percent of the process causing 80 percent of the problem (stratification) and then (2) focusing subsequent efforts to find deeper root causes on the identified 20 percent (disaggregation). In this case, the measurement process will most definitely need to be addressed by developing very clear operational definitions.

Holding the gains is a totally different issue. I see a lot of problems in organizations because data that should have been used only once for a diagnosis process have all of a sudden become "permanently temporary." After a problem is solved, the need is for only a number that is good enough. If it subsequently signals a problem, a stratification or disaggregation can suggest a *one-time* collection to diagnose the current issue, taking advantage of the fact that the process is perfectly designed to get what you are already getting.

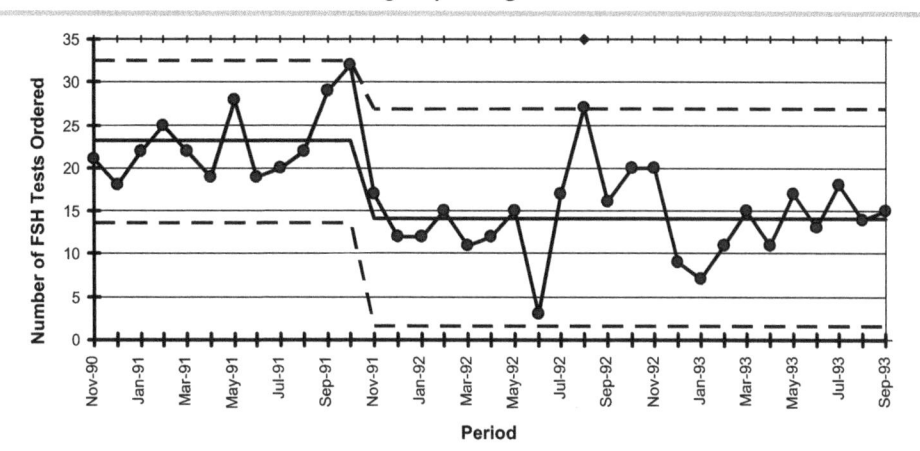

**EXHIBIT 6.19** ▪ Control Chart Showing Step Change and Common Cause Shift

*Note:* This plot recognizes the special cause in the data by showing separate needles (average) for each system. The current common cause window for this process is 2 to 27 tests in any given month.

The menopause team wisely concluded that the logistical difficulties of monthly chart reviews made the current aggregated value reported by the laboratory sufficient for their objective of simply monitoring the process. Chart reviews would be deemed necessary *only when warranted by a special cause* (as in the case of August 1992 described in the previous section). The energy that would have been routinely devoted to chart reviews for a clean number is much better spent elsewhere diagnosing other significant organizational issues.

In assessing the current gains, the process has gone from a monthly average of 23, based on the data through October 1991, to the current monthly average of 14, based on the subsequent data. Continued plotting of the monthly results monitors whether the gains are still being held.

## CONVERTING A RUN CHART INTO AN I-CHART

### Computer Information System Percentage Uptime Example

Computer uptime was a very important index to a major medical center's chief operating officer. He wanted performance to be 100 percent with no exceptions. To understand why uptime was not consistently reaching 100 percent, the data in Exhibit 6.20 were collected over a 19-month period, and a monthly meeting was held to account for the latest performance. (This is the same data contained in Lesson 5 of Chapter 2.)

When 100 percent was finally achieved in June 1989, the manager told the computer department, "Send out for pizza and send me the bill." However, the disturbing trend over the next four months made him feel the employees were taking advantage of the situation and slacking off. He decided it was time to get tough, especially after the disappointing 98.6 percent result in October. He read them the riot act, *demanding* 100 percent. When it was achieved the following month, however, there was no pizza.

The manager's actions were based on data. However, those actions presumed all variation was due to special cause. Columns of numbers say nothing. A graph is required to properly interpret the data: What can be said about the *process* producing these data?

Exhibit 6.21 shows the data sorted in ascending order. Because there are 19 numbers, the median is the 10th smallest (or, equivalently, largest) number in this sorted sequence, which is 99.3 percent.

Exhibit 6.22 shows a run chart of the computer uptime results. A quick glance yields the following conclusions:

1. No trends. The initial trend of 6 months only counts as a trend of 4 because two points (March and May) repeat exactly their preceding values. The perceived managerial trend of 100 percent down to 98.6 percent was only length 5 (four successive decreases).
2. No runs of eight or more consecutive observations either all above or below the median.

Hence, so far, what is revealed is a common cause system.

Look again at the manager's actions. In treating the initial (or any other) 100 percent month as unique, a common cause may have been treated as a special cause. In treating months 6 through 10 (only a group of five) as a perceived trend, a probable common cause was treated as a special cause. By treating the change from 98.6 percent to 100 percent as if it was due to his strong-arm action, a common cause may have been treated as a special cause.

What situations have you either observed or been involved that were handled similarly? What were the results? Did things improve or stay the same? How did the people in those processes feel and subsequently behave? What should be done differently?

Because these data passed all the rules of the run chart, one can preliminarily conclude that a consistent process produced these data; that is, it seems to have one needle. Because the run chart tells us the data all come from a single process, it is valid to calculate the overall average of 99.3, which coincidentally was the median as well. If the run chart analysis had shown evidence of two or more processes during the time period, this average of all the numbers is meaningless.

Two questions remain:

1. What are the common cause, inherent limits of this process; that is, what is the common cause variation around the average that, for any one month, indicates stable behavior?
2. How much difference between two consecutive monthly observations is "too much"?

**EXHIBIT 6.20** Computer Information System Percentage Uptime Data

| Month | Percent Uptime |
|---|---|
| January 1989 | 98.0 |
| February | 98.7 |
| March | 98.7 |
| April | 99.2 |
| May | 99.2 |
| June | 100.0 |
| July | 99.7 |
| August | 99.5 |
| September | 99.0 |
| October | 98.6 |
| November | 100.0 |
| December | 99.3 |
| January 1990 | 99.8 |
| February | 99.8 |
| March | 98.5 |
| April | 100.0 |
| May | 100.0 |
| June | 98.6 |
| July | 99.7 |
| Average | 99.3 |

EXHIBIT 6.21 ■ Computer Information System Percentage Uptime Data Sorted in Ascending Order

| Month | Percent Uptime | Order | |
|---|---|---|---|
| January 1989 | 98.0 | 1st | (Smallest) |
| March 1990 | 98.5 | 2nd | |
| October 1989 | 98.6 | 3rd | |
| June 1990 | 98.6 | 4th | |
| February 1989 | 98.7 | 5th | |
| March 1989 | 98.7 | 6th | |
| September 1989 | 99.0 | 7th | |
| April 1989 | 99.2 | 8th | |
| May 1989 | 99.2 | 9th | |
| **December 1989** | **99.3** | **10th** | **(Median)** |
| August 1989 | 99.5 | 11th | |
| July 1989 | 99.7 | 12th | |
| July 1990 | 99.7 | 13th | |
| January 1990 | 99.8 | 14th | |
| February 1990 | 99.8 | 15th | |
| June 1989 | 100.0 | 16th | |
| November 1989 | 100.0 | 17th | |
| April 1990 | 100.0 | 18th | |
| May 1990 | 100.0 | 19th | (Largest) |

EXHIBIT 6.22 ■ Run Chart of Percentage Computer Uptime Data

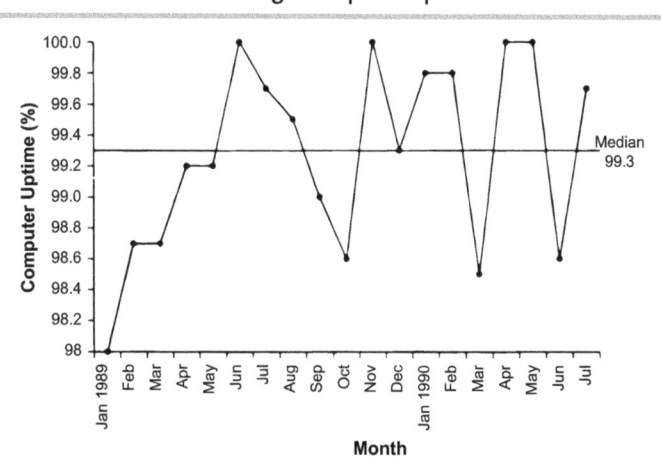

*Note:* In spite of the apparent upward trend at the beginning of the plot, no special causes can be detected with these data.

### The Median Moving Range

A very important number for the I-chart analysis is the *moving range*. Its calculation and use have an elegant simplicity that seems to be one of the few times where statistics actually seems intuitive.

The moving range is calculated from the data as a way of quantifying its variation. Appealing to your intuition, if most of the data represent a common cause system, it would seem safe to assume that two *consecutive* values in time would somehow be a good estimate of common cause variation. *It is immaterial whether the variation is positive or negative*; it is just considered variation. As it turns out, taking the absolute value of these successive differences creates some easy-to-use statistical properties.

Exhibit 6.23 demonstrates this calculation for the computer uptime data in Exhibit 6.20. To get you started, the first moving range, 0.7, is obtained by subtracting the first data point from the second (98.7 − 98.0). The next moving range, 0, is obtained similarly by subtracting the second data point from the third (98.7 − 98.7). This continues until the last moving range, 1.1, is obtained by subtracting the 18th observation from the 19th observation: (99.7 − 98.6).

From this list of moving ranges, the median is now determined. The *median moving range* ($MR_{Med}$) is the key number for understanding any process's common cause variation. *All* subsequent calculations will involve it. There are two important things to note:

1. Moving ranges are calculated from the data in its naturally occurring time order, not the sorted order; and
2. When calculating the median moving range, remember that the number of moving ranges is always one less than the number of data points.

Exhibit 6.24 contains the sorted moving ranges for the computer data.

The 19 data points yield 18 moving ranges. Because 18 is even, the $MR_{Med}$ is the average of the 9th and 10th sorted moving ranges. In this case, they both happen to be 0.5, so the $MR_{Med} = 0.5$.

### *Helpful Information*

Multiplying the $MR_{Med}$ by 3.865 (a constant derived from statistical theory) yields the maximum difference between two consecutive data points that could be attributable to common cause. If a moving range exceeds the upper limit of ($MR_{Med} \times 3.865$), $MR_{Max}$, it might be indicative of a special cause, usually either:

- A significant shift in the process average (a needle bump); or
- An outlier, usually indicated by two consecutive excessive values.

The factor 3.865 is valid for any time sequence where the median (not the average) moving range is calculated, *regardless* of the sequence length.

$MR_{Max}$ is a useful piece of information that can be used to supplement the I-chart of the actual data as the primary analysis. From my experience, I find that $MR_{Max}$ is virtually always larger than managers, executives, and boards would like it to be. So it is also a simple piece of information that may help stop potential tampering.

For the uptime data, one month's performance can differ from its previous month's performance by as much as: $(3.865 \times 0.5) = 1.9$. Remember when the manager did not like the trend down to 98.6 and came down hard on the computer system personnel, resulting in 100 percent performance the next month? Note that the difference is $(100 - 98.6) = 1.4$, which is less than 1.9 and not necessarily a special cause.

# PROCESS-ORIENTED STATISTICS

## EXHIBIT 6.23 ■ Calculating the Moving Range

The moving range is a measure of the variation between two consecutive data points. It is calculated simply as the absolute value of their difference. In other words, one value is subtracted from the other. If the result is positive, it is the moving range between the two points. If the result is negative, delete the minus sign to make it positive. The new result is the moving range between the points.

A procedure for calculating the moving range of a set of data follows:
1. List the data in time sequence.
2. Subtract the first point from the second and ignore the sign (moving ranges are *always* positive).
3. Return to step 2 and use the second and third numbers, third and fourth, etc.

The calculation of moving ranges is demonstrated below with the uptime data from Exhibit 6.20.

| Month | Data | Moving Range Calculation | |
|---|---|---|---|
| 1 | 98.0 | | |
| 2 | 98.7 | 98.7 − 98.0 = 0.7 | This is positive. The moving range is 0.7. |
| 3 | 98.7 | 98.7 − 98.7 = 0.0 | A moving range can have a value of zero. |
| 4 | 99.2 | 99.2 − 98.7 = 0.5 | |
| 5 | 99.2 | 99.2 − 99.2 = 0.0 | |
| 6 | 100.0 | 100.0 − 99.2 = 0.8 | |
| 7 | 99.7 | 99.7 − 100.0 = −0.3 | This is negative, so remove the minus sign. The moving range is 0.3. |
| ... | | | |
| 18 | 98.6 | 98.6 − 100.0 = −1.4 | |
| 19 | 99.7 | 99.7 − 98.6 = 1.1 | |

Reprinting the data and moving ranges:

| Time Order | Percent Uptime | Moving Range |
|---|---|---|
| January 1989 | 98.0 | * |
| February | 98.7 | 0.7 |
| March | 98.7 | 0.0 |
| April | 99.2 | 0.5 |
| May | 99.2 | 0.0 |
| June | 100.0 | 0.8 |
| July | 99.7 | 0.3 |
| August | 99.5 | 0.2 |
| September | 99.0 | 0.5 |
| October | 98.6 | 0.4 |
| November | 100.0 | 1.4 |
| December | 99.3 | 0.7 |
| January 1990 | 99.8 | 0.5 |
| February | 99.8 | 0.0 |
| March | 98.5 | 1.3 |
| April | 100.0 | 1.5 |
| May | 100.0 | 0.0 |
| June | 98.6 | 1.4 |
| July | 99.7 | 1.1 |

*Note that there are 19 measurements in the data but only 18 moving ranges. There will always be one less moving range than there are data points.

**EXHIBIT 6.24** ■ Percentage Computer Information System Median Moving Range Determination

| Sorted Moving Range | Order | |
|---|---|---|
| 0.0 | 1st | (Smallest) |
| 0.0 | 2nd | |
| 0.0 | 3rd | |
| 0.0 | 4th | |
| 0.2 | 5th | |
| 0.3 | 6th | |
| 0.4 | 7th | |
| 0.5 | 8th | |
| 0.5 | 9th | Median is average of 9th and 10th |
| 0.5 | 10th | |
| 0.7 | 11th | |
| 0.7 | 12th | |
| 0.8 | 13th | |
| 1.0 | 14th | |
| 1.3 | 15th | |
| 1.4 | 16th | |
| 1.4 | 17th | |
| 1.5 | 18th | (Largest) |

I also want you to note that determination of common cause comes strictly *from the data*. It does not necessarily have to end in a 0 or a 5, nor is it an arbitrary percentage (typically ±10–15 percent) of the average because that is what a manager feels it *should* be.

Many times you will discover that the variation in which you are immersed is much greater than you thought, which has a good news/bad news aspect to it. As has been repeatedly emphasized, if the process is stable (to be confirmed by further control chart analysis), one can now use a common cause strategy *regardless* of the amount of variation.

### *Obtaining the Process Performance Common Cause Limits*

To obtain the process's common cause limits, one multiplies $MR_{Med}$ by 3.14 (another constant from statistical theory to be used with the median moving range and has nothing to do with pi [$\pi$]) and adds and subtracts it to the process average. For the uptime data:

$$99.3 \pm (3.14 \times 0.5) = [97.7 - 100.9]$$

Given the natural restrictions of this situation, greater than 100 percent uptime is impossible. Exhibit 6.25 shows 100 percent as the upper limit.

This analysis confirms that attainment of 100 percent uptime is not necessarily a special cause, but well within common cause performance: There will be times when everything that can go right does go right, due to sheer good luck, resulting in a performance of 100 percent.

Something worth noting is that statistics does not understand the numerical limitations of one's process, so please use common sense and your knowledge of a situation accordingly when considering the common cause limits you obtain.

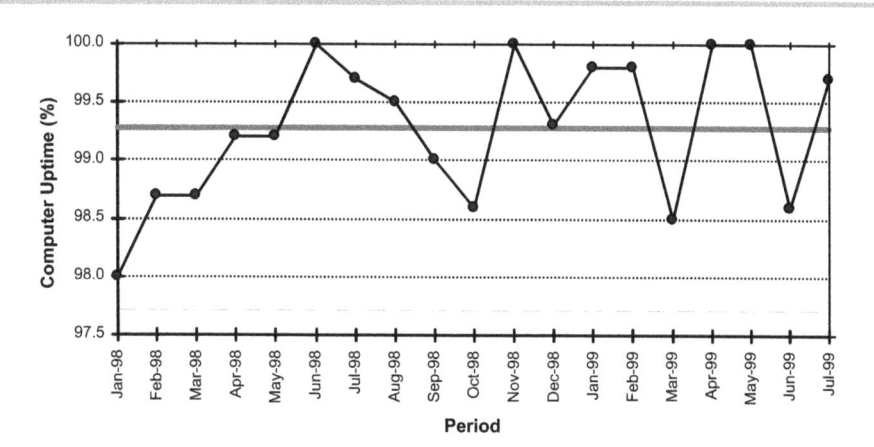

### EXHIBIT 6.25  Control Chart for Percentage Computer Uptime Data

*Note:* The control chart shows that the uptime process has been stable for the past 19 months at a performance level of 99.3 percent. 100 percent uptime will be achieved in some, but not all, months due to random luck.

This will also be encountered when charting occurrences of undesirable events (e.g., medication errors, complaints). In this case, it is not unusual for calculated lower limits to be negative, which, once again, is impossible. The lower limit will need to be set to zero. And do this if necessary before presenting any data, especially to physicians, or it is guaranteed that those darn humans will use it as a stated reason for ignoring both the validity and implications of the analysis.

On the chart, notice that its lower limit is 97.7 percent. Recall that the manager did not like the trend down to 98.6. I can guarantee that if all he does is continue to exhort, there will be a month when *everything* that can go wrong will go wrong and result in 97.7 percent performance. It will be through no fault of the workers and will be relatively rare, but it will happen. When it will happen cannot be predicted. For example, do you know when leaving the house in the morning that it is going to be the morning when you are going to encounter *all* the red lights (and a school bus and a garbage truck) on your way to work?

To summarize thus far, as shown in the MI telephone example and this example, an I-chart is a time plot of the data that includes lines added for the average and natural process variation. These limits represent a common cause range around the average where individual data points may be expected to fall if the underlying process does not change (think back to the process I described of 50 people flipping coins: Although averaging 25 heads, any individual flip will yield a number between 14 and 36).

### *What Is the Strategy for Improving This Process?*

In reaction to the monthly uptime result, there was always a scheduled meeting to discuss the past month's reasons for having downtime. This approach is tantamount to treating the current monthly result as a special cause. And notice that in Exhibit 6.25 the average amount of downtime is 0.7 percent, approximately 5 hours per month. However, because of the stability of this process, one could now use a common cause strategy to *aggregate all*

*19 months' worth of downtime* (approximately 85 hours) to analyze with a Pareto matrix. This would have a better chance of isolating some major opportunities for improvement.

When does the downtime occur? Was it certain times during the day, certain days of the week, or certain times in the month? What were the causes of downtime? Was there any pattern to when different causes occurred? Who was the system operator during downtime?

There seems to be an additional dilemma. As discussed, the goal of 100 percent is contained within the common cause variation and can easily occur in individual months without any improvement to the system. How could interventions be evaluated?

Once a control chart has determined that a system is stable, the rules used with the run chart can still be applied as more data are obtained. If an improvement team exposes opportunity by analyzing an aggregated Pareto matrix of downtime, makes an intervention, and the control chart has an immediate trend of five or six increases, a run of eight observations in a row above the current average, or seven months in a row of 100 percent performance (see Chapter 7, the "seven in a row of the same value" rule), then it could be assumed that the intervention created a special cause with a beneficial effect.

### A Warning about Arbitrary Numerical Goals

This example shows yet again the danger of arbitrary numerical goals, especially when they lie within a process's common cause variation. Immediate reaction to individual data points then risks the danger of tampering, which usually makes things worse. There is then further risk when the common cause variation in the ensuing data is now interpreted to evaluate the effects of this tampering, which are random patterns being misinterpreted as special causes according to interpreter biases.

To complicate matters, the tampering has then become an additional normal input to the process, which can actually inflate the underlying common cause variation. The difference is that variation caused by tampering is artificially created. It is inappropriate variation in addition to the normal process variation. As a matter of fact, some forms of tampering can increase the inherent common cause variation of a process by approximately 40 percent. This has the effect of not only further masking the problem, but there certainly is no resulting improvement.

This has become even more of a problem since the publication of the second edition of *Quality Improvement: Practical Applications for Medical Group Practice* in 1996 (see Resources) because of the current plague of traffic light systems featuring the red/yellow/green scheme for reporting data; any deviation from the green performance (arbitrary) goal is treated as a special cause.

Processes do not understand goals. Processes can only perform at the levels allowed by their inputs. One must study a process to understand its capability with respect to the goal. After this, one must learn whether observed variation, or failure to meet the goal, is due to special or common causes. Focus on the process, not its output, but allow the output to serve as an indicator of assessment and measurement of the progress of process improvement.

### Real Common Cause: Learn to Recognize the Underlying Sources of Variation

While teaching a class, I asked participants to create a control chart of an indicator that was important to them. A lab supervisor presented me with the chart shown in Exhibit 6.26 on the number of procedures her department performed and told me that it wasn't very

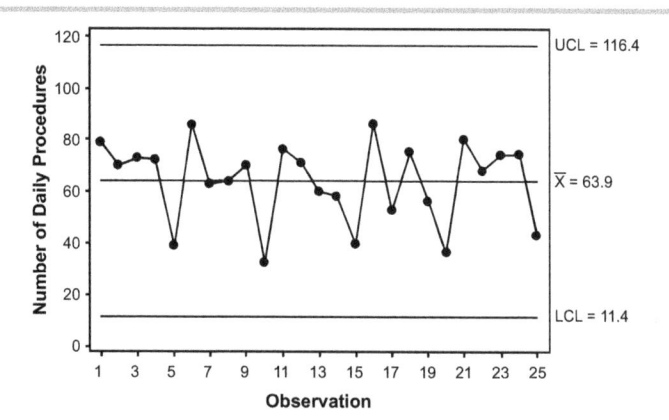

EXHIBIT 6.26 ■ Control Chart: Number of Procedures Performed

[Control chart showing Number of Daily Procedures across 25 observations, with UCL = 116.4, X̄ = 63.9, and LCL = 11.4]

Source: Davis Balestracci Jr., MS, *Quality Digest*, August 2005. www.qualitydigest.com. Reprinted with permission.

useful. She wanted to use it for staffing purposes, and the wide limits were discouraging to the point of being ridiculous.

You may have access to software with the famous eight Western Electric special cause tests programmed in. In this case, none of them were triggered. Therefore, at least so far, it's a common cause process. In addition, the data "pass" a normality test with a $p$-value of 0.092.

In situations like these, we can lose credibility as quality professionals if we're not careful. People just roll their eyes at the wide limits as we try to explain that their process is perfectly designed to have this variation, and that they're going to have to tell management they need a new process. At which point our listeners roll their eyes again and say, "Thanks," while muttering under their breath, "for nothing."

Chapter 5 described three common cause strategies: process stratification, process dissection, and experimentation. They should be approached in that order, but the typical response to common cause is to jump right to experimentation, based on the *very* common misconception that, faced with common cause, a process redesign is the only option. This is not necessarily true. Common cause just means that data points can neither be looked at individually nor compared to one to another.

First we must ask, "How were these data collected?" A lot of Six Sigma training emphasizes the need for more frequent data collection on processes being studied. But this can cause additional problems in interpretation if one isn't careful.

When I asked the lab supervisor at my class how these numbers were obtained, she told me that they represented five weeks of daily procedure counts and that the lab was closed on weekends. So it was five weeks of Monday-through-Friday data. In cases such as this, it is useful and obvious to stratify, that is, separate, the data simply by coding it by the specific day of the week. This can be easily done by coding each data point by "day of the week" to see whether there is a pattern to either *all* the high values and/or *all* the low values. Does Exhibit 6.27, in its simplicity, give some significant insight for proceeding without the added confusion of "statistics"?

**EXHIBIT 6.27** ■ Run Chart for Number of Procedures Coded by Day of the Week

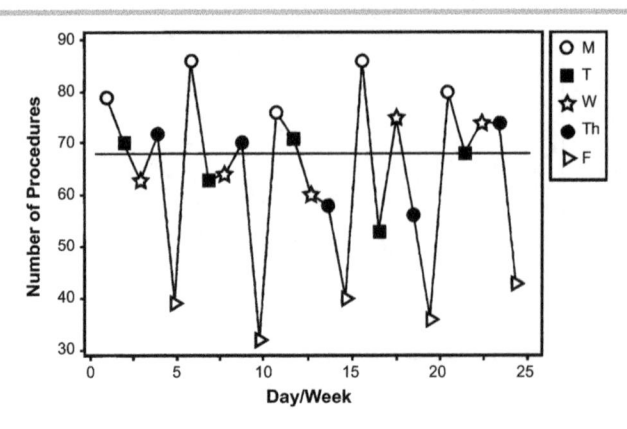

Source: Davis Balestracci Jr., MS, *Quality Digest*, August 2005. www.qualitydigest.com. Reprinted with permission.

In cases like this, I have found that a *stratified* histogram comparing the values by the days of the week is a very effective visual presentation, although the simple coding in the time plot shown has done as good a job. The stratified histogram is to continuous data what a Pareto analysis of tally counts is to count data. This is the only way I use histograms, that is, stratified. In my opinion, for a service industry such as healthcare, a good control chart with correctly calculated limits is a far more effective situation summary than a generalized histogram, which is better suited for the manufacturing industry (Exhibit 6.28).

These two displays simply and visually expose a "hidden" special cause by day of the week in these data: Mondays tend to be high, Fridays tend to be low, and Tuesdays through Thursdays are in the middle. This special cause has rendered the initial control chart and normality test *invalid* because the moving ranges between consecutive points do not all necessarily reflect *random* variation. The *nonrandom* fixed-difference special causes in the moving ranges from Mondays to Tuesdays, Thursdays to Fridays, and then Fridays to Mondays inappropriately *inflate the limits*. This could also be a lurking issue if you sample several times in one day — hourly, by shift, and so forth.

How does telling her to staff to anticipate 11–116 procedures every day compare to telling the lab supervisor to staff as follows (notice the tightened ranges compared with the initial chart): Monday: 50–103; Tuesday–Thursday: 40–80; Friday: 23–63?

Over the years, I have seen various sources make the point that for prediction such as ordering supplies or staffing, one should anticipate the "80 percent point." Statistically, this is *approximately* halfway between the average and upper limit. In this case, it would result in staffing for 90 procedures for Monday, 70 for Tuesday–Thursday, and 53 for Friday. If an ongoing control chart signals a special cause, then immediate contingency plans should be available to handle the unique situation.

By understanding the underlying sources of variation by asking *how the data were collected*, we are able to make better predictions with less variation.

Any good statistical analysis will always lead to the following question. The best advice I can give for any quality improvement effort is to be relentless in understanding the variation in a situation. This leads us to ask, "What can I ultimately predict?"

EXHIBIT 6.28 ■ Number of Procedures Stratified by Weekday

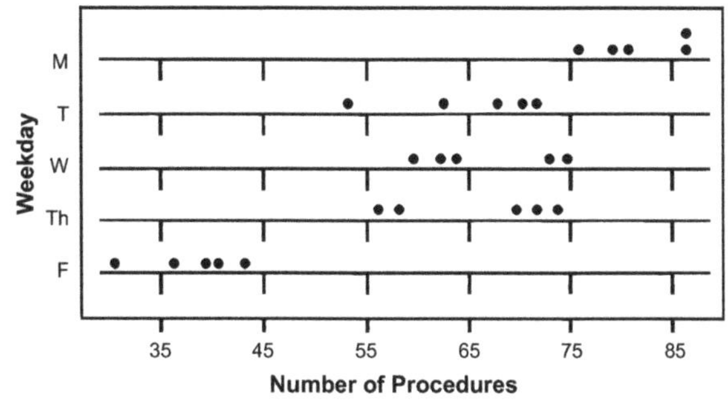

Source: Davis Balestracci Jr., MS, *Quality Digest*, August 2005. www.qualitydigest.com. Reprinted with permission.

EXHIBIT 6.29 ■ Performance Review: Year-End Review Data

| PHYSICAL THERAPY DEPARTMENT Monthly Quality Report LEAD Measures | | | | | | Interpolated Scores | | | | | | | | |
|---|---|---|---|---|---|---|---|---|---|---|---|---|---|---|
| | | | | | | 95%–100% of Target | | | 94%–85% of Target | | | ≤84% of Target | | |
| 2010 Average | 2011 YTD Average | Target | Jan | Feb | Mar | Apr | May | Jun | Jul | Aug | Sep | Oct | Nov | Dec |
| 9.40% | 10.0% | ≤10% | 9.2% | 11.8% | 8.5% | 8.5% | 10.1% | 9.4% | 13.0% | 9.7% | 9.1% | 7.9% | 9.1% | 12.10% |

## Performance Reviews That Solve Problems

How many of you dread the year-end performance review in which you account for your results vs. your goal(s)? Actually, it may not be all that bad because most people will be showing their past 12 months of results, which allows you to apply statistical thinking to these processes to get a true picture. At one facility, missed appointments were an ongoing problem. Exhibit 6.29 shows some actual data that were presented at one such year-end review. The explanation of what constituted green, yellow, or red performance is shown in Exhibit 6.30.

The national standard was 20 percent and one of your colleagues was asked to "stretch." So your colleague set a tough goal of 10 percent.

While the meeting goes off to the Milky Way discussing (1) why performance was worse this year vs. last (10 percent vs. 9.4 percent) and (2) the reasons for the yellow and red months (especially the current month's red), you can easily come up with the data table (Exhibit 6.31), then sketch the run chart below the table (Exhibit 6.32).

Even though the data are limited, nothing really looks amiss. You can now easily construct the process behavior chart (I-chart) well before the current discussion of the data ends (Exhibit 6.33).

You have entertained yourself during the meeting and can gain respect from your colleagues after the meeting.

**EXHIBIT 6.30** ■ Performance Review Table

| | |
|---|---|
| or | **Based on a Standard** (Target cell below) |
| | **Green, Yellow, or Red Status Defined in Action Plan Column for that Quality Indicator** |
| | Action Taken |
| | Responsible Party |
| | <10.5% = Green, 11.8–10.4% = Yellow, >11.9% = Red National Standard is 20% |

**EXHIBIT 6.31** ■ Performance Review: Data Table

| | |
|---|---|
| Jan-11 | 9.2% |
| Feb-11 | 11.8% |
| Mar-11 | 8.5% |
| Apr-11 | 8.5% |
| May-11 | 10.1% |
| Jun-11 | 9.4% |
| Jul-11 | 13.0% |
| Aug-11 | 9.7% |
| Sep-11 | 9.1% |
| Oct-11 | 7.9% |
| Nov-11 | 9.1% |
| Dec-11 | 12.10% |

**EXHIBIT 6.32** ■ Performance Review: Run Chart

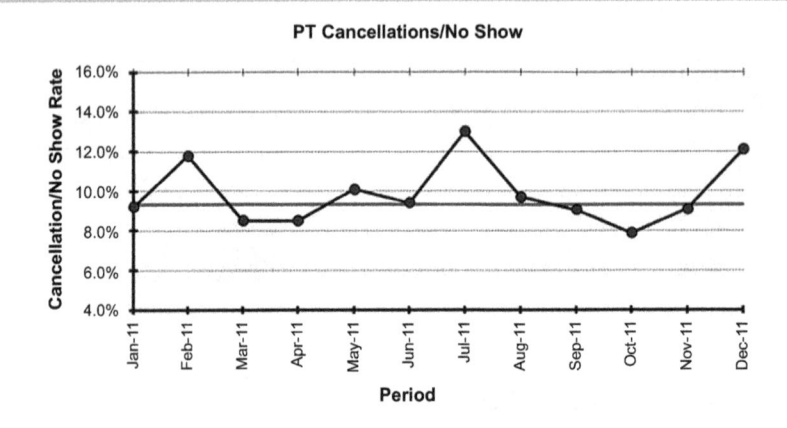

**EXHIBIT 6.33** ■ Performance Review: I-Chart

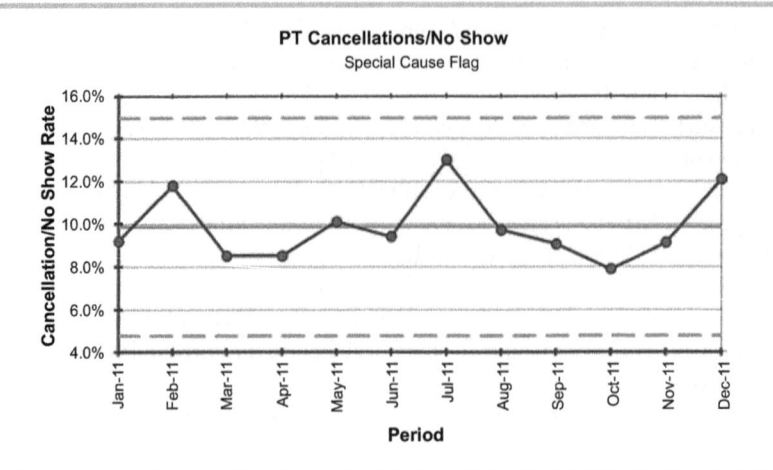

## Help Your Colleagues Look Good

If people are open to a new (and correct) way of defining performance vs. a goal, the goal your colleague has set was met all year because its average was 10 percent. And, rather than (1) treating every cancellation as a special cause and (2) treating any deviation from the goal as a special cause, especially the months greater than 10 percent, you interpret the chart for appropriate action: It's all common cause. This suggests the common cause strategy of stratification: Aggregate *all* the cancellations of the past year, then do a Pareto analysis. Your colleague could even go further to possibly include years previous to this one if they show the same behavior.

Isn't this more productive than explaining the three months above the goal, which could just as easily have been up to nine months above the goal due to random variation? Of course, talk then ensues about how "tough" your colleague should make her goal next year. Remember: 50 percent of time executives spend in meetings involving data is wasted time. Of course, speaking up like this in a meeting with the leadership team present could very well be political suicide; but I'm sure your colleague would be very grateful if you suggested this once you got outside this meeting and let your colleague have all the credit when showing an unprecedentedly low rate.

Remember that arbitrary numerical goals are not useful. What are you perfectly designed to get vis-à-vis the goal? Is the gap from the goal a common cause or special cause? With a goal rather than process focus, the goal becomes "to meet the goal." A frightened culture is very clever; it will meet goals by either distorting the process or somehow distorting the numbers.

To show the power of data sanity, start by quietly helping colleagues get real results behind the scenes that astonish the leadership team at review times. Maybe these breakthroughs in knowledge will help them refine their thinking away from the belief that "these funny-sounding statistical ideas have no place in managing and leading an organization."

## Common Traps with Percentages

To avoid the common traps with percentages, follow this advice:
- Don't treat every deviation from the goal as a special cause and fall into the traffic light trap.
- Don't treat every noncompliance as a special cause and fall into the unexpected event ("shouldn't happen") trap.
- All noncompliances are caused by the same process and a common cause strategy is required. If it's common cause, then a noncompliance on a green day or month is the same as a noncompliance on a yellow day or month, which is the same as a noncompliance on a red day or month.
- Being able to explain something after the fact does not mean it is a special cause.

# BEYOND MECHANICS

## Monthly Patient Satisfaction Survey

The following example is an excellent reminder of our key question in data collection: "How were these data collected?"

At every one of its 20 clinics, a multispecialty clinic had a table with a sign saying, "Tell Us How Your Visit Was." If patients *chose*, they had the opportunity to rank the clinic on a 1 (worst) to 5 (best) basis in nine categories. At the end of every month, these

EXHIBIT 6.34 ■ Overall Satisfaction Data and Summary for Past 19 Months

| Month | Ov_Sat | % Change | Sorted Ov_Sat Scores | |
|---|---|---|---|---|
| 1 | 4.29 | * | 4.08 | |
| 2 | 4.18 | −2.6 | 4.16 | |
| 3 | 4.08 | −2.4 | 4.18 | |
| 4 | 4.31 | 5.6 | 4.21 | |
| 5 | 4.16 | −3.5 | 4.26 | |
| 6 | 4.33 | 4.1 | 4.27 | |
| 7 | 4.27 | −1.4 | 4.27 | |
| 8 | 4.44 | 4.0 | 4.29 | |
| 9 | 4.26 | −4.1 | 4.30 | |
| 10 | 4.49 | 5.4 | 4.31 | Median |
| 11 | 4.51 | 0.5 | 4.31 | |
| 12 | 4.49 | −0.4 | 4.33 | |
| 13 | 4.35 | −3.1 | 4.35 | |
| 14 | 4.21 | −3.2 | 4.36 | |
| 15 | 4.42 | 5.0 | 4.42 | |
| 16 | 4.31 | −2.5 | 4.44 | |
| 17 | 4.36 | 1.2 | 4.49 | |
| 18 | 4.27 | −2.1 | 4.49 | |
| 19 | 4.30 | 0.7 | 4.51 | |

| Mean | Median | Tr Mean | St Dev | SE Mean |
|---|---|---|---|---|
| 4.3174 | 4.3100 | 4.3200 | 0.1168 | 0.0268 |

| Min | Max | Q1 | Q3 |
|---|---|---|---|
| 4.08 | 4.51 | 4.26 | 4.42 |

cards were collected and sent out for processing, which was an expensive process. The subsequent monthly summary statistics were then given to the clinic administrators, and they were held accountable for the results. Any clinic with a 5 percent or larger drop from the previous month had to submit a written report with an explanation along with an action plan for improving the score the following month. A 10 percent increase over the previous month *might* get you a "Good job!" or even pizza if the administration was feeling particularly generous.

Exhibit 6.34 shows one clinic's "overall satisfaction" results and summary statistics for 19 months, and Exhibit 6.35 shows the resulting run chart and its analysis.

The runs analysis shows this process to be stable, exhibiting common cause. Over the last 19 months, they have been using as a strategy a meeting discussing *that specific month's* data, which is a special cause strategy.

A control chart analysis will help answer some important additional questions:

- If nothing else changes, what is the typical *range* in the monthly performance so as to avoid overreaction?
  - Have any of the past 19 months been outside of that range, either high or low?
- How much of a difference between two *consecutive* months is considered too much? What is this difference expressed as a percentage of the mean?
  - Is the percent change from the previous month a meaningful measure?

**EXHIBIT 6.35** Run Chart and Runs Analysis of Overall Satisfaction Data: Common Cause

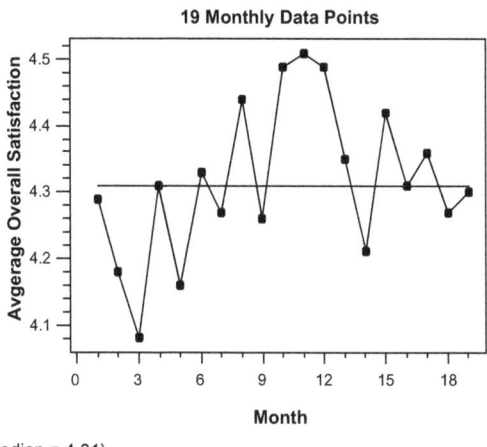

**19 Monthly Data Points**

(Median = 4.31)

No trends of 6 (less than 20 data points) and no runs of length 8.

- When everything that can possibly go wrong does go wrong (and it will), through no fault of the workers, what is the worst score one could expect from this process under normal circumstances?

The moving range and median moving range calculations are shown in Exhibit 6.36. Nineteen data points yield 18 moving ranges, so the median moving range is the average of the 9th and 10th in the sorted sequence.

Once again:

1. If, from a time-ordered sequence of data of any length, the moving ranges are calculated and the median moving range ($MR_{Med}$) is found, then multiplying $MR_{Med}$ by 3.865 (from statistical theory and valid for use with *median* moving range only) will yield the *maximum difference between two consecutive data points that could be attributable to common cause*.

    Given this process, one month can differ from its *immediately preceding* month by as much as:

    $3.865 \times 0.125 = 0.48$

    or 11 percent of the mean. Note that no month-to-month difference came even close to this value.

2. If the $MR_{Med}$ is multiplied by 3.14 (from statistical theory, and, once again, valid only for calculations involving the *median* moving range), this represents the common cause range on either side of the average:

    $4.317 \pm (3.14 \times 0.125) = (3.92 - 4.71)$

    resulting in the chart shown in Exhibit 6.37.

Nothing has changed. We have characterized the current process and know what we are perfectly designed to get, *for people who choose to fill out surveys*. Is that a useful number?

As long as the current process continues, that is, processing a biased sample of data and exhorting people according to treating-common-cause-as-special-cause arbitrary

**EXHIBIT 6.36** ■ Moving Range and Median Moving Range Calculations

| Month | Ov_Sat | MR | MR_Sort |
|---|---|---|---|
| 1 | 4.29 | — | 0.02 |
| 2 | 4.18 | 0.11* | 0.02 |
| 3 | 4.08 | 0.10 | 0.03 |
| 4 | 4.31 | 0.23 | 0.05 |
| 5 | 4.16 | 0.15 | 0.06 |
| 6 | 4.33 | 0.17 | 0.09 |
| 7 | 4.27 | 0.06 | 0.10 |
| 8 | 4.44 | 0.17 | 0.11 |
| 9 | 4.26 | 0.18 | 0.11† |
| 10 | 4.49 | 0.23 | 0.14† |
| 11 | 4.51 | 0.02 | 0.14 |
| 12 | 4.49 | 0.02 | 0.15 |
| 13 | 4.35 | 0.14 | 0.17 |
| 14 | 4.21 | 0.14 | 0.17 |
| 15 | 4.42 | 0.21 | 0.18 |
| 16 | 4.31 | 0.11 | 0.21 |
| 17 | 4.36 | 0.05 | 0.23 |
| 18 | 4.27 | 0.09 | 0.23 |
| 19 | 4.30 | 0.03 | * |

\* (4.18 − 4.29 = −0.11)
† Median Moving Range = (0.11 + 0.14)/2 = 0.125
($MR_{Avg}$ = 0.123)

Note that there are 19 measurements in the data but only 18 moving ranges. There will always be one less moving range than there are data points.

**EXHIBIT 6.37** ■ Control Chart of Overall Satisfaction Data

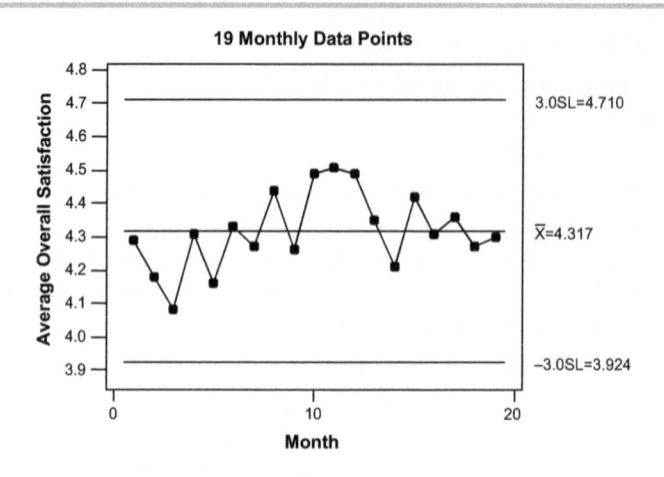

19 Monthly Data Points

3.0SL=4.710
$\bar{X}$=4.317
−3.0SL=3.924

Average Overall Satisfaction
Month

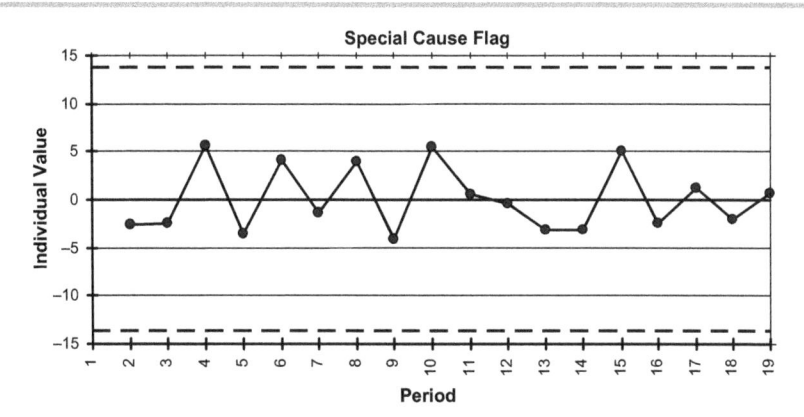

EXHIBIT 6.38 ■ Control Chart of Percentage Change from Previous Month

interpretations, a number will be calculated at the end of the month and be between 3.92 and 4.71. One month can differ from its previous month by as much as approximately 0.5 units. The exhortation has become imbedded into the process. It is *perfectly* designed to get the results it is already getting.

Exhibit 6.38 shows an I-chart of the percentage difference from month to month. Notice the average is zero. The normal monthly variation around that average is approximately 13 percent. What if management felt that things should not change more than plus or minus 5–10 percent month to month? There is high potential for tampering. This is why one should be cautious using two-point comparisons based on percent change.

### What Good Is This and Why Do They Keep Doing It?

I have come to the conclusion that this process is not very enlightening. It is also expensive and creates a lot of unnecessary confusion, conflict, complexity, and chaos (and cost), *so why continue it?* I talk about innovative ways to get customer information and useful customer satisfaction data in Chapter 10.

### Use of Median Moving Range vs. Average Moving Range

Because the process of using the moving range is so intuitive, are some of you wondering whether the *average* moving range could be used? In fact, I am willing to bet that many of you have been taught that technique in past statistical process control seminars. Many I-chart programs indeed default to using the average moving range.

Let me briefly explain the difference. The *process* for creating the chart is virtually the same. The individual moving ranges are calculated as shown before, except one now calculates their *average* instead of median. If so, *different statistical constants* must be used to convert it to the appropriate common cause. This is clarified by the summary instructions for I-chart analysis in Exhibit 6.39.

In the case of the current example using overall satisfaction data, as shown in Exhibit 6.36, the average moving range ($MR_{Avg}$) is 0.123.

- To determine the maximum moving range between two consecutive observations, the constant 3.268 is used (instead of 3.865, which is used with the median moving range).

    In this case, 3.268 × 0.123 = 0.4, the maximum difference between two consecutive months.
- To determine the common cause limits, the constant 2.66 is used (instead of 3.14, which is used with the median moving range).

    In this case, 4.317 ± (2.66 × 0.123) = (3.99 – 4.64).

Statistically, the average moving range is what is called more "efficient." It makes better use of the information in the data. However, as I will show you in the next example, if there are outliers in the data, the average moving range will then be inflated. (Remember: One bad data point produces *two* consecutive large moving ranges.) This results in an inflated estimate of the common cause, which could compromise your ability to find a special cause. The median moving range is robust to outliers.

My point is, do not bog down in mechanics. A good computer package will allow you to use both easily. As you saw in this survey data example, if there are no outliers, there really is not that much difference in the results. With outliers, you usually have no choice but to use the median moving range for the best estimation of limits.

Another thing to consider is if you are in a boring meeting and do not have your computer, the median moving range is much easier to calculate and use by hand.

With a small number of observations, say, fewer than 20, unless there are truly obvious outliers, I tend to favor the average moving range because of the efficiency issue.

I hope you have noted that I have shown you how to calculate common cause by using the moving ranges (either average or median). There has been no mention of the typical spreadsheet calculation of standard deviation that we were all taught in basic statistics. You will see why shortly in some examples (and in Chapter 7). It is important to always initially use a run chart, do not become mired in mechanics, and *think*.

## What Do the Common Cause Limits Represent?

Walter Shewhart, inventor of the control chart, originally designated that common cause limits should be drawn at three standard deviations on either side of the average. This is what results from the calculations I have shown you. They are sometimes referred to as *control limits, three standard deviation limits, three sigma limits*, or, using the numeral and Greek letter, $3\sigma$ *limits*.

In my use of control charts for more than 30 years, Shewhart's empirical wisdom has been confirmed. Astonishingly, he did not rely on elegant mathematical or statistical proofs. Deming often explained that Shewhart merely stipulated that three standard deviations seem to work very well in balancing the risk of the two errors to which I alluded in Chapter 5 and which all traditional statistical courses teach:

- Type I error — Treating a deviation as special cause when it is common cause; and
- Type II error — Failing to recognize a deviation as a special cause and treating it as common cause.

### A Common Trap

I am sure some of you are doing the math and have figured out that two-thirds of the distance between the average and the upper and lower common cause limits represents

**EXHIBIT 6.39** ■ How to Convert a Time-Ordered Sequence of Data into a Control Chart

1. Plot the data points in their naturally occurring time order, and if there are no obvious special causes, find the median and apply the run chart rules.
2. If there are special causes at this point (trends, shifts, too few or too many runs), try to identify the reasons for them. The presence of special causes could, under certain circumstances, invalidate the use of Steps 4–9 if special causes are not accounted for.
3. Compute the moving ranges (MRs) between *naturally occurring adjacent points in time*.
4. Rank these moving ranges in ascending order and determine the **median moving range ($MR_{Med}$)** (or find the average moving range [$MR_{Avg}$], especially if you have <20 data points).
5. Multiply **$MR_{Med}$** by 3.865 (or $MR_{Avg}$ by 3.268).
   - If any *individual* moving range exceeds this value, chances are your process showed a significant shift (special cause) at that point.
   - *Two consecutive* special cause moving ranges typically signal the presence of an outlier. (If this happens using the $MR_{Avg}$, it is highly advisable to redo the calculations using the $MR_{Med}$.)
6. **Only if the runs analysis showed no special causes,** calculate the average of all the data. Otherwise, calculate the appropriate average of the data based on your runs analysis.
7. Multiply **$MR_{Med}$** by 3.14 (or $MR_{Avg}$ by 2.66) and:
   - Add this quantity, that is, **3.14 × $MR_{Med}$** (or 2.66 × $MR_{Avg}$), to the average calculated in Step 6 (this is the upper control limit for common cause), then,
   - Subtract this quantity from the average calculated in Step 7 (this is the lower control limit for common cause).

   **Important: Do NOT use "3× (standard deviation of the data set)" for common cause.**

   The area between these two limits represents the region where you **expect** your data to fall if only common cause is present. They are based on 3 standard deviations, calculated correctly.

   Any point outside of these limits represents a special cause acting on the system.
8. Look for any obvious patterns or peculiarities in the pattern such as cycles, clusters close to the limits, or any other direct process influences such as known interventions.
9. *Keep using runs analysis when subsequent data points are plotted.*

*Note:* I prefer using the median moving range. As you can see, the appropriate constants for the common cause calculations using the average moving range are also shown above. Most books (and intuition) say to use the average moving range, but remember, *one bad data point produces two consecutive bad moving ranges*, potentially *inflating* the true common cause when the average of the moving ranges is taken. The *process* is the same regardless of which is used; only the statistical constants used differ. Most good programs will allow either option to be used with ease. I generally go with the one that gives me the narrower set of limits. If the number of data points is less than 20, I tend to favor the average moving range.

*Regardless, do not use the traditional standard deviation of all the data.*

two standard deviations from the average (sometimes called "two sigma limits"). *Two sigma* (sometimes also incorrectly called *95 percent confidence*) is a concept with which we are all familiar from basic statistics.

For many people, two standard deviations is an ironclad rule of thumb for declaring "significance" (*alleged* 5 percent risk of treating a common cause as if it were a special cause). It is not uncommon to see people use two standard deviations (or even one) instead of three when constructing control charts. This is not without serious risk. It dramatically increases the probability of incurring a Type I error.

People seem to forget that when they are taught decision making in a typical statistics course, they are applying a decision rule to *one decision only* from a data set designed specifically to test a difference. In this case, the 95 percent confidence strategy implicit in using two standard deviations does yield a 5 percent risk of treating a common cause as if it were special: It is the *only* decision being made.

More discussion of this issue occurs later in the section "Some Other Helpful Special Cause Rules" as well as in Chapter 7.

### Calculating the Common Cause Standard Deviation

Should you desire to know what the actual standard deviation is, it can be easily calculated from either the average moving range ($MR_{Avg}$) or median moving range ($MR_{Med}$) as follows:

$$\text{Process common cause standard deviation} = [(MR_{Med})/0.954] \text{ or } [(MR_{Avg})/1.128]$$

As with all of the other control chart constants described so far, the constants in these denominators are derived from statistical theory.

### Expect Occasional Points Near the Limits

Let me revisit the traffic light example from Chapter 2 — percentage conformance to a goal performance — to make several points in this and the next section. Exhibit 6.40 shows the control chart of percent conformance to meeting a goal of time to seeing patients.

The 10th observation is very close to the lower control limit. When I originally showed people this graph, they got defensive about that point, "But Davis, we had two doctors on leave and two of our nurses called in sick!"

As usual, people have no trouble explaining things after the fact and it was probably true; however, as I have been emphasizing, that does not necessarily make it a special cause. I then asked them, "If you have 200 people working in an emergency department, could it happen that you have two doctors out on leave and, due to sheer bad luck, it also happens that two nurses also call in sick that week? In a department of 200 people, could that happen?" They generally answer, "Yes," to which I then ask, "Can you predict when it's going to happen?" and they usually say "No." Well, it happened — the "week from hell," when everything that can go wrong did go wrong.

### Don't Forget Common Cause Strategies

Let me change Exhibit 6.40 a bit, which yields Exhibit 6.41.

I worked with a hospital that had an emergency department policy that there were never to be more than two doctors on leave at any one time. This chart has no points

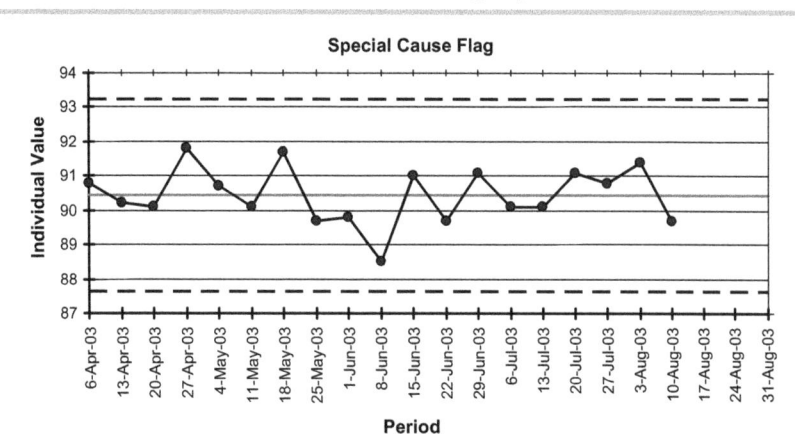

EXHIBIT 6.40 ■ Stable Process of Accident and Emergency

EXHIBIT 6.41 ■ Control Chart of Accident and Emergency Performance

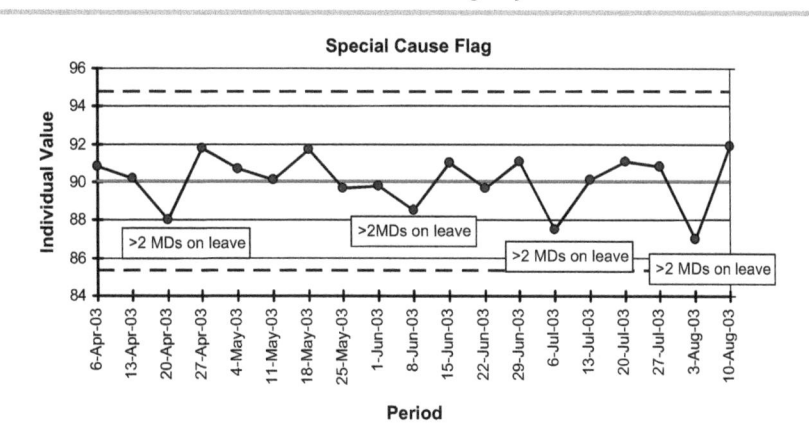

outside the limits, and none of the moving ranges exceed $MR_{Max}$, calculated from $MR_{Med}$ to be 3.2.

Suppose that, on further investigation of their low performance weeks, *every* one coincided with having more than two doctors on leave and those were the only weeks with more than two doctors on leave. In other words, there is a *pattern* to the low performance weeks; it is always the same reason. An underlying special cause has been exposed: The policy is justified, but *the process of enforcement* is not consistent.

Special causes can be present even if the points stay within the common cause limits and do not form a statistical pattern. In this instance, worker knowledge of the process was key.

**EXHIBIT 6.42** ■ Intervention: Point Outside Upper Limit

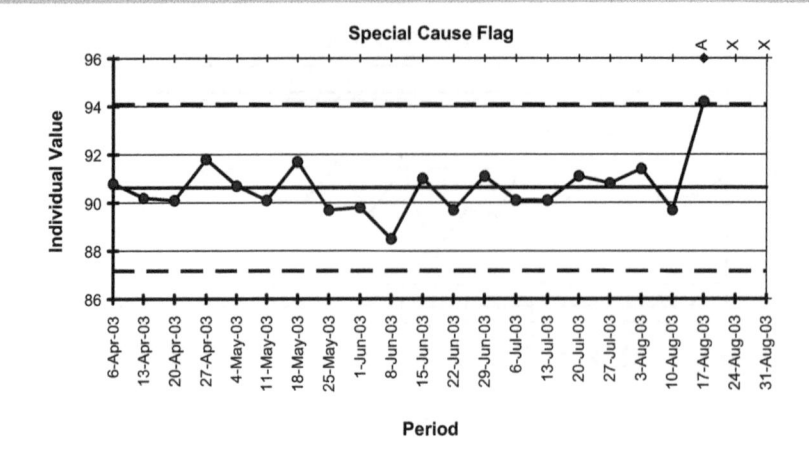

*Special Cause Flag chart showing Individual Value (y-axis, 86–96) vs Period (6-Apr-03 through 31-Aug-03). Most points hover around 90–92, with a spike to ~94 on 17-Aug-03 (flagged A) and X marks on 24-Aug-03 and 31-Aug-03.*

**EXHIBIT 6.43** ■ Intervention: Point Inside Upper Limit, but Significant Moving Range

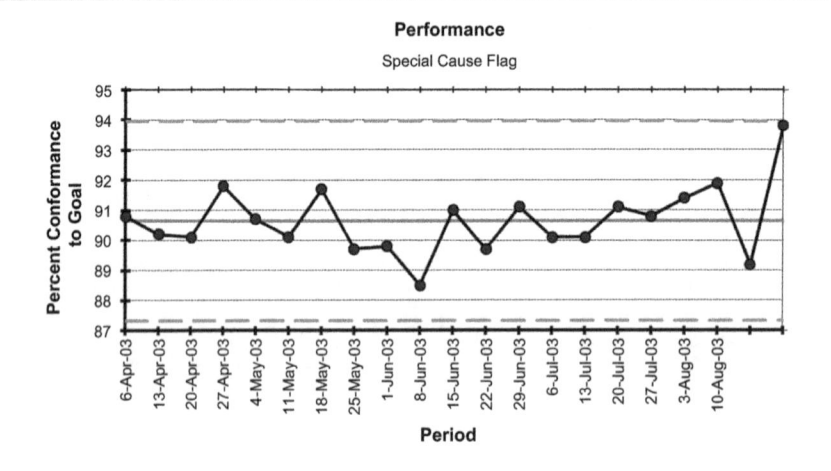

*Performance / Special Cause Flag chart showing Percent Conformance to Goal (y-axis, 87–95) vs Period (6-Apr-03 through 10-Aug-03). Values range around 88–92, ending with a rise to ~94.*

### Some Other Helpful Special Cause Rules

There are indeed other rules to declare special causes besides one observation outside of three standard deviations. They also involve less risk than merely using strictly a two standard deviations criterion. Continuing with the traffic light example, I demonstrate some other commonly used special cause tests.

The stable baseline graph was shown in Exhibit 6.40. Suppose a common cause strategy was applied to the nonconformances: there has been an intervention, and it is desired to know whether it worked as soon as possible.

Exhibit 6.42 is the best-case scenario: The week following the intervention, the result goes outside the upper limit — the desired direction — indicating a special cause, and success.

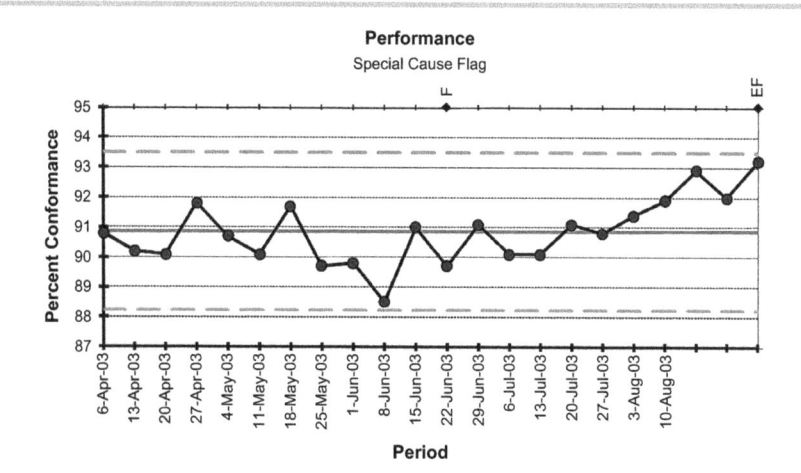

EXHIBIT 6.44 ■ Intervention: Two-out-of-Three Rule

**Performance**
Special Cause Flag

Exhibit 6.43 is also a successful scenario: Despite the fact that the result does not go outside the upper limit, its moving range relative to the previous week is greater than $MR_{Max}$. This indicates a significant shift in the desired direction, probably not due to common cause.

Exhibit 6.44 shows a very common scenario. The first week after the intervention, the result is above two standard deviations from the average. This is promising, but it could happen randomly. The next week contains a discouraging drop in performance. However, the third week's performance, although not outside the upper limit, goes back to being above two standard deviations from the average.

This is called the "two-out-of-three" rule: Two out of three consecutive data points are farther than two standard deviations away from the average. This is a strong indication that the needle has shifted in that direction. Most good control chart software programs have this rule programmed into them.

There is a more subtle version of this test that is programmed in many statistical packages. It is known as the "four-out-of-five" rule; that is observing five *consecutive* observations, four of which are greater than *one* standard deviation away from the average. In my experience, I have found this rule to occur as a false-positive quite a bit during an initial informal perusal of a data set. People also seem to find it confusing and hard to investigate. However, I have no problems using it as a primary test on data *immediately after a process intervention.*

Financial people love to play "gotcha" with me by saying, "I can't wait for seven periods to declare a trend." Well, the graph in Exhibit 6.45 shows only a trend of five (four successive increases) with all of the data still within the three standard deviation limits. However, the fact that the last two trigger the two-out-of-three rule would seem to show the intervention to be effective.

Actually, it has become acceptable over the past few years to relax the trend rule to three or four successive increases or decreases to declare a successful intervention ***only if*** the data points occur *immediately* after a formal intervention whose intent was to move the process needle *specifically* in the observed direction, which was true with this data. Similarly, one can also relax the rule of "eight in a row either all above or below the

EXHIBIT 6.45 ■ Who Says You Have to Wait for Seven or Eight?

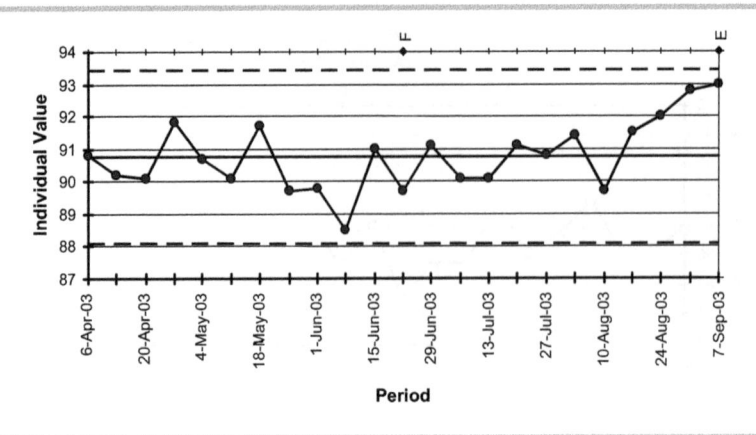

median" to "five or six in a row" above or below the median *only if* the run of five or six occurs immediately after a formal intervention whose intent was to move the process needle specifically in the observed direction.

So you see, one is not necessarily handcuffed by using three standard deviations for common cause limits as much as initially thought. It is also a way, in Shewhart's wisdom, of having an *overall* probability of error of approximately 0.05.

Think of it this way: These graphs have about 20 data points, so you are in essence making 20 simultaneous decisions. To look at it another way, ask, "What is the probability that all 20 data points would be within plus or minus two standard deviations?" It's $(0.95)^{20}$, which equals 0.358. In other words, there is an approximate 36 percent chance that all 20 data points will be within plus or minus two standard deviations, which means that there is a 64 percent chance (100 − 36 = 64) that *at least one data point* out of the 20 will be greater than two standard deviations away from the average. Would you like to take that risk of tampering?

Three standard deviation limits cover approximately 99 to 100 percent of the stable territory. In an equivalent calculation to the previous paragraph, the probability of all 20 data points being within plus or minus three standard deviations is, using normal distribution theory (which may not necessarily apply, but it is good enough), approximately $(0.997)^{20}$, which equals 0.942. So, even with the conservative three standard deviations scriterion, there is still a 6 percent chance that at least one data point out of the 20 could be greater than three standard deviations away from the average, which is pretty darn close to the gold standard of 5 percent. I talk more about the two vs. three standard deviations criterion conundrum regarding multiple simultaneous decision-making in Chapter 7.

I once again want to reiterate that, even though a control chart uses three standard deviations for its limits, this does not mean that it is equivalent to taking the standard deviation of the data (as defined in most statistical texts) and multiplying it by three. As I show in the next example, the presence of a special cause in the data has the potential to seriously inflate this typical estimate. If the common cause estimate is inflated, it will hinder the ability to find special causes in the process.

Unfortunately, this is commonly done, which results in people using two, or even one, standard deviation criteria for declaring outliers. Many times, calculating the standard deviation *correctly*, as I have shown in this chapter, yields three standard deviation limits that can actually be narrower than the one or two standard deviation limits obtained from the standard basic calculation everyone is taught.

Never use a spreadsheet calculation of the standard deviation to establish control limits. And do not even consider any computer package or freeware that uses it exclusively; this practice is more common than you would think. I show what might be considered an exception in Appendix 7A at the end of Chapter 7, but this application is for the more advanced practitioner.

The following examples are typical of everyday data I encounter that present opportunities to use statistical thinking. I hope they will show you how to go beyond techniques to get clearer insight into a situation and lead to more productive subsequent conversations and action.

### *The Medication Error Data Example*

Exhibit 6.46 shows the actual data (and resulting moving ranges) from the medication error scenario described in Chapter 2. The run chart of these data demonstrated common cause (see Exhibit 2.14), and a subsequent application of a common cause strategy saw a pattern to the high values — they all occurred in July.

This example helps make several points. I will begin by showing an alleged control chart whose limits are based on the traditional calculation of the standard deviation of all 36 observations: 12.91.

Exhibit 6.47 demonstrates the point I made in the previous section: Note that all of the data lie within the limits, which many people would incorrectly interpret (and teach) as having no special causes. This is why I like teaching run charts (as well as control charts) within a context of also teaching common cause strategies. Many seminars skip run charts and go right to control charts.

It's very easy to bog down in the technical minutiae without teaching good interpretation. Seminar participants can be left with the impression that the only rule one uses to determine special causes is whether individual data points lie outside the calculated limits. They do not know how to apply the other tests. I have seen these issues time and time again. Many seminars and statistical packages totally miss the underlying need for interpretation. As a result, confusion, poor use, and misinformation propagate.

From the run chart analysis, knowing that Julys are special causes means that the moving ranges involving Julys are not random. They reflect the difference in July's process vis-à-vis the process of the other 11 months. Hence, the six moving ranges involving Julys — (28, 49), (31, 26), and (26, 44) — seriously inflate the estimate of the standard deviation as reflected in the estimates using the usual spreadsheet calculation (12.91) and average moving range (11.97 yielding a standard deviation of 11.97/1.128 = 10.6).

Using the median moving range, 8, which is robust to these six outliers:

1. The best estimate of the underlying common cause standard deviation is (8/0.954 = 8.4), which is a reduction of more than 25 percent from the other two estimates.

2. If one calculates the maximum moving range due to common cause, (3.865 × 8 ≈ 31), it calls one's attention to the moving ranges associated with July.

3. Calculating the control limits (51 – 101), it calls attention to two of the three Julys (110, 97, 112) (Exhibit 6.48).

To the credit of the average moving range, its calculated upper control chart limit of 108 and maximum moving range of 39 (3.268 × 11.97) would also have called attention

## EXHIBIT 6.46 — Medication Error Data and Moving Ranges

|  | 2000 | MR | 2001 | MR | 2002 | MR |
|---|---|---|---|---|---|---|
| January | 74 | — | 75 | 3 | 71 | 11 |
|  | 70 | 4 | 63 | 12 | 68 | 3 |
|  | 67 | 3 | 71 | 8 | 80 | 12 |
|  | 65 | 2 | 59 | 12 | 97 | 17 |
|  | 63 | 2 | 70 | 11 | 87 | 10 |
|  | 82 | 19 | 66 | 4 | 86 | 1 |
| July | 110 | 28 | 97 | 31 | 112 | 26 |
|  | 61 | 49 | 71 | 26 | 68 | 44 |
|  | 75 | 14 | 84 | 13 | 76 | 8 |
|  | 78 | 3 | 85 | 1 | 76 | 0 |
|  | 76 | 2 | 57 | 28 | 77 | 1 |
|  | 78 | 2 | 60 | 3 | 71 | 6 |

**Descriptive Statistics**

|  | Mean | Median | St Dev | Min | Max |
|---|---|---|---|---|---|
| Med_err | 75.72 | 74.5 | 12.91 | 57 | 112 |
| MR | 11.97 | 8 | — | 0 | 49 |

## EXHIBIT 6.47 — Incorrect Control Chart of Medication Error Data Using Overall Standard Deviation

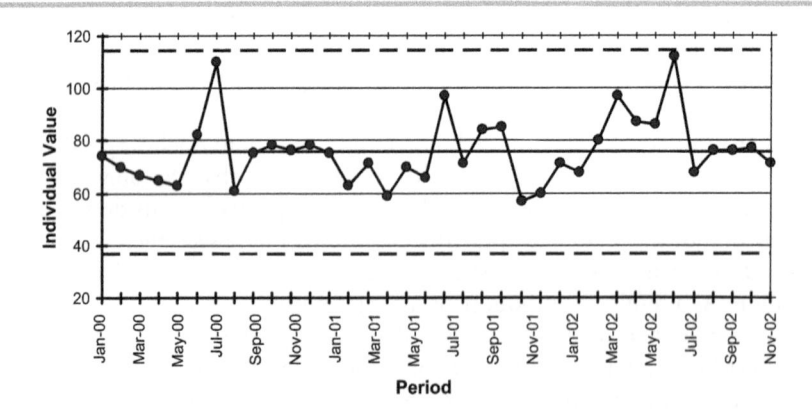

to the July data as well. This should then motivate recalculations using the median moving range.

### Another Example of Inflated Control Limits

#### The C-Section Scenario

I once attended a meeting where the quality director wanted to establish a standard because, at the time, people thought there were "too many" cesarean sections (C-sections). Four years — 48 months — of hospital C-section data was presented in the bar graph format in Exhibit 6.49. I see this often (as well as, of course, the summary stats in Exhibit 6.50). People intuitively seem to want to group the data by month and plot all the Januarys

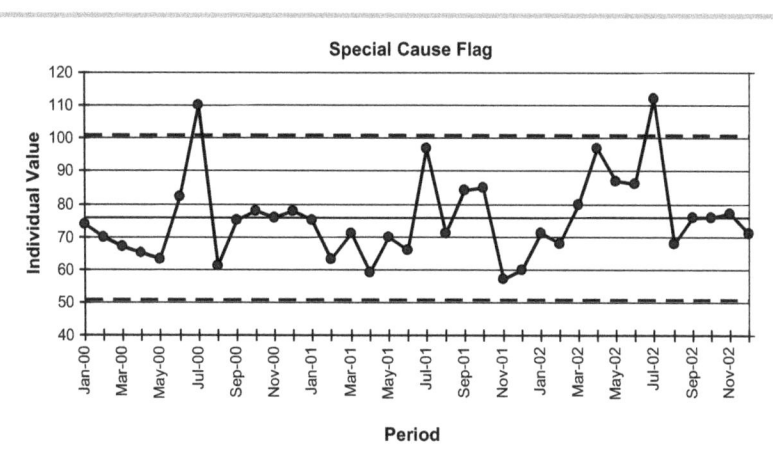

EXHIBIT 6.48 ■ Correct Control Chart of Medication Error Data Using Median Moving Range to Calculate Limits

together, all the Februarys together, and so forth, because they feel strongly that it is only fair to compare similar months. What is the theory?

When I press people who present data like this as to how this is helpful, many times with a profound look, they say in earnestness, "Seasonality" (stated reason). Instead they should say, "Because I have no idea and that's the way we've always done it" (real reason; darn humans).

Assuming the presence of seasonality in the data — certain months being consistently different from other months in the same pattern regardless of the year — implies special causes. If a smart person theorizes them to be present and looks for them, the odds of finding them are pretty high even if they are not there. Suppose there is only common cause? The potential for tampering exists again.

I will show my thought process as I approached this data, but first, I want to make you aware of some common incorrect practices that are routinely being taught by incompetent practitioners (whom Deming unabashedly called "hacks"). It's not a matter of "if" you encounter them, but "when," and you may want to bookmark sections of this chapter when one of these hacks tries to nullify your hard work and make you doubt your abilities.

### A Little Knowledge Is a Dangerous Thing

Let's say we have three quality practitioners. Practitioner 1 would like to do a control chart of this data and will base his decision to do so on the result of testing the data for normality. Since it "passes" ($p$-value of 0.412), he constructs a control chart using the average plus or minus three standard deviations ($3 \times 2.23 = 6.7$), based on the summary in Exhibit 6.50. He notices that none of the points are outside the limits, so he feels justified in now using a two standard deviations criterion (two-thirds the width of the current limits) and, as a result, declares months 9, 12, 13, and 31 as individual special causes needing investigation because they are outside the limits.

Practitioner 2 recently took a class on control charts that said the overall standard deviation of the data must *never* be used. Rather, the common cause variation should be

**EXHIBIT 6.49** ■ Typical Year-over-Year Seasonality Bar Graph of C-Section Data

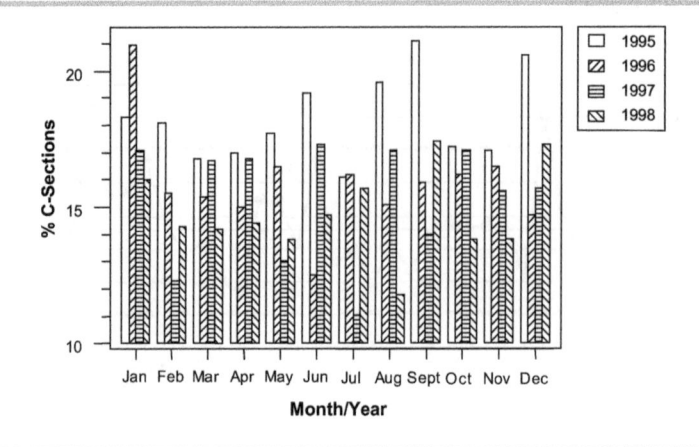

**EXHIBIT 6.50** ■ Summary Statistics of C-Section Data

|         | N  | Mean   | Median | Tr Mean | St Dev | SE Mean |
|---------|----|--------|--------|---------|--------|---------|
| % C-Sect| 48 | 16.046 | 16.150 | 16.030  | 2.230  | 0.322   |

|         | Min  | Max  | Q1     | Q3     |
|---------|------|------|--------|--------|
| % C-Sect| 11.0 | 21.1 | 14.475 | 17.175 |

based on the *average* moving range. For this data, the width of the three standard deviation limits on either side of the data average becomes (2.66 × 2.145 = 5.7). There are no points outside the control limits, so this person concludes there are no special causes.

Practitioner 3 recently read a book that said to use the *median* moving range to calculate the common cause variation, which in this case would be (3.14 × 1.5 = 4.7). Months 9, 13, and 31 are outside the limits. Practitioner 1 is confused because the conclusion based on these three standard deviation limits is almost the same as his conclusion based on two standard deviation limits.

The three charts are shown in Exhibit 6.51 in their respective order from top to bottom. All these charts and resulting conclusions are well-meaning, but wrong, as will be explained next.

*Another Incorrect Use of the Myth of Needing Normality*

Wheeler said, "Whenever the teachers lack understanding, superstitious nonsense is inevitable. Until you learn to separate myth from fact you will be fair game for those who were taught the nonsense."[2] Although the control chart constants are created under the assumption of normally distributed data, the control chart technique is essentially insensitive to this assumption. The normality of the data is neither a prerequisite nor a consequence of statistical control.

**EXHIBIT 6.51** ■ Control Chart Comparison Using Three Different Estimates of Standard Deviation

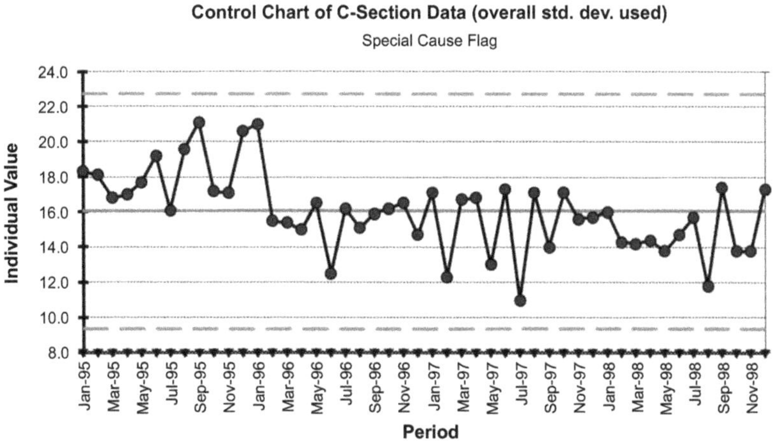

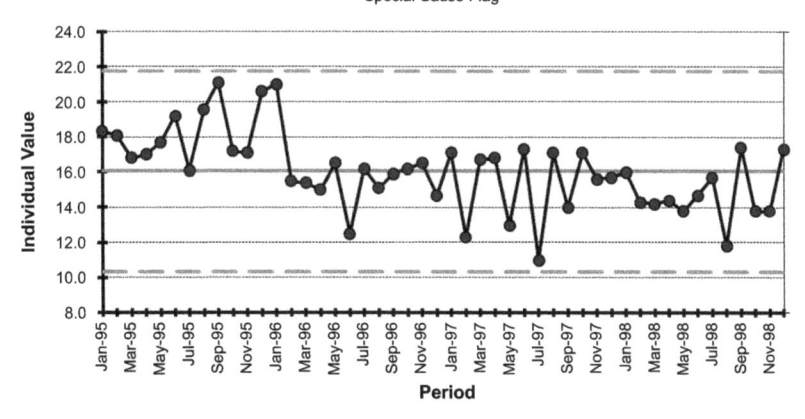

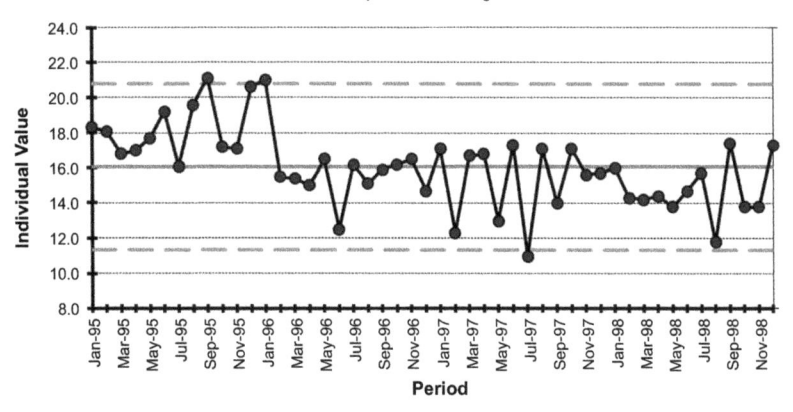

**Control Chart of C-Section Data (overall std. dev. used)**
Special Cause Flag

**Control Chart of C-Section Data (average MR used)**
Special Cause Flag

**Control Chart of C-Section Data (median MR used)**
Special Cause Flag

### The Myth of Three Standard Deviations Being Too Conservative

Shewhart, the originator of the control chart, *deliberately* chose three standard deviation limits. He is quoted by Wheeler as saying, "the justification for a technique does not depend on a fine ancestry of highbrow statistical theorems, but rather upon empirical evidence that it works."[3] He wanted limits wide enough so that people wouldn't waste time interpreting noise as signals (a Type I error). He also wanted limits narrow enough to detect an important signal that people shouldn't miss (avoiding a Type II error). In years of practice he found, *empirically*, that three standard deviation limits, *calculated correctly*, provided a satisfactory balance between these two mistakes. My experience has borne this out as well.

### The Myth of "So Let's Use Two Standard Deviations Instead"

The "two standard deviations" criterion, sometimes incorrectly called 95 percent confidence, for (alleged) significance has been drummed into peoples' heads as the gold standard for decision making. This reasoning is based on the central limit theorem (which I purposely haven't mentioned) and making *only one* decision. A chart is making as many decisions as there are data points, which is an invitation to randomness to make something look significant, as it inevitably will.

People oftentimes resort to this criterion when they have performed an incorrect calculation of the standard deviation that has (unknowingly) resulted in an inflated estimate. They typically use the readily available basic calculation taught in an introductory statistics course, which is *inappropriate* for the analytic statistics approach or, for that matter, virtually any real-world data set. I have seen people even use *one* standard deviation, calculated this way, as a criterion for outliers.

The bottom line is, don't sacrifice the rationality of data analysis to superstition. The additional myths that only the data points outside the control limits are important or that each special cause signal must be individually investigated (treating each signal as a special cause) is explained in the following sidebar, which once again debunks the myth of trends.

### Importance of the Run Chart

My analysis approach to the C-section monthly performance data will show: (1) the wisdom of first doing a run chart as opposed to jumping right to either a statistical analysis or control chart; (2) the uselessness of bar graph presentation; and (3) making the point that, to quote the wisdom of the late famous applied statistician Ellis Ott: "First you plot the data, then you plot the data, then you plot the data, then you *think*!"[4] In fact, as you will see, the issue of seasonality is moot; something else was going on.

As you know, one of the most powerful rules in analyzing a process run chart is looking for a cluster of eight consecutive data points either all above or below the median. This indicates the presence of a process shift somewhere in the data, usually somewhere at the beginning of the run of eight. However, as you will see in the run chart of the four years of monthly data in Exhibit 6.52, this isn't always necessarily true.

Observations 35–44 are below the median, but this doesn't necessarily mean that a special cause occurred there, only that the process exhibited at least one shift during the time frame. The goal is to avoid statistical dogmatism and, instead, use one's knowledge of process history to determine where an event may have occurred to cause a shift. I hope it has now become obvious to you that something happened after observation 13. Observations 1–13 did not exhibit a run of eight above the median anywhere because

## Control Charts: Simple Elegance or Legalized Torture?

For all the talk about the power of control charts, I can empathize when those taking mandated courses on quality tools are left puzzled. When I look at training materials or books, their tendency is to bog down heavily in the mechanics of construction without offering a clue about interpretation. Some seminars even teach all seven control charts. And then there is the inevitable torturous discussion of "special cause tests" (usually the eight Western Electric rules). People are then left even more confused. Does each test signal need to be individually investigated, that is, treated as a special cause? Not to worry — most people usually investigate only the points outside the control limits. The focus tends to be on individual observations. But what if there is one underlying explanation generating many of these signals that has nothing to do with individual outliers, for example, a step change?

Someone once presented me with the graph shown in Figure 1, which nearly convinces you that there is a trend.

I can almost picture Six Sigma Black Belt A scolding them: "Test the data for normality, and if it passes, you need to plot that as a control chart." Note that it does indeed pass ($p$-value = 0.507), but the test is totally inappropriate and irrelevant.

Using standard control chart software that also performs the eight Western Electric tests, the individuals' chart for percentage conformance is shown in Figure 2.

Look at all those special causes in Figure 2 shown on the top line of the graph. Sixteen of the 52 data points generate 30 signals. Where should you start? Many people would investigate the four points outside the three standard deviation limits (observations 9 and 50–52).

Then Black Belt B says, "The control chart needs to be adjusted for the trend." There's plenty of customer-friendly software that will do just that (Figure 3).

That was obviously the solution. Figure 3 shows we're down from 30 special cause signals to 7. Better still, there are no data points outside the limits. Now what? Perhaps investigate each signal, but which one do you start with? And what do we do with observations with more than one signal? As I've said many times, the computer will do anything you want.

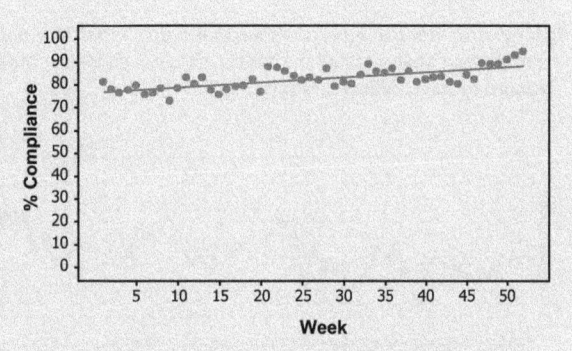

Figure 1. Trend Analysis of Percentage Goal Compliance

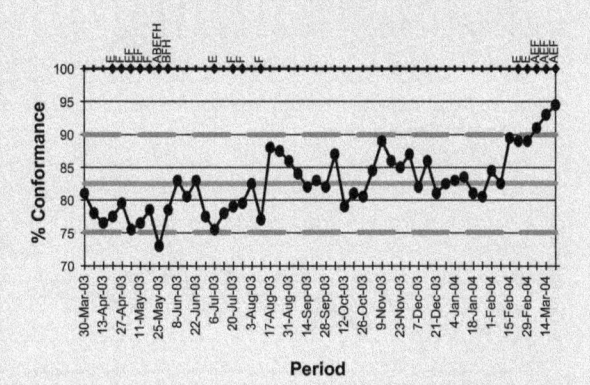

Figure 2. Individuals' Chart of Percentage Conformance to Goal

(Continues)

(Continued)

Trend lines and bar graphs seem to be the two ubiquitous tools that people use for (alleged) analysis. Regression was my favorite course in graduate school, but I rarely use it. In my 30 years as a statistical practitioner, I have never seen an appropriate use of a trend line on data from a service industry (e.g., healthcare) plotted over time.

Over the years, I have developed an increasing affection for the much-neglected run chart: a time plot of your process data with the median (not the average) drawn in as a reference. It is "filter 1" for any process data and answers the question: "Did this process have at least one shift during this time period?" (This is generally signaled by a clump of eight consecutive data points either all above or below the median.) If it did, then it makes no sense to do a control chart at this time because the overall average of all these data doesn't exist.

All the time, I hear people say, "We use run charts," but I see very few of them. It's generally taught as a boring prelude to the (allegedly) more important and powerful control chart. Usually that is left to the end of the training because it is the most difficult, which further complicates matters. So they stumble by rote through the hand calculations of each of the seven chart types and are then assured that they can now use their company's designated computer software to generate future charts, aided by the smart software add-in of guiding one to the allegedly correct chart.

Many computer packages don't generate run charts. Why not jump right to the more advanced control chart analysis of all the data? One can then look at the special cause signals and try to find reasons for each individual signal.

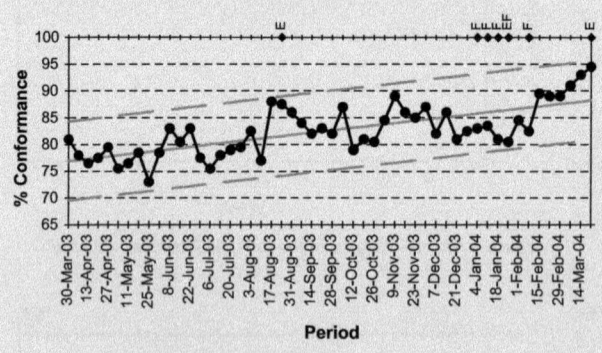

**Figure 3. Trend-Adjusted Percentage Conformance to Goal with Seven Special Cause Signals**

The run chart does not find individual special cause observations, but that is not its purpose. The control chart is "filter 2," plotting the data after the shifts have been determined, which then usually reduces the number of special cause signals and results in a lot less confusion.

What does the run chart of these data in Figure 4 tell us?

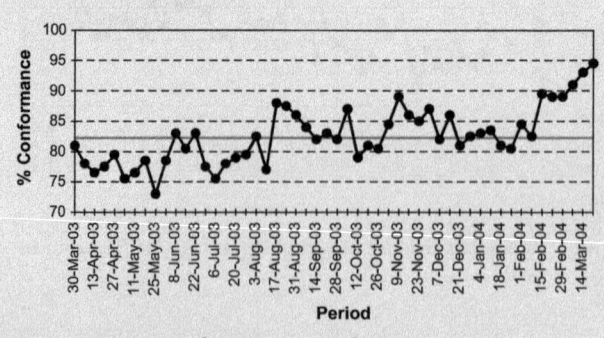

**Figure 4. Run Chart of Percentage Conformance to Goal**

With the y-axis scale a lot healthier and no control limits as a distraction, doesn't it look like the process "needle" shifted twice — around August 17 (observation 21) and February 15 (observation 47)? In fact, when I asked the clients about those two dates, they looked at me like I was a magician and asked, "How did you know?" Those dates

(Continues)

(Continued)

coincided with two major interventions to improve this process. As the chart in Figure 4 shows, they worked; two distinct needle bumps (step-change special cause), not a continuously increasing improvement trend.

In other words, a process goes from what it is "perfectly designed" to get with its original inputs and transitions to what it is "perfectly designed" to get based on the new inputs. It eventually settles in to the new average based on these inputs. This also puts the trend special cause test (six successive increases or decreases) into perspective: A step change can manifest as a trend during the transition. It won't continue.

The correct resulting control chart is shown in Figure 5, and there's not a special cause to be found (other than the programmed step changes).

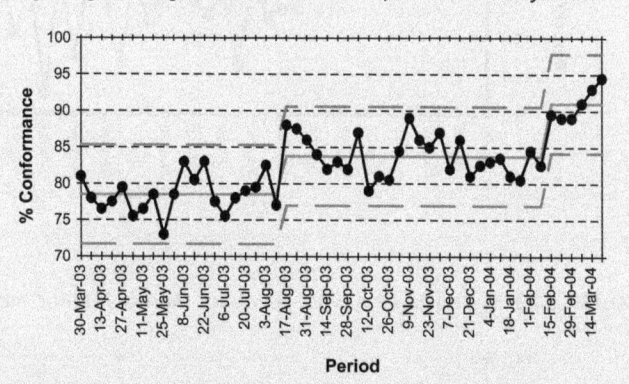

Figure 5. Percentage Conformance to Goal sans Special Cause

### Interpretation

Their original performance was 78.5 percent. Their first intervention improved the process to 83.8 percent, and their second intervention improved that further to 91 percent. They had recently started yet another intervention, and based on the last four data points, it looks relatively promising. What would indicate success?

1. There are three immediate increases. Two or three more would be good evidence (trend transition).

2. Maybe a weekly performance will go outside the upper limit (97.8%).

3. Maybe the next four to six weeks will all be above the average (91%).

4. Two out of three consecutive weeks' performances will be between 95.5 percent (two standard deviations above the average) and 97.8 percent (three standard deviations' upper limit). This is a very useful test known as the *two-out-of-three rule*.

And, not to overreact, if performance goes down from one week to the next, be advised that it could differ as much as 8.4 percent from the previous week simply due to common cause (upper limit of the moving range chart). What could be simpler if taught correctly?

Once again, I'm beginning to understand Deming's curmudgeonliness and his hatred of what he termed statistical "hacks."

How many hours are you spending in meetings looking at trends?

Source: Adapted from Davis Balestracci. 2014. "Control Charts: Simple Elegance or Legalized Torture? Once Again, I'm Beginning to Understand Deming's Hatred of Statistical 'Hacks.'" *Quality Digest* (January). www.qualitydigest.com/inside/quality-insider-column/control-charts-simple-elegance-or-legalized-torture.html.

228　　CHAPTER 6

EXHIBIT 6.52 ■ Run Chart of Monthly Department C-Section Rate (all data)

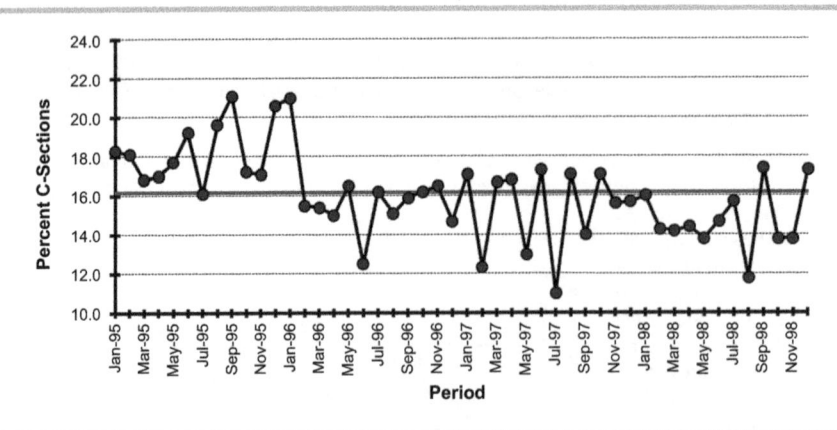

EXHIBIT 6.53 ■ Run Chart of Post-Feedback Monthly Department C-Section Rate

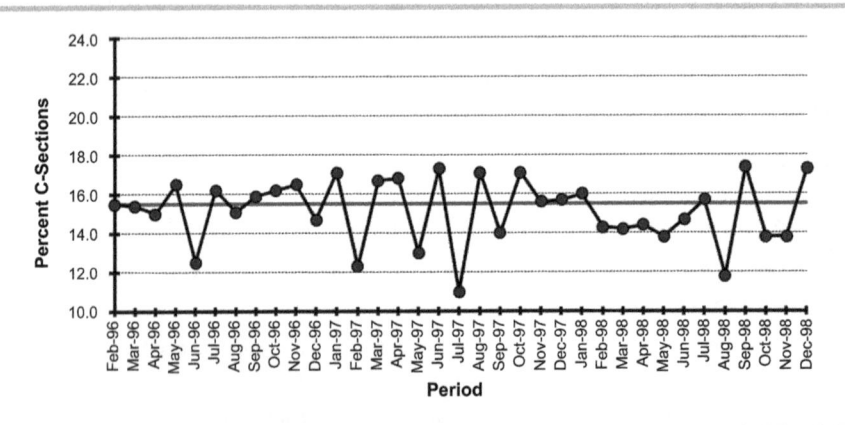

observation 7, as luck would have it, was below the median. However, the observed step change shift is such a strong signal that it manifested elsewhere.

In quality improvement, a good analysis always suggests the next question. Upon inquiry about what happened at month 13, I learned that the doctors had begun getting feedback on their individual C-section rates, which seems to have had an effect.

This process actually had two averages, which (1) rendered the initial test for normality worthless, (2) yielded three charts each with the wrong average, and (3) inflated the standard deviation calculated in the traditional manner.

Because the data exhibit the behavior of two "systems" (one of 13 months and one of 35 months), the next logical question is whether a run chart of the latter remains stable after the obvious change (Exhibit 6.53).

The process shifted in performance from 18.4 percent (average of observations 1–13) to 15.2 percent (average of observations 14–48), and Exhibit 6.54 shows it currently in statistical control, that is, stable and predictable, in an expected monthly range approximately between 10 and 20 percent.

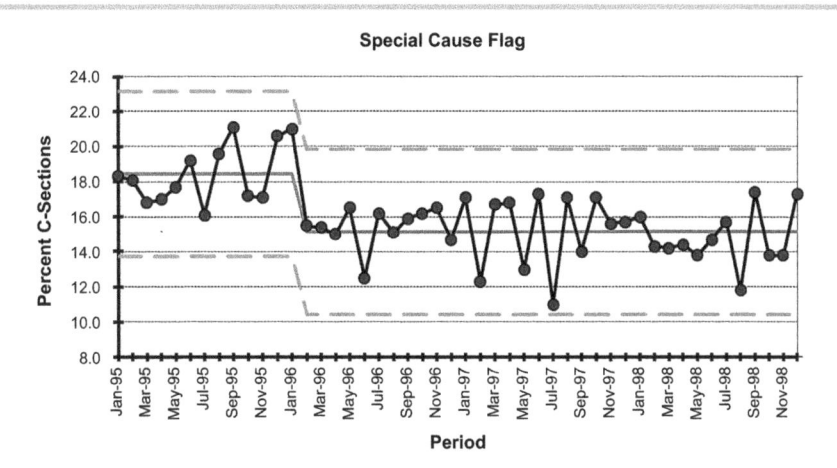

EXHIBIT 6.54 ■ Correct Control Chart Presentation of C-Section Data

*Special Cause Flag chart showing Percent C-Sections from Jan-95 to Nov-98, with a step change at approximately Jan-96, and control limits adjusted accordingly.*

Never underestimate the power of initially plotting any set of data in its naturally occurring time order and using a run chart analysis to see whether you have the privilege of calculating the average. As I hope you learned from this C-section scenario, you will begin asking different and more relevant questions. The initial question asking what the C-section standard should be is wrong. Note that consideration of this neither came up in this analysis nor, in the end, was it relevant. Bar graphs, normality tests, and static summaries are virtually worthless as initial analyses.

This C-section data set will be further analyzed and discussed in the next chapter with yet another *new conversation*. These are not the typical conversations resulting from enforcement of an arbitrarily chosen standard, which usually reacts to the latest numbers and treats deviations from the standard as special causes.

As I see so often done, I also put the data into a standard control chart package that is programmed with what are considered to be the eight standard special cause tests (sometimes called the Western Electric tests or Nelson rules; see my 2008 article titled "How Do You Treat Special-Cause Signals?" under Resources). This resulting chart gave 15 special cause signals. Yet, intelligent use of an initial run chart of the 48 observations made it clear that there was only *one* signal — the step change at observation 13.

When the data were summarized in the I-chart shown in Exhibit 6.54 allowing for that one special cause, no further special cause signals were obtained.

## Another Bar Graph and a Lesson about "Count" Data

The bar graph at the top of Exhibit 6.55 was briefly introduced in Lesson 5 of Chapter 2. It was presented during a hospital quarterly meeting to discuss hospital-acquired infections. The initial reaction of one board member was to scream, "After that downward trend in improvement the middle three years, I demand to know why it went up this past year even before we got the fourth quarter of data!" Board member number 2 was a bit more benevolent: "I understand the concern, but is the overall trend going in the right direction?" This is allegedly addressed by the bottom graph. What do you think?

**EXHIBIT 6.55** ■ Bacteremia Bar Graph and Typical Trend Analysis

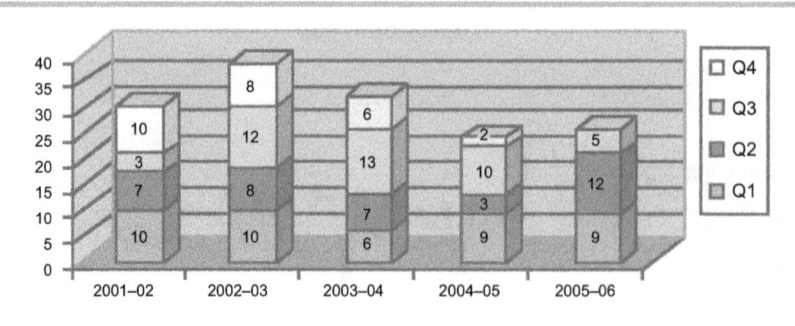

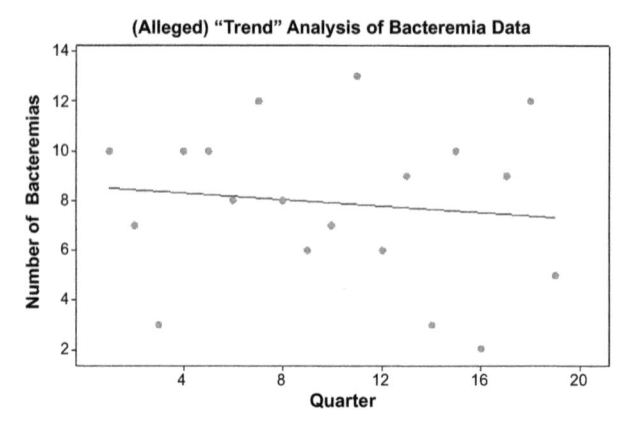

After lengthy discussions about the current trend, individual incidents from the reported quarter were considered. Because the number of infections is relatively small, there is a tendency at these meetings to pull the charts of the patients involved, look at each individually, maybe even apply a root cause analysis, and develop a solution to implement systemwide. It is a special cause strategy.

I considered the data as a 19 separate "dots" and plotted a run chart (Exhibit 6.56). The run chart shows no trends and no runs of eight in a row all above or below the median. This shows there is common cause.

It is easy to obtain the median moving range of 4 (shown in Exhibit 6.57), which yields the I-chart in Exhibit 6.58.

The chart shows an average of eight occurrences that results in any one quarter experiencing somewhere between zero and 20 bacteremias. And, from the moving range calculation, one quarter can differ from the previous quarter by as many as 15.

Obtaining a quarter of zero occurrences would not necessarily be a special cause. And they have not had the "quarter from hell" yet where, if everything that can go wrong does go wrong, they will get 20.

When I use this example in my seminars, it is not unusual to hear audible gasps. I then ask, "Is this how you deal with similar undesirable incidents in your organizations?" and

# PROCESS-ORIENTED STATISTICS

**EXHIBIT 6.56** Run Chart of 19 Quarterly Bacteremia Counts

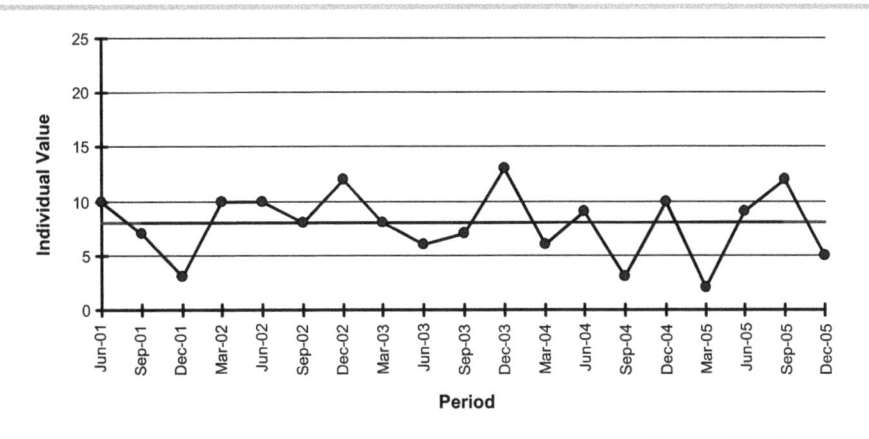

**EXHIBIT 6.57** Calculation of Moving Ranges and Median Moving Range for Bacteremia Data

| Period | No. Bacteremias | Moving Range | Sorted Moving Ranges |
|---|---|---|---|
| Q1-2001 | 10 | * | 0 |
| Q2 | 7 | 3 | 1 |
| Q3 | 3 | 4 | 2 |
| Q4 | 10 | 7 | 2 |
| Q1-2002 | 10 | 0 | 3 |
| Q2 | 8 | 2 | 3 |
| Q3 | 12 | 4 | 3 |
| Q4 | 8 | 4 | 4 |
| Q1-2003 | 6 | 2 | 4 |
| Q2 | 7 | 1 | 4 |
| Q3 | 13 | 6 | 6 |
| Q4 | 6 | 7 | 6 |
| Q1-2004 | 9 | 3 | 7 |
| Q2 | 3 | 6 | 7 |
| Q3 | 10 | 7 | 7 |
| Q4 | 2 | 8 | 7 |
| Q1-2005 | 9 | 7 | 7 |
| Q2 | 12 | 3 | 8 |
| Q3 | 5 | 7 | |

*Note that 19 data points yield 18 moving ranges. Median: average of 9th and 10th in sorted sequence (both = 4).

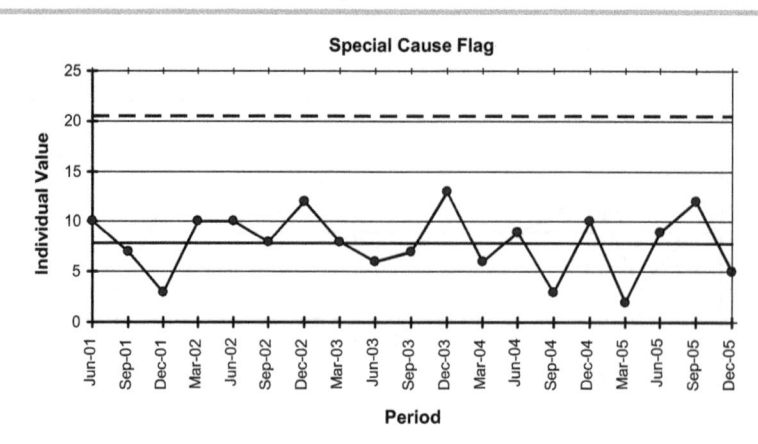

EXHIBIT 6.58 ■ Control Chart of Quarterly Bacteremia Counts

many heads nod in affirmation. I then ask, "Have you plotted your data to see whether you are dealing with common or special cause?" and even more heads shake in denial.

It is so tempting to use a special cause strategy, looking at each incident uniquely and only that quarter's small number of incidents at one time, because "We *shouldn't* have bacteremias." In this case, is the approach working? No, the chart shows no change in five years. And a lot of unnecessary complexity has no doubt been added to the process.

Should they change how they approach this issue? Yes, why not use a common cause strategy of aggregating *all 150* bacteremia cases and stratifying them via a Pareto matrix?

## SENTINEL EVENT, ROOT CAUSE ANALYSIS, AND NEAR-MISS INVESTIGATIONS

It should now be clear why I caution people about the improvement strategies noted in this section's title. The natural tendency is to treat what people call sentinel events, near misses, and, more recently, "never" events as special cause. Now, maybe things like this are so serious that one may need to do damage control, which is a temporary short-term Level 1 fix (see Chapter 1). However, one should not lose the memory of the event. If the run chart shows no progress, it would be prudent to consider a common cause strategy on the aggregated occurrences.

Remember my common cause, process-oriented definition of *incident:* a hazardous situation that was unsuccessfully avoided. The situation is always present, but, if you consider each patient experience as a piece of Swiss cheese, sometimes all of the holes line up, allowing the incident to occur. Many root cause analyses are in essence looking at the "holes" rather than the situation. Another patient could now have a different sequence of different holes that could line up.

### A Statistical Issue Regarding Incidents: The C-Chart

You will notice that I have been using one type of control chart in this chapter, the control chart for individuals, or I-chart. You may be aware that there are seven different types of control charts out there, and many books go through great lengths to create

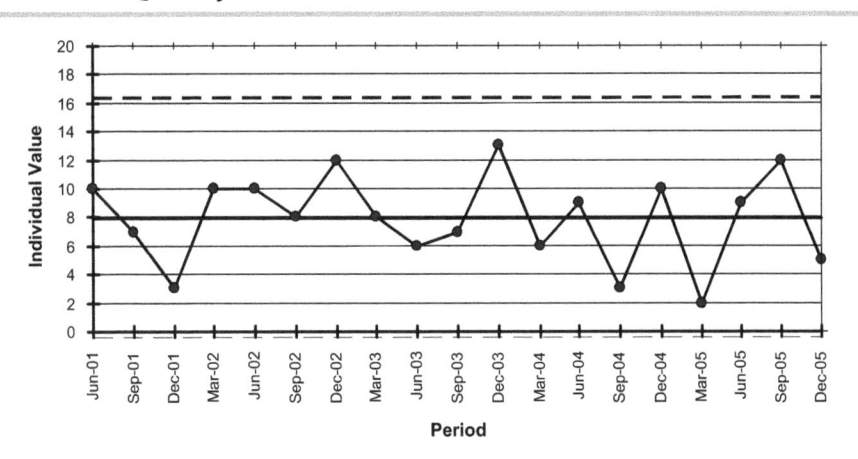

EXHIBIT 6.59 ■ Quarterly Bacteremia Data Plotted as C-Chart

tables so that you will know which chart to use for what kind of data and what situation. This is far too confusing. It is not necessary to understand this level of detail to be a good improvement practitioner (see my 2014 article called "Right Chart or Right Action?" under Resources.)

I cover two more charts in Chapter 10. But, when data are plotted over time, the I-chart I teach here is the "Swiss Army knife" of control charts. It is quite robust to the structure of the underlying data; once again, I do not mention the normal distribution as a useful consideration in analysis. The issue is not which chart to use, but making sure to apply appropriate reaction to variation.

Incident data that are random counts of things (medication errors, bacteremias, needle sticks, falls, etc.) many times follow what some of you have learned as the Poisson distribution. The technically correct chart in this case is what is known as a *c-chart*. It is still plotted with the average as the center, but the limits are calculated differently.

A complicated multiple series of random factors have converged because, for each factor, either $x = 0$ or $x = 1$. When *all* $x = 1$, an "incident" results. Using the Swiss cheese analogy once again, all the holes line up. It also helps me define *near miss*: You just did not get the last hole of the Swiss cheese.

For Poisson data, it turns out that the standard deviation of a stable process is the square root of its average. So, in the case of the bacteremia data, the technically correct limits for the c-chart (Exhibit 6.59) are:

$$7.89 \pm (3 \times \sqrt{7.89}) = 7.89 \pm (3 \times 2.8)$$
$$= (0 - 16)$$

These limits are very close to those obtained by the X-MR process: (0 – 20). Some of you might be bothered by the discrepancy. Here is my point: *The approximate chart still led to the right subsequent action to solve the problem.*

**Rule of thumb:** As long as the overall average of the count data is five or greater, the I-chart is a very good approximation (and do the run chart first).

EXHIBIT 6.60 ■ Rare Event Infection Occurrence

| Date of Infection | Day of Year | Days between Nosocomial Infections | Infections per Day | Nosocomial Infection Rate |
|---|---|---|---|---|
| 1/18/2004 | 18 | | | |
| 1/29/2004 | 29 | 11 | 0.0909 | 33.18 |
| 2/4/2004 | 35 | 6 | 0.1667 | 60.83 |
| 2/6/2004 | 37 | 2 | 0.5000 | 182.50 |
| 2/24/2004 | 55 | 18 | 0.0556 | 20.28 |
| 4/14/2004 | 104 | 49 | 0.0204 | 7.45 |
| 5/22/2004 | 142 | 38 | 0.0263 | 9.61 |
| 5/29/2004 | 149 | 7 | 0.1429 | 52.14 |
| 7/20/2004 | 201 | 52 | 0.0192 | 7.02 |
| 8/11/2004 | 222 | 21 | 0.0476 | 17.38 |
| 8/15/2004 | 226 | 4 | 0.2500 | 91.25 |
| 8/26/2004 | 237 | 11 | 0.0909 | 33.18 |
| 9/2/2004 | 244 | 7 | 0.1429 | 52.14 |
| 10/21/2004 | 293 | 49 | 0.0204 | 7.45 |
| 10/22/2004 | 294 | 1 | 1.0000 | 365.00 |
| 12/2/2004 | 336 | 42 | 0.0238 | 8.69 |
| 6/29/2005 | 180 | 210 | 0.0048 | 1.74 |
| 8/19/2005 | 231 | 51 | 0.0196 | 7.16 |
| 9/11/2005 | 254 | 23 | 0.0435 | 15.87 |
| 9/12/2005 | 255 | 1 | 1.0000 | 365.00 |
| 11/7/2005 | 311 | 56 | 0.0179 | 6.52 |

## Dealing with Rare Events

I had mixed emotions about dealing with the subject of rare events. With an increase in patient safety awareness, there has been a corresponding decrease in the public's tolerance for medical errors that cause life-threatening infections or, in extreme cases, even unnecessary deaths. Statistically, this is known as dealing with rare events (a subset of sentinel events). These are fraught with emotion and the urge to "do something." I decided I just could not ignore this topic.

This can only be considered an introduction. My purpose is to create some awareness and suggestions for preliminary analysis of data. It may allow you to focus your efforts on these unfortunate, tragic incidents to be more effective in truly eradicating them.

As you know, the tendency is to treat each occurrence of a rare event as a special cause. However, what if they are common cause — a hazardous situation (constantly in the background) that was unsuccessfully avoided? And, because of their rarity, how does one determine that the process has indeed been improved? There are some analysis approaches that are helpful.

Some real data on infections in one hospital unit are shown in Exhibit 6.60. The date is given for when an infection occurred and the second column is how many days into the year the event occurred so that column three, "Days between Nosocomial Infections," could be calculated.

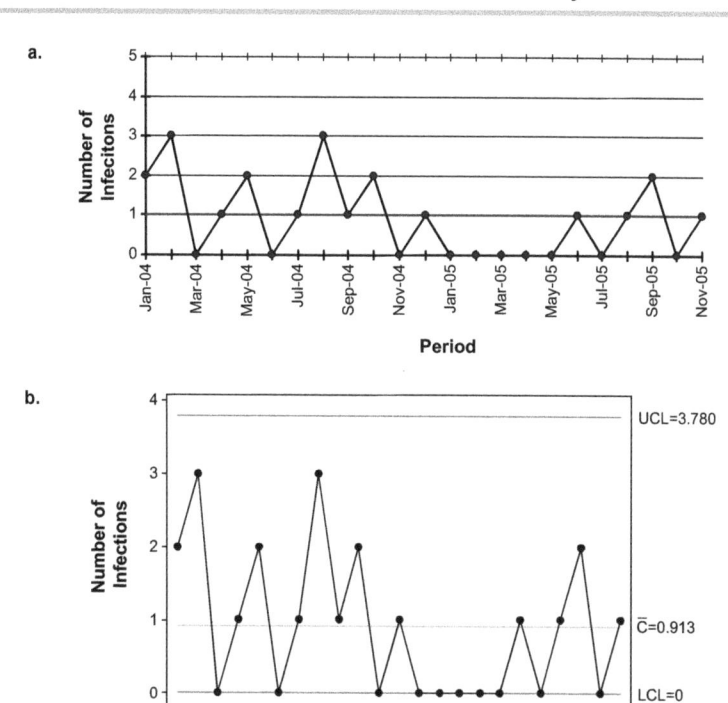

EXHIBIT 6.61 ■ Run and Control Chart for Number of Infections by Month

Some people prefer using the calculations in the next two columns. The days between infections is turned into a rate of infections per day by taking its reciprocal [1/(days between infections)]. Other people prefer to work with expected infections per year. This is easily obtained by multiplying the rate in column four by 365.

### Standard Run and Control Chart Analysis of Event Occurrence

Consider a run chart and an I-chart that look at the occurrences of infections per month (Exhibit 6.61). In the run chart of Exhibit 6.61a, observations 11 through 20 have three points on the median, resulting in a run of only seven, not eight, points below the median. There is no statistical evidence of a special cause, that is, improvement.

Considering the ensuing I-chart, the overall average of the data was less than five. As explained in my discussion of count data, I used the c-chart calculation (although using the average moving range came very close to duplicating these limits). Once again, no statistical evidence of improvement.

### Days between Events, or Rates?

I have also seen people deal with data like this using either of the two control charts shown in Exhibit 6.62: Days between consecutive events or some version of its reciprocal, which converts it to a rate (in this case, the yearly rate, i.e., an average of 67 infections per year).

EXHIBIT 6.62 ■ Control Chart of Days between Infections and Rate

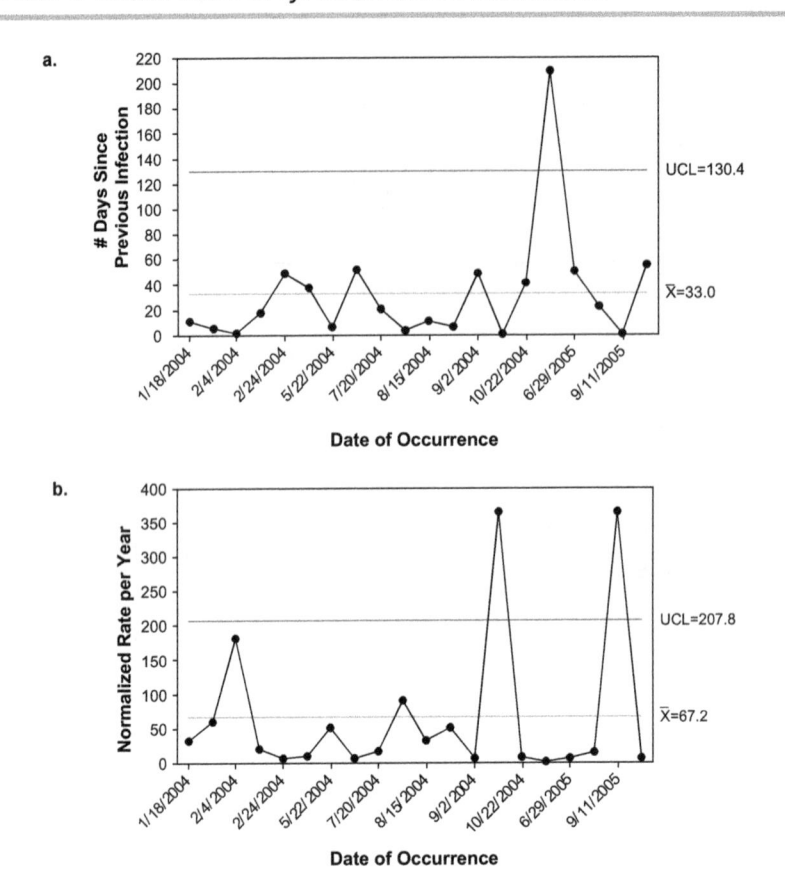

a.

UCL=130.4
X̄=33.0

b.

UCL=207.8
X̄=67.2

The latter case is sometimes used so that, in line with one's intuition, "lower is better." There is evidence of special cause, but the interpretation is not clear; are these unique occurrences or was there a needle bump in the desired direction?

### An Alternative

A suggestion from a respected colleague, Tom Nolan, might be easier to use. Nolan suggests plotting the number of occurrences of an event, but using a time spacing whereby its average is forced to be approximately *one event observed per (this time period)*. In the case of the current data set, it happens to be monthly.

His special cause rule is this: If the data are plotted with this spacing, then observing *six zeroes in a row* would indicate improvement.

Given this rule and chart, once again, there is no indication of improvement.

### Another Data Set

I recently obtained a data set from another hospital dealing with "unexpected deaths" (Exhibit 6.63).

EXHIBIT 6.63 ■ Tabulation of Unit Deaths

| Date of Death | Day of Year | Days between Deaths | Rate: Deaths per Day | Rate: Deaths per Year |
|---|---|---|---|---|
| 2/27/2000 | 58 | | | |
| 3/2/2000 | 61 | 3 | 0.3333 | 121.67 |
| 7/23/2000 | 204 | 143 | 0.0070 | 2.55 |
| 8/7/2000 | 219 | 15 | 0.0667 | 24.33 |
| 9/24/2000 | 267 | 48 | 0.0208 | 7.60 |
| 11/14/2000 | 318 | 51 | 0.0196 | 7.16 |
| 1/3/2001 | 3 | 50 | 0.0200 | 7.3 |
| 1/19/2001 | 19 | 16 | 0.0625 | 22.81 |
| 8/6/2001 | 218 | 199 | 0.005 | 1.83 |
| 9/12/2001 | 255 | 37 | 0.0270 | 9.86 |
| 11/5/2001 | 319 | 64 | 0.0156 | 5.70 |
| 5/23/2002 | 144 | 200 | 0.0050 | 1.83 |
| 6/3/2002 | 155 | 11 | 0.0909 | 33.18 |
| 6/18/2002 | 170 | 15 | 0.0667 | 24.33 |
| 10/11/2002 | 285 | 115 | 0.0087 | 3.17 |
| 1/6/2003 | 6 | 86 | 0.0115 | 4.20 |
| 3/10/2003 | 69 | 63 | 0.0159 | 5.79 |
| 5/12/2003 | 130 | 61 | 0.0163 | 5.98 |
| 10/29/2003 | 302 | 172 | 0.0058 | 2.12 |
| 3/18/2004 | 77 | 140 | 0.0071 | 2.61 |
| 6/3/2004 | 154 | 77 | 0.0130 | 4.74 |

**The usual "time between events" and "rates" analyses.** As before, Exhibit 6.64 shows the run and I-charts of days between deaths as well as its reciprocal, the rate. These are the usual time between events and rates analyses.

**"One incident per time period" analysis.** Here we consider incident occurrence per month, resulting in the c-chart of Exhibit 6.65.

Based on the average, which is 0.389 deaths per month, there seems to be one death every three months (1/0.389 = 2.57, rounded up to 3). I then grouped the data by quarter and plotted these individual three-month totals, resulting in the c-chart shown in Exhibit 6.66.

To summarize, then, testing an intervention after constructing a chart with an average of 1, five or six time periods in a row where zero events are obtained could be used to declare improvement.

There are no easy answers. And, in the case of this second data set, the organization seems perfectly designed to have this death rate for this particular type of patient. Maybe this is a case where benchmarking might help. Rare events are never easy to deal with for quick action.

My purpose in this section was to have you start questioning your current methods for dealing with rare or sentinel events. I have tried to suggest some simple alternatives for insight. But maybe the most important thing for you to consider is whether I have created some awareness in you that you may be using special cause strategies when a common cause strategy is needed.

EXHIBIT 6.64 ■ Run and Control Charts of Days between Deaths and Death Rate (365 × 1/days)

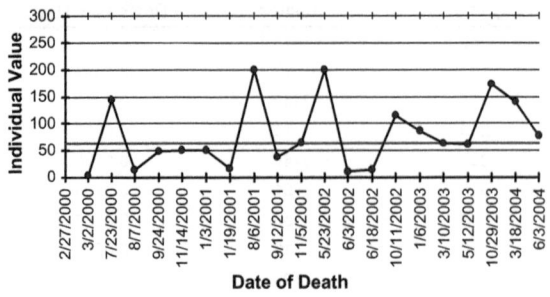

**a. Days between Deaths**

**b. Days between Deaths**

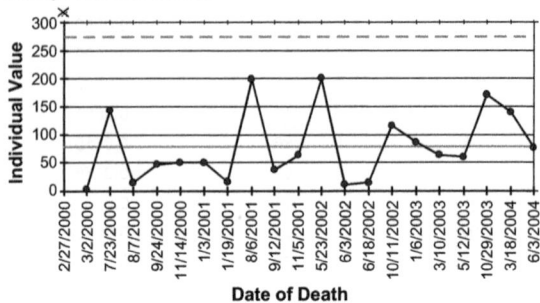

**c. Rate: Deaths per Year**

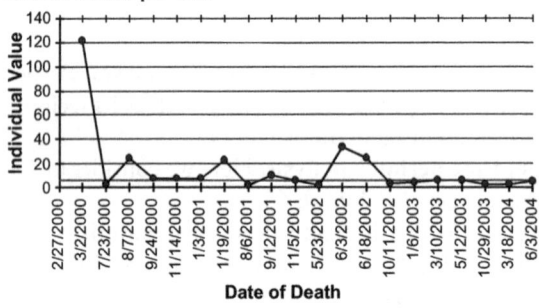

**d. Rate: Deaths per Year**

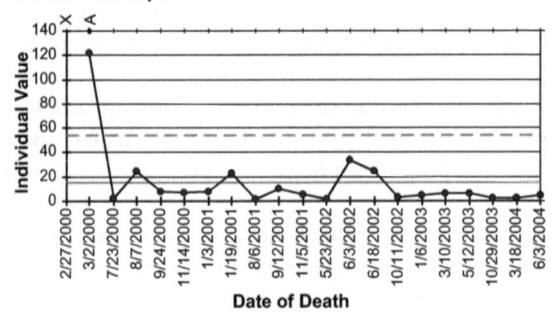

EXHIBIT 6.65 ■ Control Chart of Deaths, Plotted Monthly

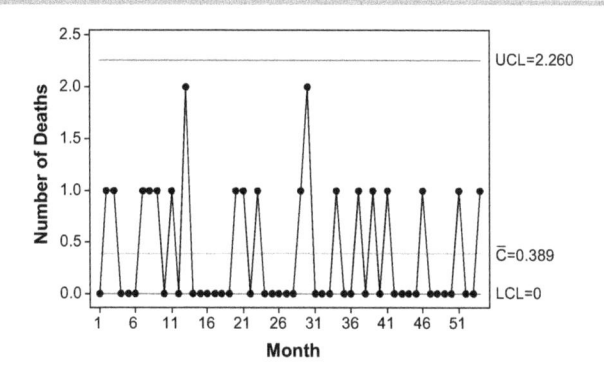

EXHIBIT 6.66 ■ Control Chart of Deaths, Aggregated Quarterly

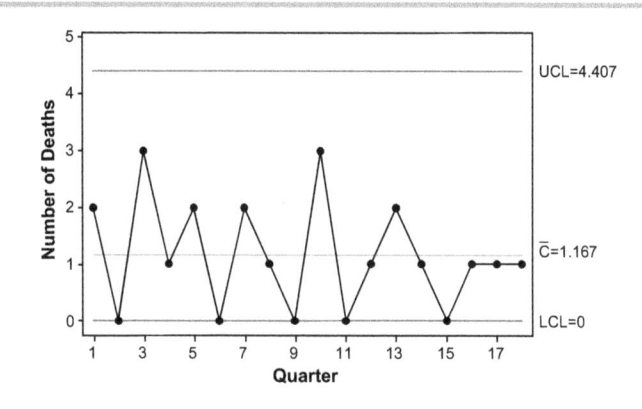

## Two Inevitable Questions

In Chapter 5 I gave you eight questions to ask when looking at a sample of any routine meeting's raw data, the last of which could be the most important of all: *Does a plot of these data in their naturally occurring time order exist? How could you construct one?*

However, rather than getting better at critical thinking, one question that seems to be of greatest concern to practitioners is: "When and how often should I recalculate my limits?" If you feel the instinct to ask that question, pause and think of how you would answer these critical-thinking questions from me instead:

1. Can you show me any existing data (or describe an actual situation) that are making you ask me this question?
2. Can you tell me why this situation is important?
3. Can you show me a run chart of these data plotted over time?
4. What ultimate actions would you like to take with these data?
5. What "big dot" in the boardroom are these data and chart going to affect? Or less tactfully, "Who cares whether the limits are correct or not?"

Knowing when to recalculate limits is somewhat useful information, but for the moment, you've got far more important things to do. Answering these questions addresses the issue of finding out what is wrong with your data to make it more useful. I hope the examples in this chapter have been useful in that regard. (For an excellent further discussion of this issue, see Wheeler's 2002 article "When Should We Compute New Limits?" under Resources.)

The time to re-compute the limits for your charts comes *when they no longer adequately reflect your experience with the process.* There are no hard and fast rules. It is mostly a matter of deep thought analyzing the way the process behaves, the way the data are collected, and the chart's purpose. Wheeler said, "Once again, tinkering with the limits misses the point. Remember, the objective is to take the right action on the process. No credit is given for finding the 'right numbers.'"[5]

You may ask how many data points you need for a good chart. My predictable, vague reply would be: "How much data do you have?" Despite the pedantic proclamations many of you have encountered in favor of waiting for anywhere from 15 to 25 data points, I have found that useful limits may be computed with much less data. As few as 6 to 10 observations are sufficient to start computing limits, especially if it's all you have, which is something that happens to me frequently. What else are you going to do? I dare you to find a more accurate way to assess the situation.

Limits do begin to solidify when 15 to 20 individual values are used in the computation. To argue semantics, when fewer data are available, the limits can be considered "temporary limits," subject to revision as additional data become available. As long as the limits are computed correctly via the moving range between consecutive observations in time order and three sigma are used, then they are "correct limits." As Wheeler pointed out, notice that the definite article is missing: They are just "correct limits," not "the correct limits."[6]

## SUMMARY

Whether or not people understand statistics, they are already using statistics. This chapter has tried to demonstrate productive use of simple statistical methods on data many of you are already routinely generating. I've also tried to make you aware of some common well-meaning errors in perceptions and applications.

Tampering, although unintentional, is rampant, and the losses it causes are incalculable. Variation is everywhere. Only through statistical thinking and the use of basic statistical theory can variation be understood so that appropriate action can be taken.

### Plot the Dots

One major change will be to move away from using highly aggregated data summaries. A quality improvement culture will substitute and consider smaller, more frequent samples taken over time. For effective analysis, these samples will need to initially be plotted in their natural time order — first as a run chart; then, depending on the runs analysis and stability, an appropriate control chart, usually an I-chart.

Think about your organization's current data collections. How many of them consist of aggregated summaries such as the accident and medication error data with no traceability to the process inputs? Do people react as though every undesirable event is a special cause requiring an explanation? Are month-to-month comparisons made as well as comparisons to the same month/time period the previous year? Do people make comparisons to goals and treat the differences as special causes?

I have tried to demonstrate how something as simple as a run chart allows an assessment of any process. This assessment and its accompanying language, based in process, help guide people toward the proper improvement actions through more productive conversations.

Control charts take the run chart one step further. There are several types. From my experience in healthcare, I have found that identifying special causes with the main control chart taught here — the I-chart — will serve most purposes, especially as an initial process analysis.

Many books and material adapted from manufacturing (where this theory originated) to healthcare have a tendency to bog down in things such as "sampling," "rational subgrouping," and mechanics of various charts. This can overwhelm people, especially in a service environment such as healthcare, and cause them to lose sight of the purpose of the charts.

Everyday use of statistics needs to become process oriented. In this context, sample size is not an issue. The choice of how frequently in time to sample, not the total number of samples, is the key issue. Other factors dictating sampling include the potential sources of variation currently being studied. The time frame can be chosen either in line with theorized occurrences of special causes or the crucial time frame within which one must be alerted to special causes. The objective is to study and assess the stability of a process, not to estimate its performance accurately.

This application is different than designing a one-shot, controlled research study. Also, many everyday organizational process outputs are not strictly designed data collections: They are routinely produced daily, weekly, monthly, or whatever, many times with the vague objective of "knowing how we're doing."

Especially for these types of data, the I-chart is almost always appropriate and the first choice (after a good run chart analysis) for an initial analysis studying process performance. In most circumstances, it is a very close approximation to what the technically "correct" chart would give. It is so robust that it is sometimes called the Swiss Army knife of control charts.

The key objective in quality improvement is to expose and reduce inappropriate significant sources of variation. Depending on the initial process analysis, a subsequent special cause strategy or common cause strategy will be required.

### React to Variation Appropriately

The human tendency is to see all variation as special cause, the naive belief being, "If I can explain it, it's a special cause." Special cause strategies do allow people to act on their theories with quick, although not necessarily appropriate, solutions.

It is virtually guaranteed that if smart people look for reasons for (alleged) special causes, they will find them. Team members will have lots of theories. But without further data collection to locate and isolate major opportunities (usually stratification of the process inputs), deep fixes will not emerge. The seductive simplicity of obvious solutions never vanishes.

There is a misconception that if a process exhibits only common cause variation, one is saddled with the current result: The belief is that any improvement will require a major redesign. However, it is not generally understood that special causes can exist in systems exhibiting common cause behavior. They aggregate predictably to create an overall appearance of common cause, and different, additional strategies are needed for exposing them.

What should be done to really differentiate common from special causes? It will take the tenacious, judicious use of run and control charts to assess a process. Common cause strategies (stratification, disaggregation, and designed experimentation, as discussed in Chapter 5) are not widely understood, but probably represent the major opportunity for lasting improvement in most projects.

### Arbitrary Numerical Goals Improve Nothing

"A goal without a method is nonsense!"[7] Improvement does not result from focusing solely on the process output. I hope the dangers of arbitrary numerical goals are becoming more apparent. Arbitrary numerical goals can cause distraction by comparing individual results to a goal and treating the difference as a special cause. They can also result in organizational fear where the goal then becomes attaining the desired number. And the human tendency is to do it through process distortion, not improvement.

This ignores the fact that an observed output is generated by a process that exhibits an inherent range of results. The assessed process performance needs to be compared to any goal and the gap seen as variation. The resulting question then needs to be, "Is the variation from desired performance a common cause or a special cause?" The answer motivates the appropriate strategy.

Goals themselves are not bad. The point is how they are used. By what method is an organization going to try to achieve a given goal? Numerical goals have a tendency to be arbitrary. Such goals tend to end in 0 or 5, with the exception of, specifically, 3. What is the theory behind this? What specific processes need to be improved?

Exhortation to achieve goals treats a culture with special causes (obvious opportunities for improvement, which are the 20 percent of the processes that have the potential for 80 percent of the improvement) as common cause (e.g., urging everyone to cut their budget 3 percent). What effect does this have on morale? What exactly are they supposed to do differently? Remember, there is no such thing as improvement in general. Deming would often remark, "If you can accomplish a goal without a method, then why were you not doing it last year?"[7]

Once any goal is defined, the fundamental question is whether the current process is capable of meeting this goal. The time plot of the data will provide an answer. However, the individual data points will not. The plot and analysis of the process variation will then drive questions that need to be asked and the strategy for improvement.

### Process-Oriented Thinking and Deep-Level Fixes Are Key

Because most problems are based in systems (85–97 percent), the data needed for improvement must be routinely collected from that perspective. It is a natural tendency to collect and react to individual results and outputs. The good news is that plotting the current output data can give baselines from which a process's capability and the improvement attempts can be assessed.

Solution implementations can be thought of as attempts to deliberately create beneficial special causes. These causes would be detectable on run charts and control charts. The other good news is that as questions are asked for stratification purposes (or any of the seven sources of problems with a process), the answers will require small, focused, simple, efficient, one-time data collections on the work while it is performed by the team (as opposed to a retrospective view).

It is not necessary to wait to form a project team before using statistics for effective problem solving. All routine data reports can be evaluated and fed back using a common, agreed-on theory: statistical theory based in statistical thinking. Statistical theory allows the reports to be placed into contexts that reduce the human variation in perceptions.

All decisions are predictions based on interpreting patterns of variation in data (real, anecdotal, or one-point comparisons to a goal). All variation is caused and can be classified into one of two categories: common cause or special cause. Work cultures tend to treat each situation requiring action as a special cause. Problems march into one's office, people are told to "do something about it," and action is taken immediately.

Everyone in an organization needs a basic knowledge of variation. As individuals learn to appropriately respond to variation, the quality of the whole improvement process itself improves.

And even with this knowledge, one cannot blindly and dogmatically apply statistical rules. I am teaching a process that is a useful complement to any employee's master knowledge of a situation. The goal is to motivate more productive conversations and actions in response to data.

The public's increasing awareness and increasing intolerance for medical errors represents a challenging context within which to use data. I have tried to give a perspective that will help you reexamine the usual tendency to treat any undesirable incident as a special cause via sentinel event and near-miss analyses.

What if your organization is perfectly designed to have these incidents occur (common cause)? I gave an introduction to a potentially promising statistical technique to analyze and deal with rare events.

In addition, routine use of ongoing run and control charts for common clinical conditions has tremendous potential. One final note: I hope you noticed how many times I mentioned the ubiquitous normal distribution assumption and subsequently used it to solve a problem — other than the three sets of hospital cardiac mortality data, where I showed the assumption of normality to be false — virtually zero.

## REFERENCES

1. Duncan, Acheson J. 1965. *Quality Control and Industrial Statistics*, p. 930. Table P: Limiting Values for Lengths of Runs on Either Side of the Median of "n" Cases. Homewood, IL: Richard D. Irwin.
2. Wheeler, Donald J. 2012. "What Is Leptokurtophobia? And Why Does It Matter?" *Quality Digest* (July 30). www.qualitydigest.com/inside/quality-insider-column/what-leptokurtophobia.html.
3. Wheeler, Donald J. 2012. "Exact Answers to the Wrong Questions: Why Statisticians Still Do Not Understand Shewhart." *Quality Digest* (March 2). www.qualitydigest.com/inside/quality-insider-article/exact-answers-wrong-questions.html.
4. Neubauer, Dean V. 2007. "Pl-Ott the Data!" *Quality Digest* (May). www.qualitydigest.com/may07/articles/05_article.shtml.
5. Wheeler, Donald J. 2012. "When Should We Compute New Limits? How to Use the Limits to Track the Process." *Quality Digest* (April 2). www.qualitydigest.com/inside/quality-insider-article/when-should-we-compute-new-limits.html.
6. Wheeler, Donald J. 1996. "When Do I Recalculate My Limits?" *spctoolkit* (May). www.qualitydigest.com/may/spctool.html.
7. Deming, W. Edwards. 1994. *The New Economics for Industry, Government, Education*, p. 41, 122. Cambridge, MA: MIT Press.

## RESOURCES

Arthur, Jay. QIMacros™. www.QIMacros.com.

Balestracci Jr., Davis. 1996. *Quality Improvement: Practical Applications for Medical Group Practice*, 2nd ed. Englewood, CO: Center for Research in Ambulatory Health Care Administration of Medical Group Management Association. First edition published 1994.

Balestracci Jr., Davis. 2006. "An Alternative to the Red Bead Experiment: Management by Flipping Coins (MBFC)." *Quality Digest* (August). http://www.qualitydigest.com/aug06/departments/spc_guide.shtml.

Balestracci Jr., Davis. 2008. "How Do You Treat Special-Cause Signals? By Using Your Brain…" *Quality Digest* (October). www.qualitydigest.com/magazine/2008/nov/department/how-do-you-treat-special-cause-signals.html

Balestracci Jr., Davis. 2008. "An Underrated Test for Run Charts: The Total Number of Runs Above and Below the Median Proves Revealing." *Quality Digest* (October). www.qualitydigest.com/magazine/2008/oct/department/underrated-test-run-charts.html.

Balestracci Jr., Davis. 2009. "The Wisdom of David Kerridge, Part 1: Back to Basics." *Quality Digest* (June). www.qualitydigest.com/inside/twitter-ed/wisdom-david-kerridge-part-1.html.

Balestracci Jr., Davis. 2009. "The Wisdom of David Kerridge — Part 2: Statistics in the Real World Aren't Quite as Tidy as Those in a Text Book." *Quality Digest* (July). www.qualitydigest.com/inside/twitter-ed/wisdom-david-kerridge-part-2.html.

Balestracci Jr., Davis. 2014. "Right Chart or Right Action? No extra credit for choosing the technically correct chart." *Quality Digest* (June). www.qualitydigest.com/inside/quality-insider-column/right-chart-or-right-action.html.

Joiner, Brian L. 1994. *Fourth Generation Management*. New York: McGraw-Hill.

Wheeler, Donald J. n.d. [Archive]. *Quality Digest*. www.qualitydigest.com/read/content_by_author/12852.

Wheeler, Donald J. 1993. *Understanding Variation: The Key to Managing Chaos*. Knoxville, TN: SPC Press.

Wheeler, Donald J. 1996. "When Do I Recalculate My Limits?" *spctoolkit* (May). www.qualitydigest.com/may/spctool.html.

Wheeler, Donald J. 1998. *Avoiding Man-Made Chaos*. Knoxville, TN: SPC Press.

Wheeler, Donald J. 2012. "Exact Answers to the Wrong Questions: Why Statisticians Still Do Not Understand Shewhart." *Quality Digest* (March). www.qualitydigest.com/inside/quality-insider-article/exact-answers-wrong-questions.html.

Wheeler, Donald J. 2012. "When Should We Compute New Limits? How to Use the Limits to Track the Process." *Quality Digest* (April). www.qualitydigest.com/inside/quality-insider-article/when-should-we-compute-new-limits.html.

Wheeler, Donald J. 2012. "Analysis Using Few Data, Part 1: Some of These Batches Are Not Like the Others…" *Quality Digest* (June). www.qualitydigest.com/inside/quality-insider-article/analysis-using-few-data-part-1.html.

Wheeler, Donald J. 2012. "What Is Leptokurtophobia? And Why Does It Matter?" *Quality Digest* (July). www.qualitydigest.com/inside/quality-insider-column/what-leptokurtophobia.html.

Wheeler, Donald J. 2013. "But the Limits Are Too Wide! When the *XmR* Chart Doesn't Seem to Work." *Quality Digest* (January 2). www.qualitydigest.com/inside/quality-insider-column/limits-are-too-wide.html.

Wheeler, Donald J. 2013. "Contra Two Sigma: The Consequences of Using the Wrong Limits." *Quality Digest* (May). www.qualitydigest.com/inside/quality-insider-column/contra-two-sigma.html.

CHAPTER 7

# Statistical Stratification: Analysis of Means

## KEY IDEAS

- When looking at improvement opportunities, the mind-set must change from "comparisons of individual performances" to "comparison of individual performances to their inherent 'system.'"
- Analysis of means (ANOM) is a powerful, objective technique that assesses a current system and exposes potential opportunity.
- By identifying an individual as "outside" the system, all one can conclude is that the process is different than the other individuals; one cannot necessarily question the "methods" (competence) input. Collegial discussion and data will determine whether the special cause is appropriate, inappropriate, and/or unintended.
- The control charts used to assess individual performance and obtain the summary data for the ANOM are also powerful individual feedback tools. They can assess an individual's efforts to improve.
- Common cause limits for the ANOM are obtained strictly from the data. There is no guarantee of finding special causes. One should not approach a problem with an a priori assumption that there should be a given percentage of special causes. There may not even be quartiles in the data.
- Rankings are ludicrous as a means for motivating improvement. People inside the system are indistinguishable from one another and *cannot be ranked*.
- Typical displays of percentage data are extremely deceptive.
- Any graphical display of numbers (except a Pareto bar graph) needs a context of common cause variation for proper interpretation.
- There are advanced statistical techniques based on normal distribution theory. However, simpler, robust alternatives are available that work just as well. They are also easier to apply and explain.

## REVISITING QUALITY ASSURANCE VS. QUALITY IMPROVEMENT

Traditional quality assurance (QA) data would be more helpful if presented in some type of control chart form. This is far superior to the usual aggregate summaries, bar graphs, and rankings that are many times compared to arbitrary numerical goals and standards.

Rankings usually do not help to understand variation and root causes and, unfortunately, usually result in tampering. People tend to automatically assume that the highest and lowest ranked performances of that time period are special causes, and then the familiar exhortations start, "If they can do it, you can do it. Let's have results instead of alibis."

A common defensive reaction to those being ranked (particularly among those ranked near the bottom) is, "It can't be me, the data are obviously at fault" (or the classic cliché by doctors, "My patients are sicker").

Before any analysis, it may be useful to start with finding out what is wrong with the numbers to better understand them. In applying these methods, there will initially need to be intense examination of operational definitions while asking whether these are even fair comparisons. Even if they are, how should the observed variation be interpreted? What represents true special cause? What is the process for using these data?

Most importantly, if improvement is needed, how does the analysis propose to answer someone's natural question, "Well, then, what should I do differently from what I'm doing now?" Any comparison is the equivalent of a benchmark and must result in process-oriented questions. Most of the time, the issue is much deeper than assuming it is a matter of competence ("methods"); the variation is probably unintended or even appropriate.

Performance numbers tend to be viewed in a vacuum as sacrosanct with no context of variation within which to interpret them. As stated in my discussion in Chapter 2, given a set of numbers, 10 percent will be the top 10 percent. There is neither an appropriate yardstick of common cause provided to interpret the observed variation properly nor is there even a perceived need to do so.

I also many times encounter data presentations of traditional (incorrect) 95 percent confidence intervals around each individual performance's average. In an improvement context, this is neither appropriate nor helpful. The purpose of improvement analyses is to expose hidden special causes, which may or may not already be there. The underlying assumption is that everyone is following a similar process. So, the results should initially be considered equivalent.

## A Different Context from Research

Contrast this with research in which differences are *intentionally* created for *each* group under consideration. One knows up front that the processes are different; however, subsequent analysis has to determine whether these differences are big enough to warrant action. Contrast these two objectives: an analysis to find an unknown beneficial hidden opportunity vs. proactively creating several alternatives to choose the best one.

Regardless, from my experience with both of these scenarios, the issue of incorrect calculation of common cause variation via the standard deviation still arises. And as demonstrated in Chapter 6, this calculation (usually taught in most basic courses) can be seriously inflated. Depending on the type of data being analyzed, it can also be grossly inappropriate.

Because of what is taught in most basic statistics courses, there is an almost universal (inappropriate) use of two standard deviations as a gold standard outlier criterion, and more recently, I am seeing the increasing use of one standard deviation.

## ANALYSIS OF MEANS VS. RESEARCH

In exposing common causes for quality improvement, any comparisons assume that the performances form an inherent system, which has an overall average around which is a band of common cause. The performances within this band are statistically indistinguishable and cannot be ranked. (Think back to the coin flip example of Chapter 2 to introduce this concept, flipping a fair coin 50 times will result in a number of heads ranging from 14 to 36.)

Analysis of means (ANOM) is a control chart–based technique for assessing a current system. This results in appropriately exposing improvement opportunities, when present, beyond the common cause band. It was invented by Ellis Ott (see *Process Quality Control* by Ott and colleagues in Resources) and can be used with most data types. This chapter will explain and contrast its application to count data (rates and percentage) and continuous data.

## Analyzing Rates and Percentages with Analysis of Means

Before I begin by explaining the analysis of count data, I would like to summarize some of its key concepts. There are two key questions:

1. What should you include in your count?
2. What area of opportunity would you use to adjust the counts to make them comparable?

First, make sure the operational definition is clear. What's the threshold whereby something goes from a "nonissue" (i.e., a value of 0) to an "issue" (i.e., a value of 1)? Are there distinct criteria so that two or more people assessing the situation concur that the issue had occurred? As you will see, getting good numbers is only half of the job.

For example, consider complaints. How do you count them? Do you count the number of complaints received each month? Or do you count the number of customers who complained? This will need careful consideration before you can begin to collect useful count data.

Let's consider a facility where the numbers of complaints reported for one period of 21 months were, respectively, 20, 22, 9, 12, 13, 20, 8, 23, 16, 11, 14, 9, 11, 3, 5, 7, 3, 2, 1, 7, and 6. But even though you know the counts, you don't know the whole story because you don't know the context for the counts. Before anyone can make sense of these counts, certain questions must be answered. How is *complaint* defined? Are these actual customer complaints or internally generated counts? Does a complaint about a chilly reception room count?

In addition, all count data have an implicit denominator that's defined by the "area of opportunity" for that count. If you don't know the area of opportunity for a count, you don't know how to interpret that count. It depends on what's being counted, how it's being counted, and what possible restrictions there might be on the count. There needs to be some logical connection between the size of the area of opportunity and the size of the count. It also needs to be clear how to measure or count the area of opportunity, and it must bear some clear relationship to the incident being recorded. Any one count may have several possible ways to characterize the area of opportunity. In the case of a medical practice, some examples are by the number of office visits, procedures performed, or hours worked by primary caregivers.

In many cases, it is not unusual for the area of opportunity to change over time, as in the bypass survival rate example later in this chapter. In that case, the counts themselves will not be comparable. To obtain comparable values when the area of opportunity changes, one must then divide each count by its area of opportunity.

When this is done, there are two ways a resulting number can manifest – either as a rate or a percentage. In the case of a rate, *exposure to a process is constant*, and the longer there is exposure to the situation, the more likely there is to be a countable event, for example, central-line infections per 1,000 central-line days. Percentages result when a process opportunity occurs *in discrete events* whereby something either happens or it doesn't, for example, cesarean section, or C-section (per delivery).

In the case of complaints, one could look at the number of visits in which *at least one complaint* was reported, which makes it a percentage. But if one were more concerned about the actual number of complaints and multiple complaints are possible for one visit, then that now becomes a rate. A choice of the best area of opportunity to define will be necessary. (For more on count data, see "Collecting Good Count Data" in Resources.)

Note that because varying areas of opportunity tend to be the rule and not the exception, the following ANOM calculations are cumbersome to do by hand. There are many computer software packages, however, that can do them, and it is highly recommended that you have access to one, such as Minitab, SAS, JMP, or Statgraphics. QIMacros is an inexpensive package that acts as a Microsoft Excel add-in (see Arthur in Resources). They are powerful ways to stratify performance.

### Analysis of Means for Rates: The U-Chart

I introduced the use of the Pareto matrix in Lesson 3 of Chapter 2 using the accident data from Lesson 2. Many times, this matrix presentation is all one needs to identify and act on major, previously hidden special cause sources of variation.

However, let's reconsider those same departmental accident totals as if they were hospital infection numbers from specific units, only this time, each unit has a different area of opportunity, as shown in Exhibit 7.1 by the number of central-line days for each unit.

The denominator is crucial for properly defining the situation and subsequently interpreting the differences in the resulting rates. Because of this, one needs to initially compare the rates instead of the raw counts — a more formal statistical stratification, if you will.

In the instance of rate data, the statistical u-chart is appropriate to answer everyone's basic question: For this situation, are the three above-average units truly above average?

ANOM begins with the assumption that these six units form a comparable peer group "system" and that each is performing equivalently at a rate of the *six-unit system average*, 12.2/1,000 central-line days. Based on this system average, ANOM calculates a common-cause *expected* range of performance for each unit, given its specific number of

**EXHIBIT 7.1** Central Line–Associated Infection Data

| Unit | No. of Infections | No. of Central-Line Days | Infection Rate/1,000 Days |
|---|---|---|---|
| 1 | 6 | 412 | 14.6 |
| 2 | 19 | 670 | 28.4 |
| 3 | 7 | 903 | 7.8 |
| 4 | 3 | 663 | 4.5 |
| 5 | 35 | 1,793 | 19.5 |
| 6 | 7 | 1,870 | 3.7 |
| Total | 77 | 6,311 | 12.2 ($u_{avg}$) |

Source: Davis Balestracci Jr., MS, *Quality Digest*, November 2005. www.qualitydigest.com. Reprinted with permission.

**EXHIBIT 7.2** ■ Analysis of Means for Central Line–Associated Blood Infections by Unit

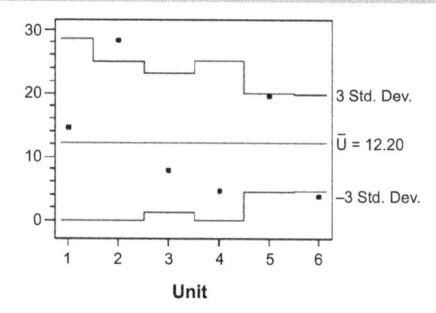

Source: Davis Balestracci Jr., MS, *Quality Digest*, November 2005. www.qualitydigest.com. Reprinted with permission.

central-line days. It is only when an individual performance falls outside of the limits that it can be declared, statistically, above or below average.

The general formula for the common-cause range of rates is:

$$U_{avg} \pm 3 \times \sqrt{U_{avg}/\text{window of opportunity}}$$

The 3 stands for 3 standard deviations as shown in the "Why Three Standard Deviations?" sidebar. For this specific scenario, the formula is:

$$12.2 \pm 3 \times \sqrt{12.2/(\text{unit's 1,000 central-line days})}$$

(Note that the *only* difference for each unit is the number of central-line days.) This results in the following chart shown in Exhibit 7.2.

One unit is truly above average (Unit 2), and one unit is truly below average (Unit 6). The others, based on this data, are indistinguishable *from each other and 12.2.*

Always be aware of how the data were collected. The raw-count numbers might be useful, but considering area of opportunity issues and, when necessary, putting them in their statistical context can many times present another critical view of a situation.

## Are You Using SWAGs? A Common Misapplication of the Normal Distribution

I am not a fan of required statistics courses. Most are taught from an inherent research perspective and are nothing short of legalized torture resulting in participants learning to turn any wild a** guess (WAG) into a statistical wild a** guess (SWAG). For example, published rankings with feedback are often used as a cost-cutting measure to identify and motivate "bad apples."

In a class of drugs, certain specific drugs are deemed more acceptable than others for reasons of cost, effectiveness, and so forth. Two common ranking scenarios are studying physician patterns of prescribing generic drugs and monitoring the use of the most expensive drug within a class of drugs; certain arbitrary targets are deemed desirable for appropriate prescriptive use. Individual performances are judged vis-à-vis these targets.

A concerned individual gave me an antibiotic managed care protocol that was going to be used on physician groups (Exhibit 7.3). It also contained an example of its use with a real data set consisting of 51 physicians' performances. While designed with the best intentions, it bore no resemblance to any theoretically sound statistical methodology.

> **EXHIBIT 7.3** ■ Antibiotic Managed Care Protocol
>
> For any given diagnosis or for any therapeutic class of drugs, there are usually several choices of drug therapy. This study is designed to compare physician's selection of antibiotics when several choices are available. This is accomplished by comparing the antibiotic-specific prescribing behavior of physicians who see similar types of patients and identifying those physicians that deviate from the established norm or standard.
>
> **Identification of Outliers**
> 1. Data will be tested for normal distribution.
> 2. *If distribution is normal* — Physicians whose prescribing deviates greater than one or two standard deviations from the mean are identified as outliers.
> 3. *If distribution is not normal* — Examine distribution of data and establish an arbitrary cutoff point above which physicians should receive feedback (this cutoff point is subjective and variable based on the distribution of ratio data).
>
> **Intervention**
> 1. Report results to local Pharmacy & Therapeutics Committee and/or medical director.
> 2. Provide feedback to outlier physicians in the form of the following material:
>    - Summary details of the physician's antibiotic prescribing sorted by antibiotic class;
>    - Summary of study results and brief explanation of how they were identified as an outlier;
>    - Patient antibiotic medication profiles for those patients receiving target antibiotics; and
>    - Educational document reviewing the standard antibiotic therapy for disease states for which the target antibiotics are commonly prescribed.

Many statistics courses impart to their students an obsession with the normal distribution. In the case of Exhibit 7.3, *it is not appropriate* because as each individual prescription is evaluated, it can only fall into one of two classes: It is either a member of the target population, $x = 1$, or it is not, $x = 0$. Technically speaking, these data form a *binomial* distribution with the additional and more serious problem of the denominators varying widely (30–217). In this protocol the test for normality is moot and inappropriate, despite the fact that the computer will do it. Interestingly, it passed with a $p$-value of 0.277.

By definition of the normal distribution, approximately one-third of the individuals will be further than one standard deviation away from the mean, and approximately 5 percent will be beyond two standard deviations. They are probably not outliers, but just common cause variation. Thus, if the data passed the test for normality, the existence of outliers could not be proven.

This also assumes that the standard deviation is calculated correctly. The commonly taught calculation in most basic courses is incorrect. The estimate will be seriously inflated if special causes are present. To deal with this (unknown) inflation, people have a naive tendency to arbitrarily use lower thresholds to determine alleged significance, as in this case, using one standard deviation.

Given this data collection and analysis process, what are the odds of tampering? What have been your experiences with this type of process? I can ask the physicians reading this if you have ever received such helpful feedback. How was it received? Did it truly motivate you to want to change your behavior? When this example is presented to audiences of physicians, they often respond with a collective synchronized pantomime of what appears to be throwing something in the garbage.

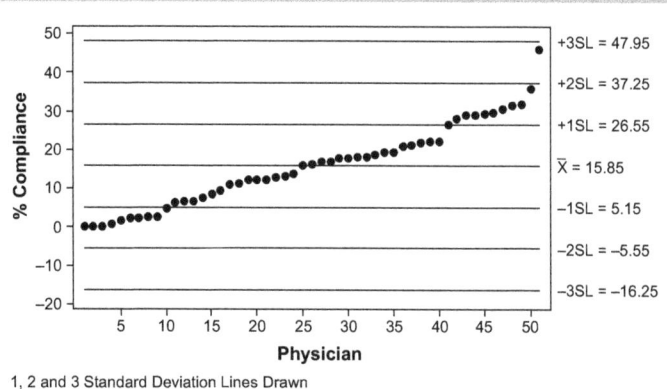

EXHIBIT 7.4 ▪ Incorrect Proposed Protocol Analysis of Target Drug Compliance

[Chart showing % Compliance vs Physician (1-50), with horizontal lines at:
+3SL = 47.95
+2SL = 37.25
+1SL = 26.55
$\bar{X}$ = 15.85
−1SL = 5.15
−2SL = −5.55
−3SL = −16.25

1, 2 and 3 Standard Deviation Lines Drawn
Standard Deviation = 10.7]

The scary issue here is the proposed ensuing analysis resulting from the results of the normality test. If data are normally distributed, doesn't that mean there are no outliers? But suppose outliers are present. In that case they are atypical and their presence would inflate the traditional calculation of standard deviation. But wait, the data passed the normality test; it is all so confusing.

Yet that does not seem to stop our quality police from lowering the "gotcha" threshold to two or even one standard deviation to find outliers (a common practice I have observed). The sidebar "Why Three Standard Deviations?" explains why three standard deviations (calculated correctly) are used as an outlier criterion.

Returning to the protocol in Exhibit 7.3, even scarier is what is proposed if the distribution is not normal: Establish an *arbitrary* cutoff point (i.e., one that's subjective and variable).

The protocol's proposed analysis of its data is given in Exhibit 7.4. Because the data passed the test for normality, the analysis shows one, two, and three standard deviation lines drawn in around the mean. (The data are sorted in ascending order. The standard deviation of the 51 performances using the traditional calculation yields a value of 10.7.)

## ANOM for Percentages: The P-Chart

### Applying ANOM to the Drug Utilization Data

Given that each physician's number of prescriptions can be analyzed and one can then count the number that were the target drug as well as the number that were not the target drug, this is considered percentage data — each prescription occurrence is discrete.

During this time period, these 51 physicians had written 4,032 prescriptions, of which 596 were for the target drugs — an overall rate of 14.8 percent. The goal of ANOM is to compare a group of physicians who have what should be similar practice types, a relatively homogenous "system," if you will. Each is compared to their system's overall average. Variation is exposed and then there is conversation to discuss the variation, then reduce the inappropriate and unintended variation.

## Why Three Standard Deviations?

Analysis of means (ANOM) is a statistical approach to stratification that offers a way to address real improvement. It was invented by Ellis Ott and explained beautifully in the book *Process Quality Control* (see Resources). ANOM should be a bread-and-butter tool of any statistical practitioner.

Most academic-based statistics courses give the impression that two standard deviations (which many consider "95 percent confidence") is the gold standard of comparison. However, you might notice that in most academic exercises, only one decision is made. The analyses in this chapter are making multiple, simultaneous decisions: six in the u-chart ANOM of the infection rate data and 51 in the p-chart ANOM of the pharmacy utilization data.

Both of these situations represent systems where, theoretically, there should be no differences among the units being compared. The assumption is that all units being compared are equivalent until proven otherwise, and they represent a system with an average performance. Each unit's performance will also be considered average unless the data show otherwise.

Given that, suppose one used the common, two-standard-deviations comparison? One must now consider, if there were no differences among the units, what's the probability that all of them would be within two standard deviations? The answer is $(0.95)^n$, where "$n$" is the number of units being simultaneously compared. For our three examples, $(0.95)^6 = 0.735$ and $(0.95)^{51} = 0.073$, respectively.

In other words, using two standard deviations means that one would run the following risks of accidentally declaring *at least one* of the units as an outlier when it actually isn't: (100 percent − 73.5 percent) = 26.5 percent and, similarly, 92.7 percent, respectively.

To more precisely determine a 5 percent risk, one must use the Z- (i.e., normal distribution) or t-value corresponding to an overall probability risk of 0.05, which is $e^{\ln(0.975)/n}$. For our scenarios, one would need to use limits comparable not to 0.95, but 0.996 and 0.9995, respectively. (Note: $0.996^6 \sim 0.975$ and $0.9995^{51} \sim 0.975$.) I used 0.975 in the calculation and not 0.95 because I'm using a two-sided test (which is how you obtained the "two" in two standard deviations in the first place).

Let's keep things simple and use the normal approximation. This corresponds to Z-scores of 2.63 and 3.29, respectively.

Unfortunately, these are not the final multipliers. Ideally, in considering each unit as a potential outlier, wouldn't you like to eliminate each data point's influence on the overall calculations, replot the data, and see whether they now fall within the remaining units' system? There's a statistical sleight of hand that does this by adjusting these limits via a factor using the "weight" of each observation. For the simplest case of equal sample sizes, this becomes

$$\sqrt{\frac{(n-1)}{n}}$$

where $n$ is the number of units being compared.

If our units had equal sample sizes (and they don't), the actual limits used for an overall risk of 5 percent would be 2.41 and 3.26, respectively.

If I were to do a statistically exact analysis for every unit, I would have to calculate different limits for each because the sample sizes aren't equal. In this case, the adjustment factor becomes

(Continues)

> (Continued)
>
> $$\sqrt{1-\frac{n_{unit}}{N_{unit}}}$$
>
> When looking for opportunities for improvement, that is, exposing inappropriate or unintended variation, I hope this has convinced you that using three standard deviations along with an estimate of the standard deviation that's calculated appropriately is good enough.
>
> W. Edwards Deming uses the three standard deviations criterion in his red bead experiment analysis and Brian Joiner (a student of Ellis Ott) told me that Ott used three as well. In the world of analytic statistics, the use of probability to make decisions, which is the backbone of enumerative statistics, is rendered questionable. Empirical evidence by Deming's mentor Walter Shewhart demonstrated that three standard deviations (calculated correctly) adequately balances the occurrence of two risks: (1) claiming significance when there is none and (2) claiming no significance when there is.
>
> If you wanted to *approximate* the overall risk you're taking in using three standard deviations, you could calculate $1 - (0.997)^n$ (the 0.997 from control-chart theory, which uses three standard deviations, but based on the normal distribution, *which, more often than not, isn't true*). This translates to risks of 1.8 percent and 14.4 percent, respectively, for our $n = 6$ and 51. This is conservative in the first case and more risky when comparing the 51 physicians, *but it gets a more productive conversation started*.
>
> Successfully using a three standard deviations criterion for more than 25 years has certainly convinced me of its value.
>
> Source: Adapted from Davis Balestracci Jr. 2006. "Why Three Standard Deviations? Analysis of Means Offers a Way to Address Real Improvements." *Quality Digest* (February). www.qualitydigest.com. Reprinted with permission.

For each individual physician's performance, one calculates the common-cause limits of what would be expected due to statistical variation from the system's 14.8 percent target prescription rate. Based on the appropriate statistical theory for percentage data based on counts (i.e., binomial), a standard deviation must be calculated separately for each physician because each wrote a different number of total prescriptions. Note that this is similar to what was done for the u-chart ANOM for rates.

The calculation for the p-chart ANOM is as follows:

$$p_{avg} \pm 3 \times \sqrt{\frac{p_{avg} \times (1 - p_{avg})}{\text{total number of opportunities for event to occur}}}$$

(*Note:* this formula and analysis work regardless of whether you use the literal proportions (range of 0 to 1) or the actual percentages (range of 0 to 100). Just be consistent in your units.)

Note its similarity to the u-chart calculation, both in its structure and the importance of the overall system average to determine common cause, as well as the philosophy of its use. They differ only in their respective calculations of the common cause band.

As with the u-chart, this result of the square root is then multiplied by three (for "three standard deviations"), then added and subtracted to the overall mean. For the prescription data, the average of 14.8 percent translates to $p_{avg} = 0.148$:

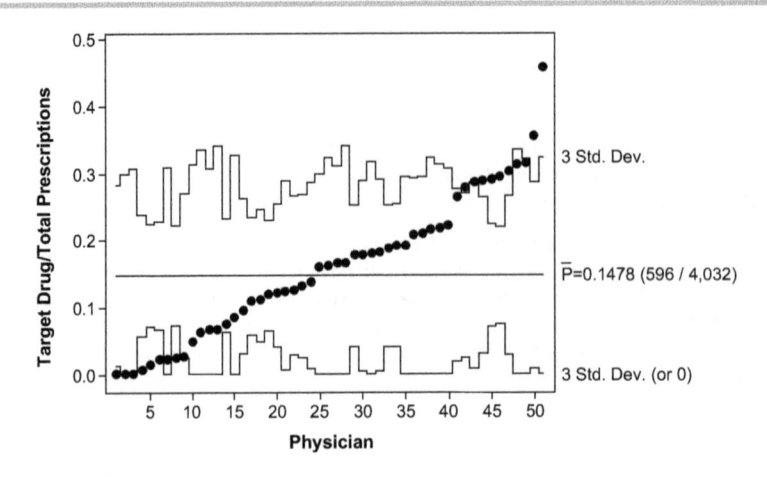

**EXHIBIT 7.5** ■ Correct Analysis for Target Drug Compliance

$$0.148 \pm 3 \times \sqrt{\frac{0.148 \times (1 - 0.148)}{\text{total number of prescriptions written}}}$$

The resulting chart will determine whether the actual value for an individual physician is in the range of this expected variation, given an assumed rate of 14.8 percent.

Compare the resulting ANOM p-chart (Exhibit 7.5) to the previous SWAG analysis.

- Note the width of the allegedly conservative three standard deviation limits.
  - Because the standard deviation was calculated appropriately, these three sigma limits are approximately equivalent to 1.5 times the incorrect (inflated) standard deviation of the SWAG analysis.
- The correct overall system average obtained from the aggregated summed numerators and denominators of the 51 physicians was 14.78 percent.
  - This is different from merely taking the average of the 51 percentages (15.85 percent) as in the SWAG analysis.
- There are eight "above average" performers (42–47 and 50–51).
- The performance of physicians 48 and 49 could still be indicative of individual processes at 14.78 percent.
  - Given the number of prescriptions written by each, their performances could just be statistical variation on 14.78 percent.
- This p-chart ANOM also found five doctors whose prescribing behavior was statistically lower than the average (participants 1, 4, 5, 6, and 8).
  - The SWAG analysis was not clear on whether it was concerned with finding below-average performers or whether its one or two standard deviations criteria would be applied to do this.
- In the SWAG analysis, depending on the analyst's mood and the standard deviation criterion subjectively selected, he or she could claim to find 1 or 10

(two inappropriate) upper outliers. The fact that it somewhat matched the correct analysis is sheer dumb luck.

### What Are the Appropriate Conclusions?

What are the correct conclusions drawn from Exhibit 7.5? Only that the eight above-average and five below-average outlier physicians have a different process than their colleagues for prescribing this particular drug. Seventy-four percent of the physicians (38 out of 51 with compliance between their individual two ANOM limits) display average behavior.

For some of the eight above-average physicians, this variation may be appropriate because of the type of patient they treat, and for others it may be inappropriate (or unintended) because of their methods of prescription, but they may not currently know it.

Maybe collegial discussion (including the five outliers whose performances are below average) using this graph as a starting point would be more productive than public blaming and shaming.

### A Quick Review of the Statistical Issues

To review, the vertical bands differ for each physician because each wrote a varying number of prescriptions (the denominator of the percent). For example, if a coin is flipped four times and no heads are obtained, do you really want to call the coin unfair? Conversely, if the same coin is flipped 16 times without obtaining any heads, how do you feel now about calling the coin unfair?

With increasing flips one becomes more confident of the coin's fairness or lack thereof. You can also estimate the coin's "true" probability better with more flips. In other words, assuming a fair coin, zero heads obtained from a window of opportunity of four flips could be common cause. However, zero heads obtained from a window of opportunity of 16 flips is a special cause. Similarly, we will be more certain whether physicians' deviations from the system average represent special cause variation as they write an increasing number of prescriptions.

A good summary of the process of prescribing the targeted drug seems to be that its use within its class has resulted in a process that is perfectly designed to have 14.8 percent use of the target drug (known as the *process capability*): Approximately 16 percent of the physicians display above-average prescribing behavior in prescribing this particular drug and 10 percent display below-average prescribing behavior.

### Reconsidering the Issue of Arbitrary Goals

What if it had been arbitrarily declared, "The target drug should not be more than 15 percent of prescriptions in this class"? Actually, based on the average of the p-chart being 14.8 percent, *the process is meeting this goal*. The process does, however, have eight physicians who are "above average" in their performance, which is outside their individual common cause limits. But in addition to these above-average physicians, who are truly special causes, 19 physicians are literally above the goal but within the upper limit of their individual common cause band.

If just the "no more than 15 percent" goal (a WAG) were arbitrarily used as a cutoff, 27 physicians would inappropriately receive feedback: They are statistically neither different from the goal nor are they different from the 19 physicians who happened to "win the lottery" and end up in the common cause band below the average.

**EXHIBIT 7.6** ■ P-Chart of Bypass Survival Rate

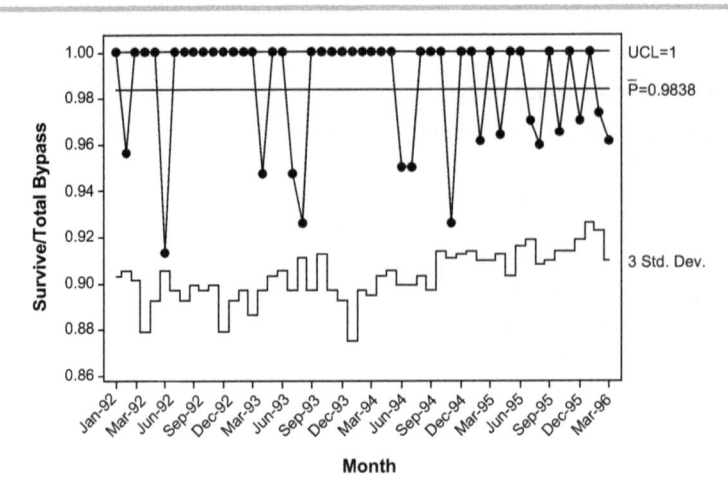

Suppose the goal had arbitrarily been set at 10 percent? The process as currently designed cannot attain it: It is designed for 14.8 percent performance and does not understand goals.

However, in treating *any* positive deviation from the desired 10 percent performance as a special cause (and given the fact that the underlying process variation gap from the desired goal is common cause), even more tampering (albeit well meaning) would result. This process, as it currently exists and operates, is not capable of meeting a goal of 10 percent.

Short term, one could use a strategy of getting the above-average physicians, where appropriate, to lower their rates to the current process average, an improvement of sorts. But, ultimately, there would need to be a fundamental change in *all* physician behavior.

This is a case where studying the physicians who are special causes below average could maybe yield some appropriate behaviors that could lead to such improvement or even decide, based on outcome analyses, that they are underutilizing the target drug and 10 percent is not a good goal for clinical reasons.

This whole analysis could be summarized with one more law of improvement: A process is what it is. The first task is to find out what it is.

## Another Example of Percentage Deceptiveness

The chart shown in Exhibit 7.6, calculated as a p-chart, was presented to a hospital's upper management. It describes the fraction of patients who were successfully treated and discharged following a primary procedure of coronary artery bypass.

The data represent four years of monthly performance. Numerators and denominators were available. The limits were calculated by the p-chart procedure described earlier in this chapter. Even though this is not a formal ANOM, it is sometimes valid to apply this calculation to a time plot of the data.

A member of the executive team was familiar with run and control charts and became concerned when looking at the graph. Even though all the data points were between the limits, he felt that somewhere in 1994 the survival rate started to worsen, with the trend continuing until the present. What do you think?

## *P-Chart vs. I-Chart?*

Exhibit 7.6 is different from what would result using the I-chart "Swiss Army knife" approximation presented in Chapter 6. Given the structure of this bypass data, the p-chart is probably superior in this case. It is only when the denominators of percentages are large (approaching 50) that the I-chart becomes a good approximation.

In this case, the denominators ranged from the teens to low thirties, which might tax this approximation.

Donald Wheeler argues in his book, *Understanding Variation* (see Resources) that the p-chart may not even necessarily be correct in this situation. He makes a convincing argument that one may have no choice but to use the I-chart approximation in any case. The argument is subtle, and most of the time I agree with him.

In fact, I generally find this issue more problematic when the denominators are very large as in 1,000s. I have found that using the p-chart in this case creates an overabundance of special cause outliers and there is no choice but to use the I-chart.

In any case, I believe that Wheeler's warning does not apply to this particular example, and it allows me to make some elegant points about dealing with percentage-type data (true "counts/counts" data).

## *Another Test for Special Causes*

There is another special cause rule that was mentioned briefly in Chapter 6, and it seems to apply here: A special cause exists if one observes at least *seven in a row of the same data value*.

Note in this case (see Exhibit 7.6) that it happens twice: Observations 7 through 15 are all 100 percent, as are observations 21 through 29. This test can sometimes signal an issue in the data collection process.

Because the data are percentages, with both numerators and denominators, a run chart of the denominators can sometimes provide further insight. Exhibit 7.7 contains the run chart for the survival rate denominators.

It is clear that the *process* had indeed changed, but not necessarily the percent survival. Is it the "methods" input, which is competence, or, as indicated by the run chart, the "people" input, which is volume?

With a 98.4 percent survival rate and a window of opportunity — the denominator — typically, 12 to 30 (first stable process), it was unusual to see any deviant events in a given month. Virtually everyone survived.

In other words, given the current survival rate and typical number of operations performed, monthly data are not discriminating enough for meaningful analysis of process stability. However, as of month 34, the typical number of operations increased by 10 per month (changed "people" process input). The new window of opportunity of 22 to 40 operations, combined with a survival rate of 98.4 percent, is indeed now sufficient to allow monthly data to assess the ongoing stability of the process.

If you still have any doubts about the process being stable for the entire 51 months, it is easy to compare the results of months 1 through 33 (637 survivals out of 646 operations: 98.6 percent) vs. months 34 through 51 (520 survivals out of 530 operations: 98.1 percent).

**EXHIBIT 7.7** ■ Run Chart of Bypass Survival Rate Denominators (number of procedures performed)

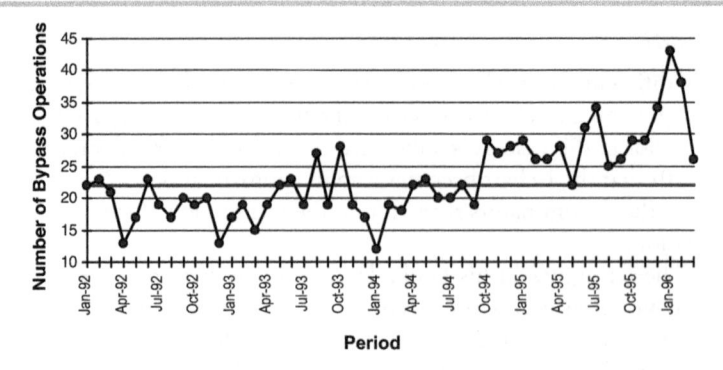

*Note:* The survival rate appears to be declining (or at least more variable) toward the end of this time period. The lower limit varies because of the different number of procedures performed in a given month.

**EXHIBIT 7.8** ■ Bypass Survival Rate Data Separated into Its Two Processes

|  | Deaths | Survivals | Total |
|---|---|---|---|
| Months 1–33 | 9 | 637 | 646 |
| Months 34–51 | 10 | 520 | 530 |
| Total | 19 | 1,157 | 1,176 |

**EXHIBIT 7.9** ■ Generic Data Structure to Compare Two Percentages

|  | Events | Nonevents | Total |
|---|---|---|---|
| Comparison 1 | a | b | a + b |
| Comparison 2 | c | d | c + d |
| Totals | a + c | b + d | N = a + b + c + d |

## A HANDY TECHNIQUE TO HAVE IN YOUR BACK POCKET

Here is a handy technique for comparing two percentages based on counts. I could use ANOM for the bypass survival data to compare the two rates. In this case, because of only one decision being made, the three standard deviation limits would be conservative. In addition, the problem of unequal denominators negates using ANOM's more exact limits (1.39 standard deviations) for a comparison at a 5 percent significance level. In cases like this, there is a nice alternative usually available in most good statistical computer packages.

One can create what is called a "2 × 2 table" as shown for the bypass survival data in Exhibit 7.8. The generic structure of such data is provided in Exhibit 7.9 so that you can understand the needed statistical calculation.

## EXHIBIT 7.10  Bypass Survival Rate Data Altered to Produce a Significant Result

|  | Deaths | Survivals | Total |
|---|---|---|---|
| Months 1–33 | 9 | 637 | 646 |
| Months 34–51 | 18 | 512 | 530 |
| Total | 27 | 1,149 | 1,176 |

The following formula results in a chi-square statistic with one degree of freedom. (The calculation looks worse than it is, but your computer package should have something akin to a 2 × 2 table chi-square analysis or contained as an option within "cross-tabs" procedures. The interpretation, however, is quite simple.)

$$X_c^2 = N \times \{(\text{absolute value } [(a \times d) - (b \times c)] - N/2)\}^2 / [(a + b) \times (c + d) \times (a + c) \times (b + d)]$$

where $N$ is the sum $(a + b + c + d)$, the total number of observations.

So, for the data above:

$$X_c^2 = 1,176 \times [\text{absolute value } (4,680 - 6,370) - 588]^2 / [(646) \times (530) \times (19) \times (1,157)]$$

$$= 0.193$$

To test the obtained statistic from this analysis (and any future analysis using this technique) for statistical significance:

- For 5 percent risk or less (of declaring common cause as special cause): >3.64; and
- For 1 percent risk or less (of declaring common cause as special cause): >6.63.

In other words, if your $X_c^2$ value is *greater than* these values, there is a good chance that the difference is real; the larger the value, the less your risk of declaring the difference as real when it is not. Obviously, with a value of 0.193 (which is much less than 3.64) for the bypass survival data, there is no evidence of a real difference.

(*Note:* If you try to reproduce these results with your package, which I highly recommend, it might give the $X_c^2$ value to be 0.446 instead of 0.193. My calculation is technically the correct one because it adjusts for the fact that these data are counts and not continuous data. This is called the *correction for continuity* and is especially important if you have small sample sizes, which is not true in this case. Regardless, the interpretation is the same.)

Now, we change this data a bit in Exhibit 7.10, keeping the original data for months 1–33 and 98.6 percent survival. Note that I have changed the result of months 34–51 to 512 survivals out of 530 operations: 96.6 percent survival (a 2 percent decrease).

Applying the preceding formula yields an $X_c^2$ of 4.35 (5.21 uncorrected), which, if one were to declare a difference, would have a risk of between 1 and 5 percent of being wrong. So, in this case, there would be good evidence that the survival had indeed gotten worse.

EXHIBIT 7.11 ■ Ventricular Fibrillation Data from Chapter 2

|  | Vfib | Non-Vfib | Total |
|---|---|---|---|
| Year 1 | 81 | 180 | 261 |
| Year 2 | 71 | 204 | 275 |
| Total | 152 | 384 | 536 |

Source: Davis Balestracci Jr. 2005. "When Processes Moonlight as Trends." *Quality Digest* (June). www.qualitydigest.com. Used with permission.

The data from Lesson 4 in Chapter 2 are reproduced for this analysis in Exhibit 7.11. Applying this calculation:

$X_c^2 = 1.546$     (1.793 uncorrected)

Because this is less than 3.64, one concludes no statistical evidence of a difference, just as was concluded from the run chart analysis.

Watch out for small table cell counts. This calculation is an approximation and will suffice in most cases. It can break down when testing data contains truly rare events. The danger begins when there are less than five occurrences in one of the table cells (the smallest value in Exhibit 7.10 was 9).

With small counts, one needs to use what is called *Fisher's exact test*. It is a messy calculation and beyond the scope of this book. For an example of undesirable medical events, see the following sidebar "Analyzing Rare Occurrences of Events." But, once again, any good basic statistical package should have it available as an option. I applied it to these two data sets and easily came to the same conclusions as the approximations I demonstrated and discussed.

## Summary Example for Percentages

Reviewing the C-section scenario presented in Chapter 6, four years of C-section performance showed a change in performance (lowered rate) as of month 13. This was the month that individual performances were shared with the practicing physicians so they could each blindly compare their performance with that of their peers. The subsequent 35 months showed no change, but at least the initial gains were held.

The doctor in charge of QA wanted to dig further to see whether any deeper opportunities existed. There were 16 physicians practicing at this hospital, so I asked the QA director for the individual performances of each physician *for the recent 35-month stable period* (number of deliveries and number of resulting C-sections). I eventually eliminated one physician's data from the analysis (to be explained later), and for your amusement, Exhibit 7.12 shows a bar graph of rates of the remaining 15 practicing physicians. The raw data and limits for a p-chart ANOM analysis are given in Exhibit 7.13.

The system value is determined as the total number of C-sections by the 15 physicians divided by the *total number* of deliveries performed by the 15 physicians (693/4,568 = 15.17 percent). It is exactly the same as the average of the past 35 months of control chart performance. I am aggregating the 35 months of data that produced that average, then disaggregating it by physician — a statistical stratification.

## Analyzing Rare Occurrences of Events

Eighty-four doctors treated 2,973 patients, and an undesirable incident occurred in 13 of the treatments (11 doctors with one incident and 1 doctor with two incidents), a rate of 0.437 percent. A p-chart analysis of means (ANOM) for these data is shown in Figure 1.

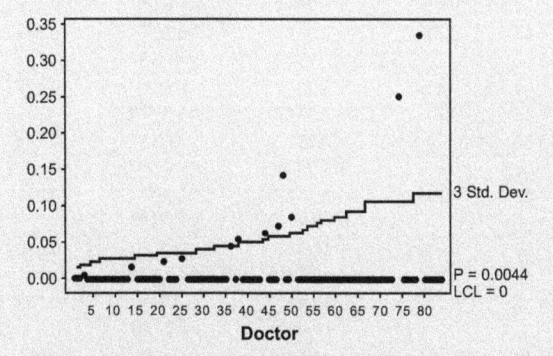

Figure 1. P-Chart of Undesirable Incident Rate

This analysis is dubious. A good rule of thumb is that multiplying the overall average rate by the number of cases for an individual should yield the possibility of at least five cases. Each doctor would need 1,000 cases to even begin to come close to this.

The table in Figure 2 uses the technique of calculating both "uncorrected" and "corrected" chi-square values. Similar to the philosophy of ANOM, I take each doctor's performance out of the aggregate and compare it to those remaining to see whether they are statistically different. For example, in Figure 2, during the first doctor's performance, one patient in the 199 patient treatments had the incident occur. So I compared his rate of 1/199 to the remaining 12/2,774.

Things break down very quickly as the denominator size decreases, especially the gap between the uncorrected and corrected chi-square values. With data like these, one has no option but to use the technique known as *Fisher's exact test* (available in most good statistical packages). Its resulting *p*-value is shown in the far right column of Figure 2. Using the example of the doctor with one incident out of 199 patients, one has to ask, "If I have a population where 13 out of 2,973 patients experienced an incident, and if I grabbed a random sample of 199 of these 2,973 patients, what is the probability that I would have at least one patient who had an incident?" As you can see in Figure 2, in the first row of the Fisher's exact test column, it is 0.594 (~60 percent), which is not unusual.

Figure 3 sets up the calculation for the only doctor for whom two patients had the event occur (out of 14 patients). So, one is comparing 2/14 vs. 11/2,959. To find the probability of obtaining two or more events in this sample caused by sheer randomness, calculate the exact probabilities of randomly obtaining zero ($p_0$) and one ($p_1$) event in a random sample of 14, then calculate $(1 - (p_0 + p_1))$. As you see from the table in Figure 2, the answer is 0.0016 (~0.2 percent).

To find out what constitutes an outlier, I'm going to use the technique discussed in the preceding sidebar "Why Three Standard Deviations?" to see what the threshold of probability might be for *overall* risks of 0.05 and 0.10 (one-tailed).

(Continues)

(Continued)

| Patients | Incident "Occurs" | Chi-squared (uncorrected) p-value | Chi-squared (corrected) p-value | Fisher's Exact Test p-value |
|---|---|---|---|---|
| 199 | 1 | 0.021 $p = 0.885$ | 0.170 $p = 0.681$ | 0.594 |
| 61 | 1 | 2.067 $p = 0.151$ | 0.209 $p = 0.647$ | 0.237 |
| 44 | 1 | 3.456 $p = 0.063$ | 0.501 $p = 0.479$ | 0.177 |
| 38 | 1 | 4.257 $p = 0.039$ | 0.682 $p = 0.409$ | 0.154 |
| 23 | 1 | 8.142 $p = 0.0043$ | 1.61 $p = 0.205$ | 0.096 |
| 19 | 1 | 10.23 $p = 0.0014$ | 2.11 $p = 0.146$ | 0.080 |
| 16 | 1 | 12.48 $p = 0.0004$ | 2.67 $p = 0.102$ | 0.068 |
| 14 | 1 | 14.53 $p = 0.00014$ | 3.17 $p = 0.075$ | 0.060 |
| 14 | 2 | 61.96 $p < 0.0001$ | 34.12 $p < 0.0001$ | 0.0016 |
| 12 | 1 | 17.26 $p < 0.0001$ | 3.85 $p = 0.05$ | 0.051 |
| 4 | 1 | 55.51 $p < 0.0001$ | 13.39 $p = 0.00025$ | 0.017 |
| 3 | 1 | 74.64 $p < 0.0001$ | 18.17 $p = 0.00002$ | 0.013 |

**Figure 2. Chi Square vs. Fisher's Exact Test**

$$\frac{\frac{13!}{0!\,13!} \times \frac{2{,}960!}{14!\,2{,}946!}}{\frac{2{,}973!}{14!\,2{,}959!}} = p_0 \qquad \frac{\frac{13!}{1!\,12!} \times \frac{2{,}960!}{13!\,2{,}947!}}{\frac{2{,}973!}{14!\,2{,}959!}} = p_1$$

Note: 0! = 1

The probability of randomly obtaining no events and one event, respectively, in a random sample of 14 taken from a population of 2,973 containing 13 events

**Figure 3. Probability of Zero or One Event**

In this case of 84 simultaneous decisions:

- Overall 5 percent risk = $p < 0.00061$ to declare significance
- Overall 10 percent risk = $p < 0.00125$

Only the 2/14 is close when compared with these criteria, but barely at the 10 percent risk level.

There are never any easy answers when rates of rare adverse events regarding human life are being compared and someone's professional reputation is at stake. Tread carefully.

Source: Adapted from Davis Balestracci Jr. 2008. "Analyzing Rare Occurrences of Events: When to Use Fisher's Exact Test." *Quality Digest* (August). www.qualitydigest.com. Reprinted with permission.

EXHIBIT 7.12 ■ Bar Graph Presentation of 15 Physicians' C-Section Performance

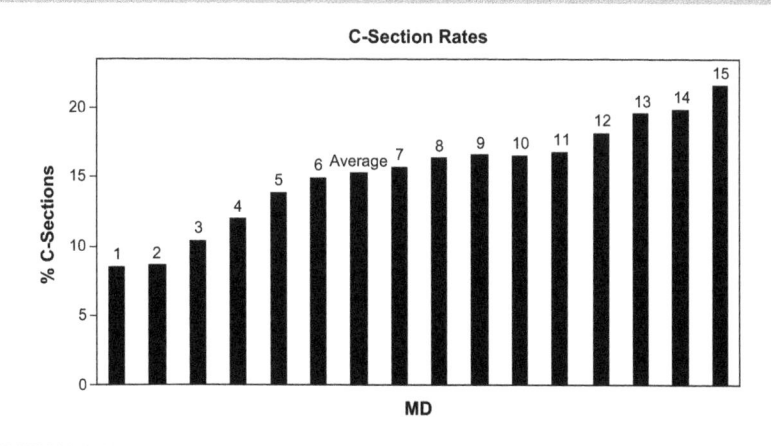

**C-Section Rates**

EXHIBIT 7.13 ■ C-Section Performance of 35-Month Baseline Stratified by Individual Physician

| MD | C-Sections | Deliveries | % C-Sections | ANOM Lower Limit | ANOM Upper Limit |
|---|---|---|---|---|---|
| 1 | 27 | 317 | 8.52 | 9.13 | 21.22 |
| 2 | 29 | 337 | 8.61 | 9.31 | 21.03 |
| 3 | 38 | 364 | 10.44 | 9.53 | 20.81 |
| 4 | 38 | 317 | 11.99 | 9.13 | 21.22 |
| 5 | 38 | 274 | 13.87 | 8.67 | 21.67 |
| 6 | 36 | 241 | 14.94 | 8.24 | 22.10 |
| 7 | 32 | 204 | 15.69 | 7.64 | 22.71 |
| 8 | 59 | 361 | 16.34 | 9.51 | 20.84 |
| 9 | 37 | 223 | 16.59 | 7.96 | 22.38 |
| 10 | 49 | 296 | 16.55 | 8.92 | 21.43 |
| 11 | 61 | 364 | 16.76 | 9.53 | 20.81 |
| 12 | 65 | 358 | 18.16 | 9.48 | 20.86 |
| 13 | 70 | 358 | 19.55 | 9.48 | 20.86 |
| 14 | 62 | 313 | 19.81 | 9.09 | 21.25 |
| 15 | 52 | 241 | 21.58 | 8.24 | 22.10 |
| Total | 693 | 4,568 | | | |
| Average | | | 15.17 | | |

Each physician is presumed "innocent" at this level of 15.17 percent unless his or her individual data show otherwise. One must now put three standard deviations on either side of this system average to see whether an individual physician's result is inside the system or outside the system.

Each physician's common cause range as shown in the data table was calculated by the p-chart formula:

EXHIBIT 7.14 ■ *p*-Chart ANOM by Physician

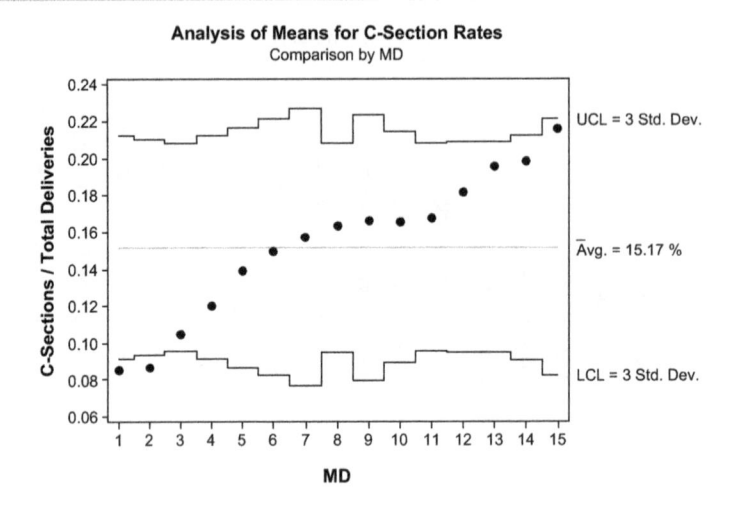

**Analysis of Means for C-Section Rates**
Comparison by MD

$$15.17 \pm 3 \sqrt{\frac{15.17 \times (100 - 15.17)}{(\text{total deliveries by MD})}}$$

and it yields the p-chart ANOM shown in Exhibit 7.14.

This data originally contained the performance of 16 physicians. The initial analysis resulted in one performance that was obviously above the upper limit. In showing it to the physician QA director, he said, "Wait a minute, is that Dr. X?" It was, to which he replied, "Well, that makes sense. She's our perinatologist." Yes indeed, a different process, using a different "people" input, and we see variation from the average that is most likely appropriate and has nothing to do with competence.

*Did you notice that there are no statistically above-average performers?* The only special causes are Physicians 1 and 2, who seem to have lower C-section rates than their colleagues. When the QA physician asked who they were and I told him, he smiled and said, "Consideration of the customer." These two physicians had reputations as being caring (and their practices may have even been closed) and word was out: If you are going to have a baby and want to do everything possible to deliver naturally, these are the guys you want. Very importantly, further analysis showed no difference vis-à-vis their colleagues in terms of their fetal outcomes.

Do you also notice that this analysis yields no individual performances that can be declared in the top, second, or third quartiles (or even fourth quartile), just two outliers?

### A Simple Intervention and Assessment of Results

Based on this analysis and the fortunate result that there were no high outliers, the QA physician wanted to present this data at a department meeting, identify the two below-average performers (who had no idea about their performances), and have them collegially discuss how they handle labor.

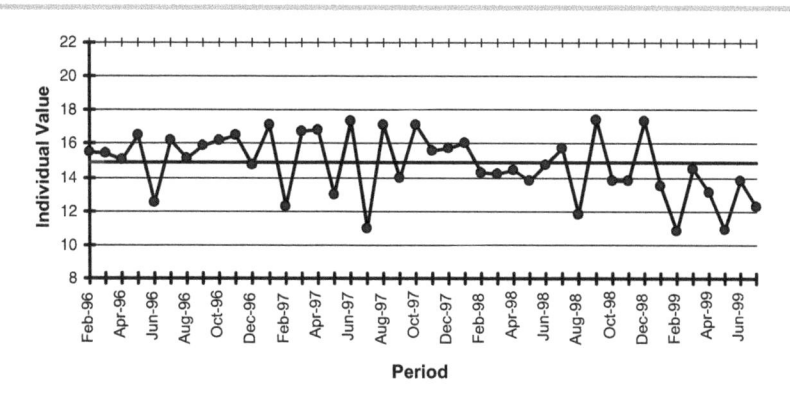

EXHIBIT 7.15 ◼ C-Section Data with Seven Months of Post-Intervention Data

EXHIBIT 7.16 ◼ Baseline and Post-Intervention Performances

|  | C-Sections | Non-C-Sections | Total Deliveries |
|---|---|---|---|
| 35-Month Baseline | 693 | 3,875 | 4,568 |
| 7-Month Follow-up | 237 | 1,624 | 1,861 |
| Total | 930 | 5,499 | 6,429 |

This was done and the last data I ever got on this situation were the seven months following this meeting. I added it to the previous stable baseline of months 14–48 (the recent stable history aggregated for this analysis) and calculated the new median. It resulted in the run chart shown in Exhibit 7.15. What do you notice about the post-meeting data?

Before the intervention, the performance was (693/4,568) = 15.2 percent, and the seven months' post-meeting aggregated performance was (237/1,861) = 12.7 percent. Is this 2.5 percent drop significant, as is strongly hinted by the run chart?

It has become acceptable to relax the run chart criterion of "eight in a row either all above or below the median" to declare a special cause, which, in this case, would be a successful intervention. One can use "five or six in a row" above or below the median *only if* the data points occur immediately after a formal intervention whose intent was to move the process needle specifically in the observed direction, which was true with this data.

Let's use the 2 × 2 table technique with these data, shown in Exhibit 7.16.

The obtained $X_c^2$ is 6.14 (6.34 uncorrected, which is not very different because of the very large denominators), and being close to the 1 percent risk value of 6.63, it is clearly a significant difference — essentially a 1 percent risk of being wrong.

## ANALYSIS OF MEANS FOR CONTINUOUS DATA

Applying ANOM to continuous data is every bit as valuable as what has been demonstrated in the u-chart and p-chart analyses. However, it is not as clean cut as those two applications, and my experience has been that it is a confusing concept for an audience,

EXHIBIT 7.17 ■ Regional Target Monitor (Goal: >90 percent)

| Period | Region 1 | Region 2 | Region 3 | Region 4 | Region 5 |
|---|---|---|---|---|---|
| 4/6/2003 | 85.1% | 96.4% | **83.5%** | 88.0% | 86.6% |
| 4/13/2003 | **83.9%** | 94.7% | **84.3%** | 89.0% | 85.4% |
| 4/20/2003 | 85.1% | 94.6% | **81.4%** | **84.0%** | 86.0% |
| 4/27/2003 | 85.2% | 92.2% | **84.0%** | 85.6% | **84.8%** |
| 5/4/2003 | **84.9%** | 93.9% | **82.3%** | **83.9%** | 86.0% |

| Period | Region 1 | Region 2 | Region 3 | Region 4 | Region 5 |
|---|---|---|---|---|---|
| 8/31/2003 | 88.0% | 96.1% | 86.5% | **84.5%** | 90.9% |
| 9/7/2003 | 91.4% | 92.1% | 85.7% | 85.5% | 93.5% |
| 9/14/2003 | 90.0% | 94.4% | 88.2% | 89.9% | 91.6% |
| 9/21/2003 | 89.6% | 92.9% | 86.3% | 91.0% | 92.1% |
| 9/28/2003 | 89.6% | 94.1% | 89.1% | 89.2% | 92.2% |

Key: ≥ 90% = Green, 85%–89% = Yellow, < 85% = **Red**

Source: Davis Balestracci Jr., MS, *Quality Digest*, July 2007. www.qualitydigest.com. Reprinted with permission.

even those with Six Sigma belts. For purposes of this book and its audience, I have made it less mathematical, more intuitively graphical, and more typical of the data and analyses I encounter in the everyday work of healthcare. For readers who are interested, I explain a few advanced concepts in Lesson 3 of Appendix 7A.

The following example is an intuitive explanation of ANOM that applies and adapts what you already know about run and control charts.

Take a look at the data in Exhibit 7.17. This chart was sent to a government agency every week for monitoring an arbitrary target that had been set. There were 28 regions. I've chosen five of them and given the first and last five weeks of data so you'll have an idea of what was presented at the meetings, which was a 26-by-28 matrix of numbers.

You might think that a comparative histogram would be a better alternative. See Exhibit 7.18, which the computer easily does, but is actually of no value.

Because I first plotted the dots of each region to assess their process performances and found out that not all of them were stable, this graph is invalid, and any attempt to use it or do an analysis of variance (ANOVA) using *all* the data would also be invalid.

Exhibit 7.19 is much better. An initial control chart analysis was used for each region to assess whether special causes were present. Most of the special causes were distinct process shifts in performance, and the data are shown as control charts adjusted for these. But more important, *all five regions are on the same scale.*

Note the difference of the histograms in Exhibit 7.18 with those in Exhibit 7.20 that uses the most recent stable history (Region 1, last 13 observations; Region 2, all the data; Region 3, last 13 observations; Region 4, all the data; and Region 5, last 13 observations). This, along with the control chart analysis in Exhibit 7.19, provides an excellent summary.

I've used ANOM to look for differences in performance with data expressed as aggregated percentages or rates. Unlike rates or percentages, with continuous data, things are unclear because, as the control charts in the exhibits show, it takes some thought to

EXHIBIT 7.18  Stratified Histograms of Performance vs. Region

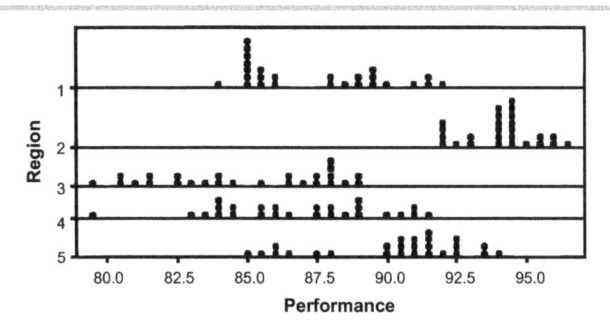

Source: Davis Balestracci Jr., MS, *Quality Digest*, July 2007. www.qualitydigest.com. Reprinted with permission.

EXHIBIT 7.19  Control Chart Comparison of Five Regions

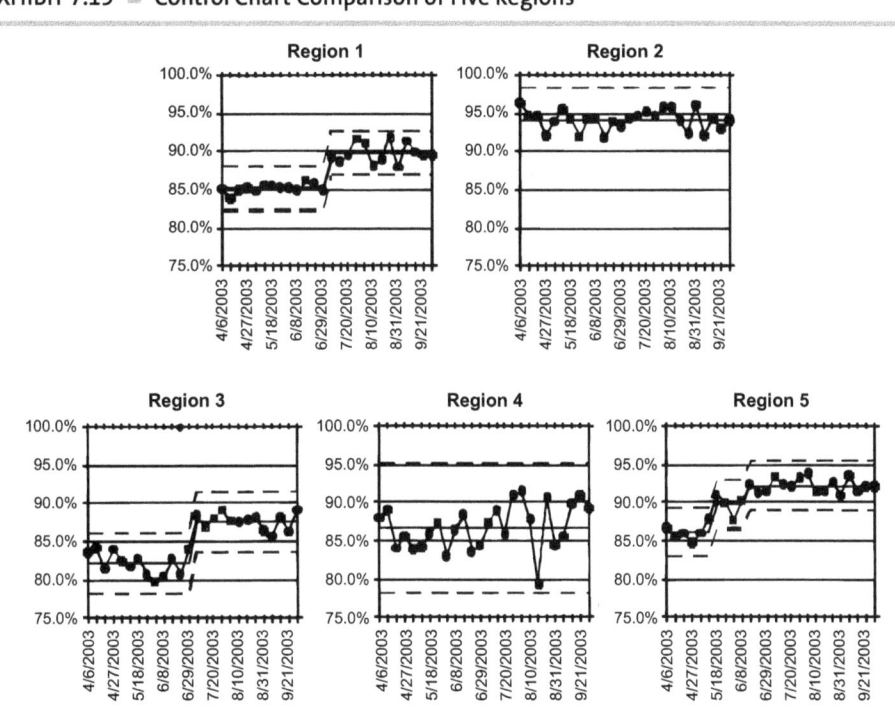

Source: Davis Balestracci Jr., MS, *Quality Digest*, July 2007. www.qualitydigest.com. Reprinted with permission.

aggregate, appropriately, a time sequence of continuous data into a calculated average. This is what you might call a "partial" ANOM because there is no formal analysis carried out using common cause limits to compare the individual averages (see Lesson 3 in Appendix 7A for issues involved in the ANOM analysis and its resulting approximate graph). I say "approximate" because, if you notice from the control charts, Region 4's performance has 2.5 times more variation than the other four regions. This common problem of unequal

EXHIBIT 7.20  Stratified Histograms Comparing Most Recent Stable Behaviors

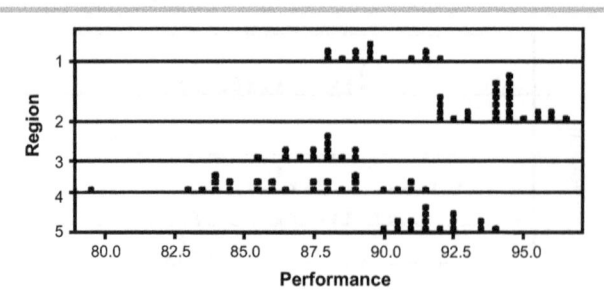

Source: Davis Balestracci Jr., MS, *Quality Digest*, July 2007. www.qualitydigest.com. Reprinted with permission

variations with continuous data can make it difficult to apply standard comparison summary techniques. This is yet another reason why the intuitive nature of staying visual by plotting the dots is a good idea and simpler to explain.

## CASE STUDY: USING ANALYSIS OF MEANS AS A DIAGNOSTIC TOOL

### Emergency Department Unpredictable Admit Data

The supervisor of inpatient admissions at a hospital was troubled. From 6 p.m. to 11 p.m., her people had to handle "unexpected" admissions to the emergency department (and she was quite adamant when she gave me these data: "We're not supposed to have these!"). This was a disturbance to the other work they also had to do. (Does this supervisor see "unexpected" admissions as a common cause or a special cause to her system of inpatient admissions? What do you think?)

She decided to collect some data on the situation, that is, study the current process. Her staff worked Monday through Friday. She collected hourly data (6–7 p.m., 7–8 p.m., 8–9 p.m., 9–10 p.m., 10–11 p.m.) for 31 consecutive days. The data are shown in their time order in Exhibit 7.21 and labeled by the particular day of the week on which they were collected.

Before doing any more formal statistical analysis, a few simple macro-level pictures might answer some natural questions about this process to be subsequently confirmed by plotting the dots. First, do there seem to be any special causes by day of the week? Second, are there any special causes by hourly period? Two stratified histograms are shown in Exhibits 7.22 and 7.23. The first separates the data by day. The second separates the data by hourly interval. What one is looking for here is whether there seem to be significant aggregate shifts of the data clusters in each histogram by day and time of night, respectively.

These are histogram presentations known as *dot plots*, with each dot representing specifically one occurrence of a particular data value. For example, looking at the six Mondays' data, each with five time periods, taken from Exhibit 7.21 and plotted on the corresponding "Monday" axis in Exhibit 7.22, these 30 hourly time periods had:

- 1 period with 1 admit
- 2 periods with 2 admits
- 4 periods with 3 admits

# STATISTICAL STRATIFICATION

**EXHIBIT 7.21** Emergency Department Unexpected Admit Data

| | Hour of Day | | | | |
|---|---|---|---|---|---|
| Day of Week | 6–7 p.m. | 7–8 p.m. | 8–9 p.m. | 9–10 p.m. | 10–11 p.m. |
| Wed | 2 | 8 | 7 | 8 | 8 |
| Thu | 8 | 4 | 11 | 6 | 5 |
| Fri | 5 | 6 | 5 | 6 | 2 |
| Mon | 3 | 5 | 7 | 9 | 11 |
| Tue | 3 | 5 | 7 | 7 | 8 |
| Wed | 9 | 4 | 5 | 8 | 1 |
| Thu | 2 | 3 | 7 | 10 | 3 |
| Fri | 1 | 2 | 5 | 6 | 3 |
| Mon | 5 | 4 | 10 | 11 | 6 |
| Tue | 4 | 2 | 3 | 7 | 6 |
| Wed | 1 | 3 | 8 | 9 | 6 |
| Thu | 4 | 4 | 8 | 6 | 6 |
| Fri | 3 | 5 | 6 | 8 | 6 |
| Mon | 4 | 1 | 5 | 13 | 6 |
| Tue | 9 | 7 | 9 | 7 | 6 |
| Wed | 4 | 6 | 11 | 9 | 6 |
| Thu | 3 | 4 | 9 | 8 | 4 |
| Fri | 2 | 3 | 5 | 5 | 6 |
| Mon | 7 | 10 | 10 | 12 | 6 |
| Tue | 1 | 5 | 8 | 6 | 5 |
| Wed | 2 | 5 | 1 | 11 | 8 |
| Thu | 5 | 2 | 7 | 4 | 5 |
| Fri | 4 | 3 | 9 | 8 | 6 |
| Mon | 2 | 5 | 4 | 5 | 4 |
| Tue | 6 | 2 | 8 | 7 | 5 |
| Wed | 3 | 5 | 1 | 9 | 10 |
| Thu | 3 | 1 | 5 | 4 | 7 |
| Fri | 4 | 5 | 6 | 9 | 9 |
| Mon | 3 | 2 | 3 | 11 | 3 |
| Tue | 4 | 7 | 6 | 15 | 4 |
| Wed | 6 | 5 | 12 | 3 | 8 |

- 4 periods with 4 admits
- 5 periods with 5 admits
- 3 periods with 6 admits
- 2 periods with 7 admits
- 0 periods with 8 admits
- 1 period with 9 admits
- 3 periods with 10 admits
- 3 periods with 11 admits
- 1 period with 12 admits
- 1 period with 13 admits

EXHIBIT 7.22 ■ Stratified Histogram of Hourly Unexpected Patient Admits by Day of the Week

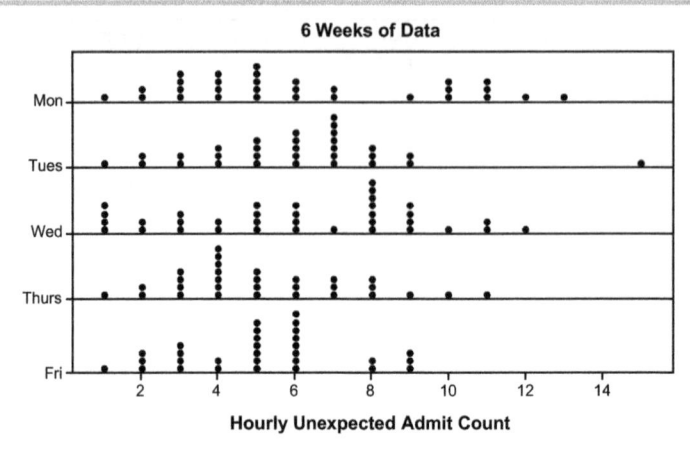

**6 Weeks of Data**

[Dot plot showing Hourly Unexpected Admit Count (x-axis: 2, 4, 6, 8, 10, 12, 14) stratified by day (Mon, Tues, Wed, Thurs, Fri)]

6–7 p.m., 7–8 p.m., 8–9 p.m., 9–10 p.m., 10–11 p.m. data aggregated

*Note:* There appear to be no blatant differences between days of the week.

Note that the data have lost their "hour of the day" identity.

Giving each a quick perusal, there seem to be no glaring differences by day of the week. However, Monday's data has a wider spread than the other days and calls attention to what appears to be an interesting separate clump of nine observations with high values. This might be useful in subsequent analysis or it might not.

The second histogram is far more interesting (see Exhibit 7.23). Distinct differences can be observed. The first two time periods seem indistinguishable from each other and on the average, lower than the other three. It also looks as if the 9–10 p.m. hour has, on average, a tendency toward higher rates of emergency department admissions.

ANOM will now be used to statistically gain more insight into the situation. After the ANOM, any conclusions will be confirmed (or disputed) by time plotting of the original data as suggested by the analysis. As stated previously, any data set has an implicit time element, which must be considered sooner or later.

The first ANOM will compare totals by day of the week. In other words, at this point, there is no concern for the hourly pattern. The question is a macro one: Do some weekdays tend to have more admissions on the whole than other days, regardless of their hourly pattern?

The hourly totals were added to get a daily total. Exhibit 7.24 shows the data for each day of the week grouped with its corresponding and subsequent weekly data. (Note that there are seven observations for Wednesdays.)

A simplified approximation to ANOM analysis by day of the week is shown in Exhibit 7.25.

The overall average of 28.7 for all 31 daily admit totals was forced in as the average for each control chart (and they all have the same scale) to see whether that day's performance generated special causes in relation to that overall average. Because of the small number of observations, I let the control chart program default to the average moving range to calculate each day's limits. Regardless, there are no obvious special causes.

# STATISTICAL STRATIFICATION

EXHIBIT 7.23 ■ Stratified Histogram of Hourly Unexpected Patient Admits by Time of Evening

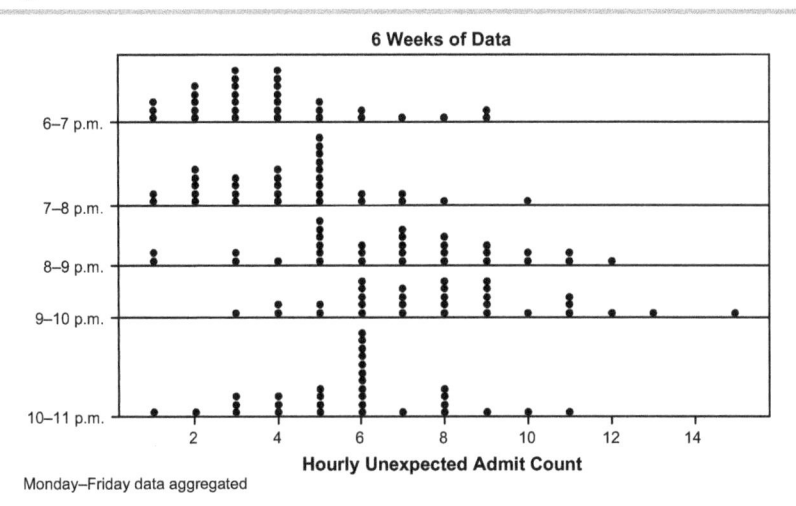

**6 Weeks of Data**

(Dot plot showing hourly unexpected admit counts stratified by time: 6–7 p.m., 7–8 p.m., 8–9 p.m., 9–10 p.m., 10–11 p.m.; x-axis: Hourly Unexpected Admit Count from 2 to 14)

Monday–Friday data aggregated

*Note:* While there appear to be no differences between days of the week, the time of night does seem to make a difference.

EXHIBIT 7.24 ■ Emergency Department Admission Data Daily Totals

| Week | Mon | Tue | Wed | Thu | Fri |
|------|-----|-----|-----|-----|-----|
| 1 | 35 | 30 | 33 | 34 | 24 |
| 2 | 36 | 22 | 27 | 25 | 17 |
| 3 | 29 | 38 | 27 | 28 | 28 |
| 4 | 45 | 25 | 36 | 28 | 21 |
| 5 | 20 | 28 | 27 | 23 | 30 |
| 6 | 22 | 36 | 28 | 20 | 33 |
| 7 |    |    | 34 |    |    |

As discussed earlier in this chapter, I can make a case that these are count data, which allows more exact calculations. It allows one to use a u-chart to compare the daily averages, as shown in Exhibit 7.26, which uses the rate formula discussed earlier this chapter.

$U_{avg}$ in this case is 28.7, and the window of opportunity is how many observations were averaged to get an individual data point: 6 (days) for Monday, Tuesday, Thursday, and Friday and 7 (days) for Wednesday.

The five daily averages all fall within the common cause band. The band is slightly tighter for Wednesday because its average contains seven observations vs. six for the other days. Thus the ANOM confirmed our intuitive analyses via the stratified histogram and simultaneous control chart presentation with the overall average forced in. Even though Mondays have the highest average and Fridays the lowest, there is no statistical difference between them, based on this small amount of data.

**EXHIBIT 7.25** ■ Graphical Equivalent ANOM Comparing Day of the Week via Forced Common Average

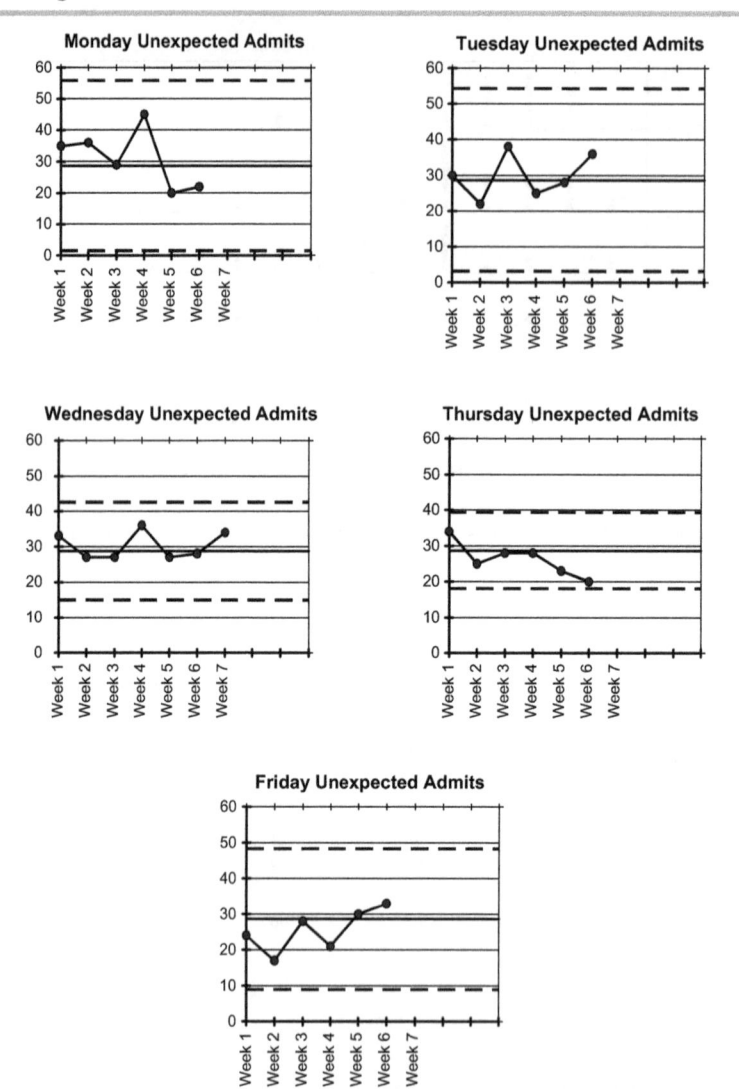

Because there are no apparent differences by day of the week, these 31 daily totals could be considered from the same process. They are plotted in run and control charts (Exhibit 7.27). The run chart is unremarkable.

Comparing the I-chart to the c-chart (Exhibit 7.27b and 7.27c), you can see just how good the I-chart approximation is to the true answer using count data. Because it is count data, the standard deviation of the c-chart is the square root of the average (28.7), which equals 5.4. The I-chart standard deviation of 6.8 was obtained using the average moving range. Note that the interpretations do not differ and in the c-chart, one point is right at the upper limit. But that is occasionally expected.

EXHIBIT 7.26 ■ Formal Analysis of Means Comparing Unexpected Admits by Day of the Week

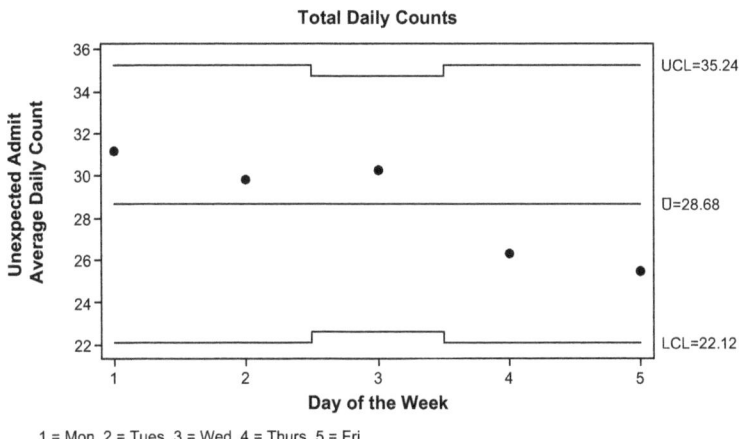

Total Daily Counts

[Chart: Unexpected Admit Average Daily Count vs Day of the Week, with UCL=35.24, Ū=28.68, LCL=22.12]

1 = Mon, 2 = Tues, 3 = Wed, 4 = Thurs, 5 = Fri
3 Standard Deviation Limits

Note: There are no statistically detectable differences between days of the week.

To conclude so far, this unpredictable process is actually quite predictable. On any given weekday night, this process averages 29 unexpected emergency department admits. Occasionally, one may have as few as 10, but there may also be the night everyone dreads, with 50 unexpected admits. Why? Just because: Given the evidence of the chart, such a night should not be reacted to with an immediate adjustment for the following night. After such a night, subsequent plotting would be useful to either confirm whether it was just a common cause event or that a process change has really taken place. The "two out of three" rule along with the "eight consecutive observations above the average" rule should be watched closely. But we must still solve the issue of the best way to plot this data for everyday use.

Consider the more interesting question of differences among the five hourly periods.

Having a reasonable amount of data, we do a run chart first on the same scale to make sure control charts are appropriate (shown in Exhibit 7.28). Because these run charts look stable, we try an approximate analysis of means by converting them to control charts. Each hour's chart average will be forced in as the overall data average of 5.73 unexpected admits per hour so that the control limits are centered on the process average of all five days of the week. At this point, I will let each hour's performance set its own control limit width using the average moving range (Exhibit 7.29).

Once again using the count calculation, the standard deviation of this data is the square root of the average (5.73), which equals 2.39. Let's revise the preceding figure a bit by using that as a common standard deviation. Exhibit 7.30 is a graphical equivalent of the usual ANOM, the summary version of which is shown in Exhibit 7.31.

These confirm our intuition from the stratified histograms: 6–7 p.m. and 7–8 p.m. tend to be below average, 8–9 p.m. and 10–11 p.m. tend to be average, and 9–10 p.m. is above average.

EXHIBIT 7.27 ■ Run Chart, I-Chart, and C-Chart of Daily Unexpected Admit Counts

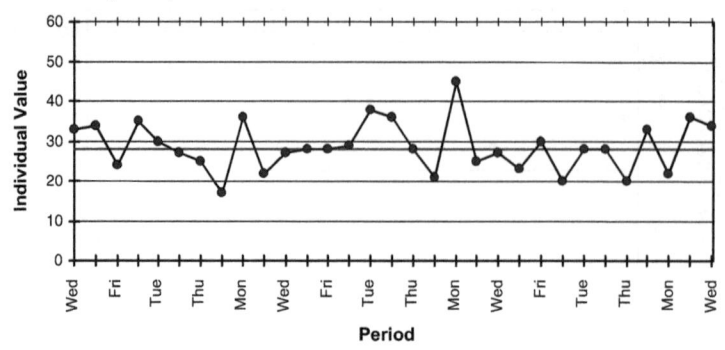

**a. Total Daily Unexpected Admits**

**b. Total Daily Unexpected Admits — I-Chart**

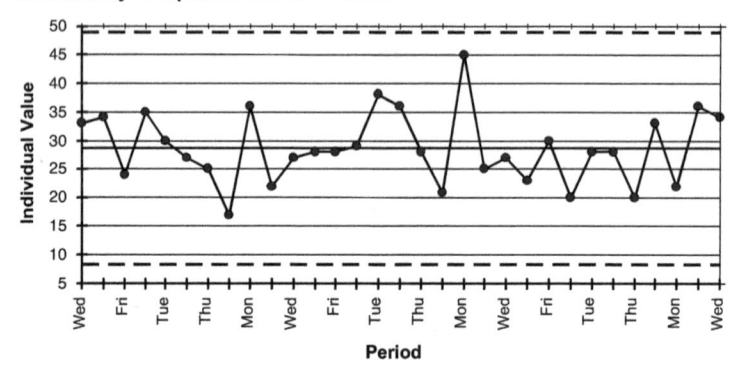

**c. Total Daily Unexpected Admits — C-Chart**

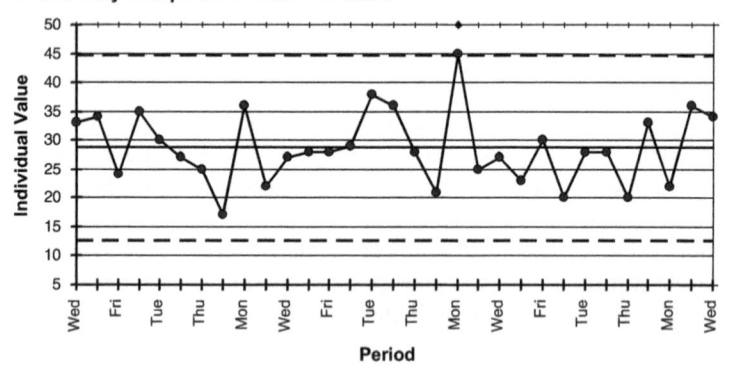

To summarize, in Exhibit 7.29, the limits were calculated separately for each control chart, and they are all quite similar. The next analysis (see Exhibit 7.30) forced in the count calculation of 2.39 for the standard deviation (this was the value used in Exhibit 7.31 in the more usual version of the ANOM). The control charts in Exhibit 7.30 have equivalent limits, but, notice once again that the I-charts were very good approximations.

EXHIBIT 7.28 ▪ Run Chart Comparison of Hour of Day

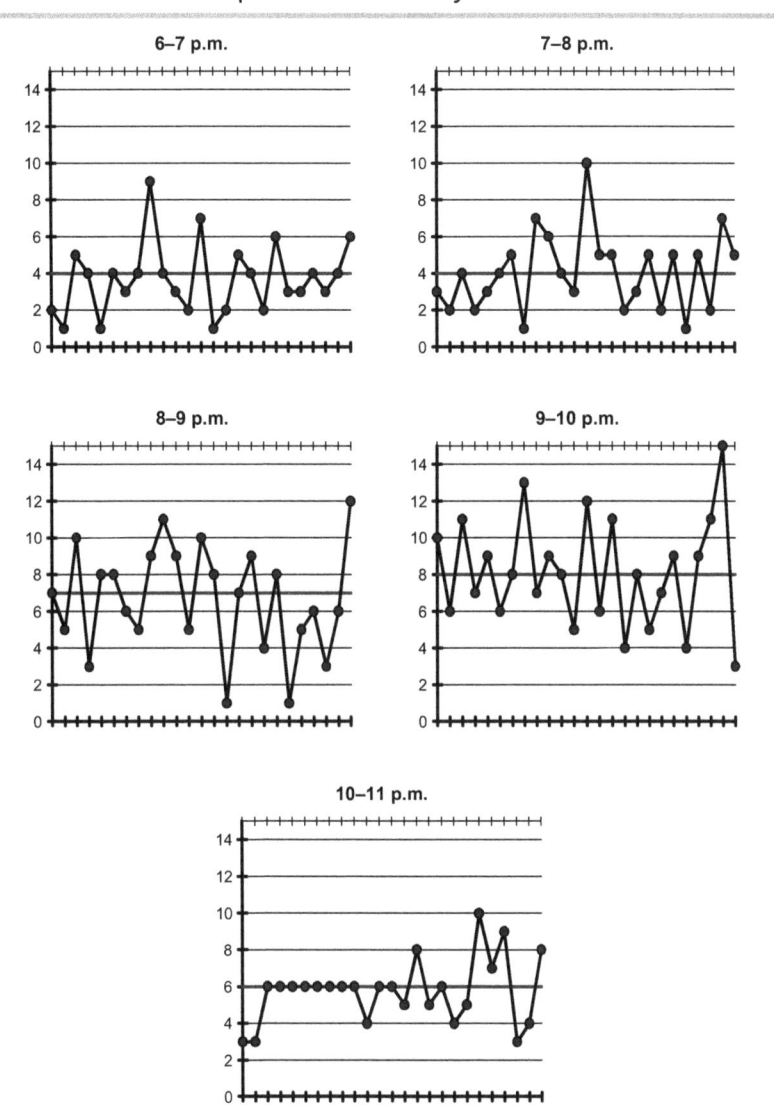

Here are some good points that this example has demonstrated so far:
1. The lack of data to compare the day of the week caused problems as do *any* data with small sample sizes. The control charts were not very helpful. Even the ANOM was not enlightening. The most powerful statistics in the world cannot help you if you do not have enough information for what you want to compare.
2. Comparing the time of evening, each hourly class has 31 observations, which is a good amount of data. If the ANOM calculations are confusing to you, *plot the dots via a control chart that forces in the overall common average of what you are comparing.*

**EXHIBIT 7.29** ■ Graphical ANOM Approximation Comparing Time of Day via Forced Common Average (default individual standard deviation)

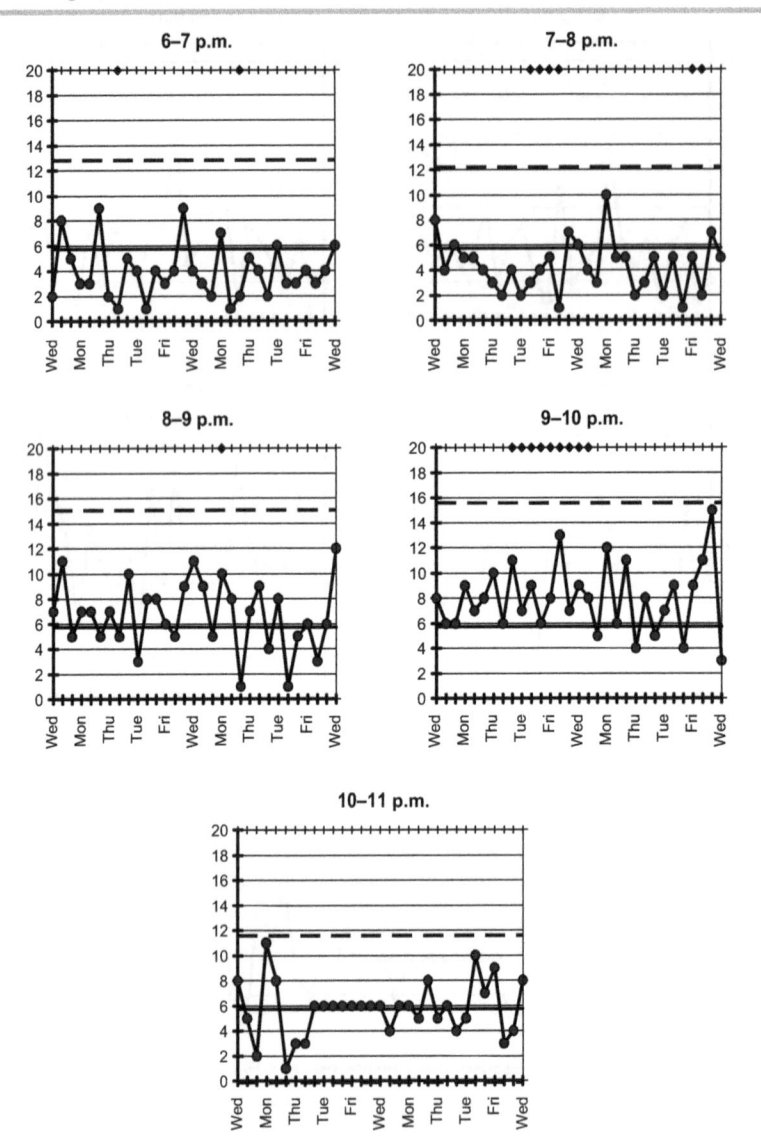

3. Even if point 2 confuses you, as long as you do initial run charts *and the data are stable*, you can then try a visual interpretation from the stratified histogram.
4. Knowing how the data were collected is very important to effectively use all the information potentially available. Note how many different graphical slices and comparisons were possible.
5. Despite the fact that the data are probably best analyzed as count data, a much simpler, more intuitive analysis was possible through judicious plotting via

# STATISTICAL STRATIFICATION

**EXHIBIT 7.30** Graphical Equivalent of ANOM Comparing Time of Day via Forced Common Average and Standard Deviation (based on count data assumption)

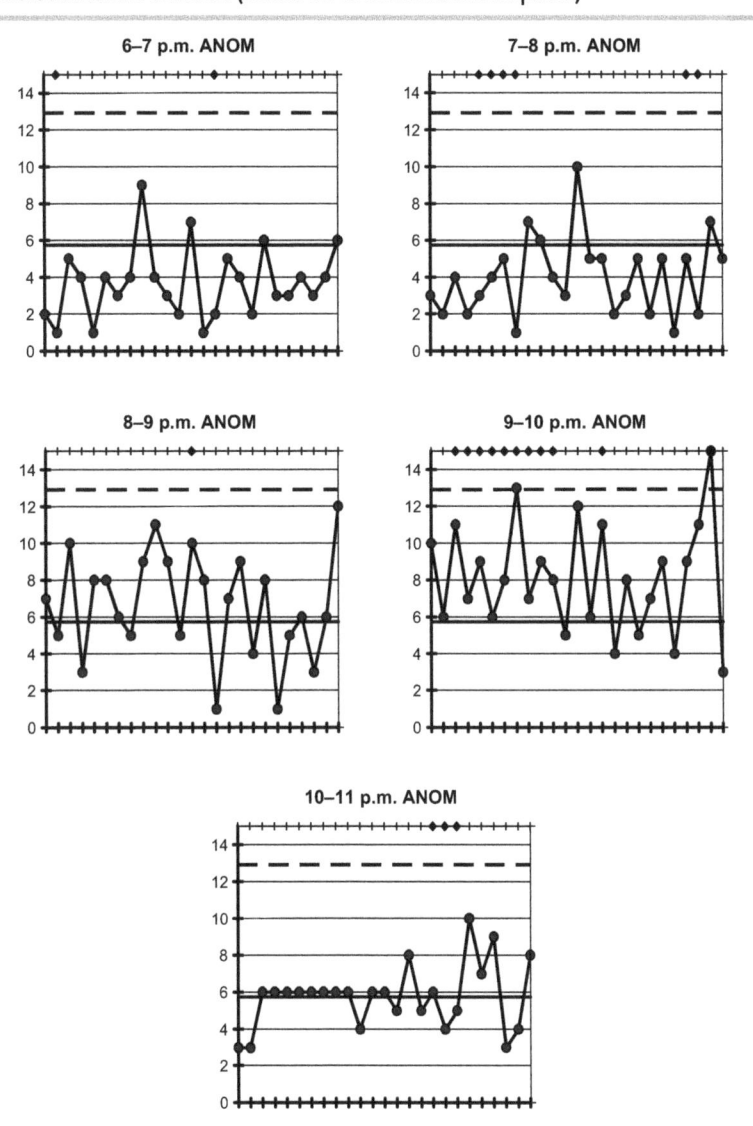

*Note:* There are distinct differences in admissions at different times of the evening.

stratified histograms, run charts, and control charts. The I-chart also showed itself once again to be a good, simple, robust approximation that leads to the right questions and action.

Although weeknight totals are indistinguishable, there is a special cause, predictable pattern within each night that could have staffing implications. The original data can now be replotted using the information gained from the ANOM to study this model's predictive ability.

EXHIBIT 7.31 ■ Usual ANOM Presentation Summary Comparing Unexpected Admits by Hour of Day

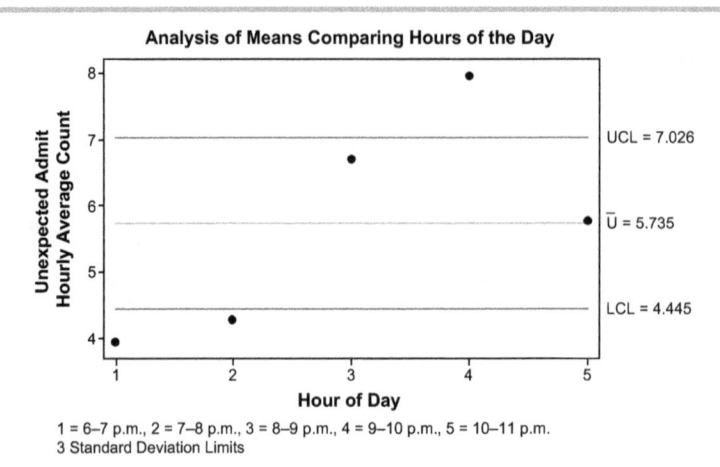

Analysis of Means Comparing Hours of the Day

UCL = 7.026
$\bar{U}$ = 5.735
LCL = 4.445

Hour of Day
1 = 6–7 p.m., 2 = 7–8 p.m., 3 = 8–9 p.m., 4 = 9–10 p.m., 5 = 10–11 p.m.
3 Standard Deviation Limits

Note: This is the more usual ANOM presentation and is the summary version of Exhibit 7.30.

The data were rearranged in their literal time order for each group of time periods. To do this, we take the data as presented in Exhibit 7.21 and put it into three columns, shown in Exhibit 7.32. They are those suggested by the ANOM by time of night:

- The data for 6–7 p.m. and 7–8 p.m. (62 observations: 2 data points per day × 31 days);
- The data for 8–9 p.m. and 10–11 p.m. (62 observations); and
- The data for 9–10 p.m. (31 observations: 1 observation per day × 31 days).

Fortunately, because there was no difference by day of the week, these did not need to be further subdivided by a special cause pattern inherent in the week. The control chart for each process is shown in Exhibits 7.33 through 7.35.

This allegedly unpredictable system is once again shown to be quite predictable. The data reasonably fit the model proposed by the two ANOMs. As is true for count data, one can also observe that the standard deviation is larger as the average gets larger.

This analysis was relatively straightforward and simplified by the fact that the relationships between the hourly patterns were statistically identical regardless of the day of the week. However, in many cases, this is not so. There can be what is called an *interaction* between the slicing and dicing factors. In the case of the current data set, this would mean that the hourly pattern relationships would be different *depending on the day of the week*.

For example, in analyzing incoming phone call data, many times Mondays especially seem to have their own hourly pattern fingerprint that is uniquely different from those of Tuesday through Friday. In analyzing emergency department admit data, weekends tend to have their own unique patterns vis-à-vis weekdays.

It is beyond the scope of this book to show how to *statistically* identify such interactive relationships formally. Even the simplest method is rather awkward, which is creating a separate stratified histogram or ANOM for each day of the week to expose obvious

## EXHIBIT 7.32  Time of Night Data Sorted into Three Systems

| Day | Time | Admits | Day | Time | Admits | Day | Time | Admits |
|---|---|---|---|---|---|---|---|---|
| 1 | 6–7 p.m. | 2 | 1 | 8–9 p.m. | 7 | 1 | 9–10 p.m. | 8 |
| 1 | 7–8 p.m. | 8 | 1 | 10–11 p.m. | 8 | 2 | 9–10 p.m. | 6 |
| 2 | 6–7 p.m. | 8 | 2 | 8–9 p.m. | 11 | 3 | 9–10 p.m. | 6 |
| 2 | 7–8 p.m. | 4 | 2 | 10–11 p.m. | 5 | 4 | 9–10 p.m. | 9 |
| 3 | 6–7 p.m. | 5 | 3 | 8–9 p.m. | 5 | 5 | 9–10 p.m. | 7 |
| 3 | 7–8 p.m. | 6 | 3 | 10–11 p.m. | 2 | 6 | 9–10 p.m. | 8 |
| 4 | 6–7 p.m. | 3 | 4 | 8–9 p.m. | 7 | 7 | 9–10 p.m. | 10 |
| 4 | 7–8 p.m. | 5 | 4 | 10–11 p.m. | 11 | 8 | 9–10 p.m. | 6 |
| 5 | 6–7 p.m. | 3 | 5 | 8–9 p.m. | 7 | 9 | 9–10 p.m. | 11 |
| 5 | 7–8 p.m. | 5 | 5 | 10–11 p.m. | 8 | 10 | 9–10 p.m. | 7 |
| 6 | 6–7 p.m. | 9 | 6 | 8–9 p.m. | 5 | 11 | 9–10 p.m. | 9 |
| 6 | 7–8 p.m. | 4 | 6 | 10–11 p.m. | 1 | 12 | 9–10 p.m. | 6 |
| 7 | 6–7 p.m. | 2 | 7 | 8–9 p.m. | 7 | 13 | 9–10 p.m. | 8 |
| 7 | 7–8 p.m. | 3 | 7 | 10–11 p.m. | 3 | 14 | 9–10 p.m. | 13 |
| 8 | 6–7 p.m. | 1 | 8 | 8–9 p.m. | 5 | 15 | 9–10 p.m. | 7 |
| 8 | 7–8 p.m. | 2 | 8 | 10–11 p.m. | 3 | 16 | 9–10 p.m. | 9 |
| 9 | 6–7 p.m. | 5 | 9 | 8–9 p.m. | 10 | 17 | 9–10 p.m. | 8 |
| 9 | 7–8 p.m. | 4 | 9 | 10–11 p.m. | 6 | 18 | 9–10 p.m. | 5 |
| 10 | 6–7 p.m. | 4 | 10 | 8–9 p.m. | 3 | 19 | 9–10 p.m. | 12 |
| 10 | 7–8 p.m. | 2 | 10 | 10–11 p.m. | 6 | 20 | 9–10 p.m. | 6 |
| 11 | 6–7 p.m. | 1 | 11 | 8–9 p.m. | 8 | 21 | 9–10 p.m. | 11 |
| 11 | 7–8 p.m. | 3 | 11 | 10–11 p.m. | 6 | 22 | 9–10 p.m. | 4 |
| 12 | 6–7 p.m. | 4 | 12 | 8–9 p.m. | 8 | 23 | 9–10 p.m. | 8 |
| 12 | 7–8 p.m. | 4 | 12 | 10–11 p.m. | 6 | 24 | 9–10 p.m. | 5 |
| 13 | 6–7 p.m. | 3 | 13 | 8–9 p.m. | 6 | 25 | 9–10 p.m. | 7 |
| 13 | 7–8 p.m. | 5 | 13 | 10–11 p.m. | 6 | 26 | 9–10 p.m. | 9 |
| 14 | 6–7 p.m. | 4 | 14 | 8–9 p.m. | 5 | 27 | 9–10 p.m. | 4 |
| 14 | 7–8 p.m. | 1 | 14 | 10–11 p.m. | 6 | 28 | 9–10 p.m. | 9 |
| 15 | 6–7 p.m. | 9 | 15 | 8–9 p.m. | 9 | 29 | 9–10 p.m. | 11 |
| 15 | 7–8 p.m. | 7 | 15 | 10–11 p.m. | 6 | 30 | 9–10 p.m. | 15 |
| 16 | 6–7 p.m. | 4 | 16 | 8–9 p.m. | 11 | 31 | 9–10 p.m. | 3 |
| 16 | 7–8 p.m. | 6 | 16 | 10–11 p.m. | 6 | | | |
| 17 | 6–7 p.m. | 3 | 17 | 8–9 p.m. | 9 | | | |
| 17 | 7–8 p.m. | 4 | 17 | 10–11 p.m. | 4 | | | |
| 18 | 6–7 p.m. | 2 | 18 | 8–9 p.m. | 5 | | | |
| 18 | 7–8 p.m. | 3 | 18 | 10–11 p.m. | 6 | | | |
| 19 | 6–7 p.m. | 7 | 19 | 8–9 p.m. | 10 | | | |
| 19 | 7–8 p.m. | 10 | 19 | 10–11 p.m. | 6 | | | |
| 20 | 6–7 p.m. | 1 | 20 | 8–9 p.m. | 8 | | | |
| 20 | 7–8 p.m. | 5 | 20 | 10–11 p.m. | 5 | | | |
| 21 | 6–7 p.m. | 2 | 21 | 8–9 p.m. | 1 | | | |
| 21 | 7–8 p.m. | 5 | 21 | 10–11 p.m. | 8 | | | |
| 22 | 6–7 p.m. | 5 | 22 | 8–9 p.m. | 7 | | | |
| 22 | 7–8 p.m. | 2 | 22 | 10–11 p.m. | 5 | | | |
| 23 | 6–7 p.m. | 4 | 23 | 8–9 p.m. | 9 | | | |
| 23 | 7–8 p.m. | 3 | 23 | 10–11 p.m. | 6 | | | |
| 24 | 6–7 p.m. | 2 | 24 | 8–9 p.m. | 4 | | | |
| 24 | 7–8 p.m. | 5 | 24 | 10–11 p.m. | 4 | | | |
| 25 | 6–7 p.m. | 6 | 25 | 8–9 p.m. | 8 | | | |
| 25 | 7–8 p.m. | 2 | 25 | 10–11 p.m. | 5 | | | |
| 26 | 6–7 p.m. | 3 | 26 | 8–9 p.m. | 1 | | | |
| 26 | 7–8 p.m. | 5 | 26 | 10–11 p.m. | 10 | | | |
| 27 | 6–7 p.m. | 3 | 27 | 8–9 p.m. | 5 | | | |
| 27 | 7–8 p.m. | 1 | 27 | 10–11 p.m. | 7 | | | |
| 28 | 6–7 p.m. | 4 | 28 | 8–9 p.m. | 6 | | | |
| 28 | 7–8 p.m. | 5 | 28 | 10–11 p.m. | 9 | | | |
| 29 | 6–7 p.m. | 3 | 29 | 8–9 p.m. | 3 | | | |
| 29 | 7–8 p.m. | 2 | 29 | 10–11 p.m. | 3 | | | |
| 30 | 6–7 p.m. | 4 | 30 | 8–9 p.m. | 6 | | | |
| 30 | 7–8 p.m. | 7 | 30 | 10–11 p.m. | 4 | | | |
| 31 | 6–7 p.m. | 6 | 31 | 8–9 p.m. | 12 | | | |
| 31 | 7–8 p.m. | 5 | 31 | 10–11 p.m. | 8 | | | |

EXHIBIT 7.33 ■ Control Chart of Unexpected Patient Admits: Process 1

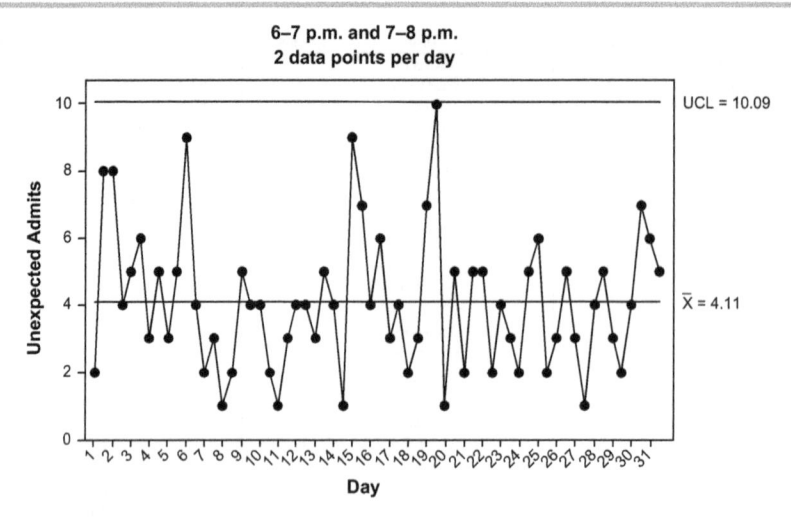

**6–7 p.m. and 7–8 p.m.
2 data points per day**

*Note:* While the averages vary among the different hourly groupings, the admissions within these particular time periods are consistent and predictable.

EXHIBIT 7.34 ■ Control Chart of Unexpected Patient Admits: Process 2

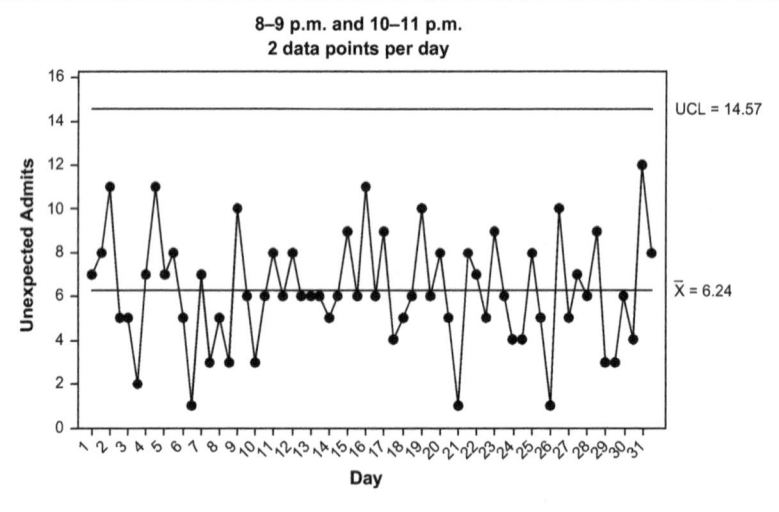

**8–9 p.m. and 10–11 p.m.
2 data points per day**

*Note:* While the averages vary among the different hourly groupings, the admissions within the time periods are consistent and predictable.

differences in the hourly patterns. This once again runs the risk of having small amounts of data as you subdivide it into more factors.

If one has a theory as to a certain inherent relationship in the data, judicious use of plotting and identifying the suspected factors on the plot may allow one to see the pattern. For example, when the data were plotted at the end of the previous analysis to confirm the

EXHIBIT 7.35  Control Chart of Unexpected Patient Admits: Process 3

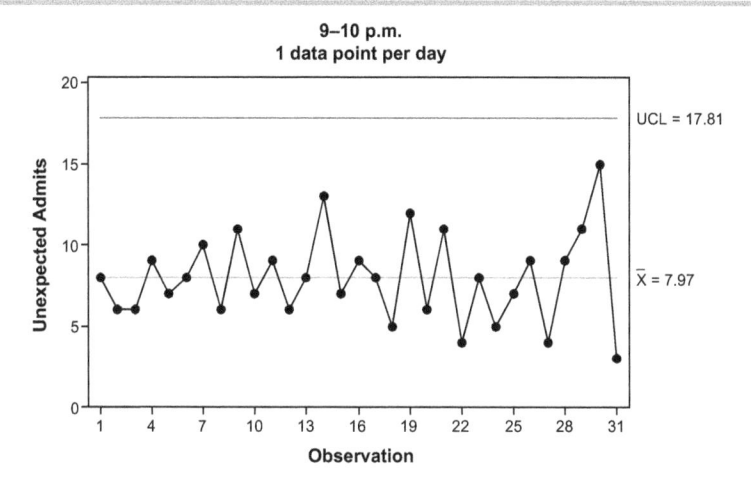

**9–10 p.m.**
**1 data point per day**

UCL = 17.81
$\bar{X}$ = 7.97

*Note:* While the averages vary among the different hourly groupings, the admissions within the time periods are consistent and predictable.

predictive ability of the suggested ANOM model, identification of the days of the week or hourly intervals on the plots would have shown a random pattern.

Suppose that Fridays for some reason had a consistently heavier flow of patient emergency department traffic than Monday through Thursday. In that case, the Friday data points would virtually always appear to be above average on the combined 6–7 p.m./7–8 p.m. and the 8–9 p.m./10–11 p.m. plots. This would be caused by the fact that the Friday pattern was different and typically higher than the Monday–Thursday pattern. Ott would always insist that his students plot the data. It is important when possible to complement any statistical analysis with one's master knowledge of a situation through some type of plotting.

## SUMMARY

I hope I have convinced you that you do not need to be a statistician to do a good analysis. Under most conditions, what has been done here is a valid, legitimate approach with reasonable statistical approximation. The objective needed in everyday application is the ability to expose the vital 20 percent of special causes in a vague situation, to be confirmed with subsequent plotting of the data via run and control charts.

People desiring more information on specific techniques and when to use them are referred to these particular items in the Resources list (see also Resources in Chapter 9):

- Executive Learning's excellent tool summary with exclusive healthcare examples, *Handbook for Improvement*; and
- Hoerl and Snee's book, *Statistical Thinking*, which is practical and gives skeletal basic traditional statistical theory for those desiring more depth.

These examples should have demonstrated the enormous versatility of the ANOM technique, both for count data (rates and percentages) and continuous data. It is amazing how often, through judicious identification of special causes present in systems, what was thought to be an unpredictable situation, process, or system is suddenly found to be quite predictable. This prediction potential inherent in the use of these simple, process-oriented statistical methods has tremendous implications in terms of:

- Budgeting;
- Forecasting;
- Measurements of performance relative to goals; and
- Subsequent identification of strategies (special cause or common cause) to achieve organizational aims.

Perspective needs to shift from comparisons of individual performance numbers in a vacuum to comparing them relative to the inherent system they form and work in. This creates a culture that is truly poised to use the power of statistical thinking: Only then can the danger of arbitrary numerical goals be fully grasped. Now people can truly work together to understand the organization's current state and plan for a future that will achieve a worthwhile mission, vision, and values.

## A Final Word on Tools and Charts

Regarding the tools, techniques, and charts presented so far, this book is designed for the everyday quality practitioner who may not have access to a statistician. I have tried to present a robust approach with methods that are sound approximations to the statistically accurate ones.

Most people neither have the time nor interest to appreciate the subtle differences among I-charts, p-charts, np-charts, c-charts, u-charts, X-bar charts, MR-charts, R-charts, S-charts, and so forth. As has been consistently shown in the examples in the text, just plotting the dots of one's data over time accomplishes more than half of any analysis in and of itself, with ensuing conversation that is so much more productive.

Lists, grids, and explanations that are intent on helping people use the right chart in the right situation, in my opinion, just cause more confusion and create opportunities to use more tools incorrectly. Remember, the overall objective is to understand variation and react to it appropriately. To paraphrase a wise axiom from my respected colleague Donald Wheeler, the purpose is not to have charts. The purpose is to use the charts. You get no credit for computing the right number – only for taking the right action. Without the follow-through of taking the right action, the computation of the right number is meaningless.

I stand behind the "good enough" philosophy of this book and have kept the emphasis on the *thinking* needed to use the analyses correctly. The tools presented have tried to keep it simple within a robust context to allow people to go down the correct path in analyzing a situation.

## APPENDIX 7A: DEEPER ISSUES AND ADVANCED STATISTICAL CONCEPTS

This appendix is not for the statistically fainthearted. My hidden agenda in writing this appendix is to scare you into using simple graphs and trusting your intuition while not relying so heavily on "turn the crank" statistical packages and rules.

If your palms are sweating and you are reading this because you feel you have to, you can now heave a huge sigh of relief. The following four lessons might be interesting, and you will no doubt glean some valuable nuggets from reading them. If while reading

EXHIBIT 7A.1 ◼ Individual County Ranking Scores

| Attr1 | Attr2 | Attr3 | Attr4 | Attr5 | Attr6 | Attr7 | Attr8 | Attr9 | Attr10 | Sum | |
|---|---|---|---|---|---|---|---|---|---|---|---|
| 6 | 4 | 3 | 8 | 2 | 1 | 3 | 2 | 1 | 12 | 42 | County1 |
| 13 | 17 | 1 | 5 | 4 | 2 | 10 | 1 | 8 | 15 | 76 | County2 |
| 9 | 8 | 12 | 3 | 19 | 7 | 14 | 6 | 3 | 3 | 84 | County3 |
| 10 | 9 | 4 | 11 | 1 | 9 | 7 | 11 | 14 | 11 | 87 | County4 |
| 2 | 5 | 10 | 14 | 14 | 12 | 11 | 5 | 11 | 8 | 92 | County5 |
| 15 | 13 | 8 | 2 | 5 | 16 | 8 | 10 | 2 | 20 | 99 | County6 |
| 1 | 3 | 18 | 4 | 9 | 18 | 15 | 14 | 18 | 1 | 101 | County7 |
| 4 | 1 | 14 | 10 | 16 | 6 | 12 | 12 | 13 | 14 | 102 | County8 |
| 18 | 15 | 6 | 1 | 11 | 10 | 13 | 7 | 7 | 17 | 105 | County9 |
| 21 | 16 | 2 | 6 | 6 | 13 | 6 | 9 | 5 | 21 | 105 | County10 |
| 12 | 14 | 9 | 13 | 15 | 8 | 2 | 13 | 17 | 4 | 107 | County11 |
| 5 | 6 | 19 | 19 | 20 | 4 | 16 | 8 | 9 | 2 | 108 | County12 |
| 14 | 12 | 5 | 9 | 12 | 11 | 4 | 19 | 21 | 5 | 112 | County13 |
| 8 | 7 | 20 | 20 | 17 | 20 | 5 | 3 | 6 | 7 | 113 | County14 |
| 7 | 2 | 16 | 17 | 18 | 14 | 1 | 4 | 16 | 19 | 114 | County15 |
| 11 | 10 | 13 | 7 | 3 | 17 | 17 | 15 | 15 | 13 | 121 | County16 |
| 17 | 18 | 15 | 12 | 8 | 19 | 9 | 17 | 4 | 9 | 128 | County17 |
| 16 | 19 | 11 | 16 | 7 | 3 | 19 | 18 | 12 | 10 | 131 | County18 |
| 19 | 20 | 7 | 18 | 10 | 5 | 18 | 20 | 10 | 18 | 145 | County19 |
| 3 | 11 | 21 | 15 | 21 | 15 | 20 | 16 | 19 | 16 | 157 | County20 |
| 20 | 21 | 17 | 21 | 13 | 21 | 21 | 21 | 20 | 6 | 181 | County21 |

them you find yourself confused, relax and do not worry about deep understanding. Keep reading for "Aha!" moments.

If your palms are not sweating and you are ready to dive in, congratulations. Either you already have an advanced degree in statistics, or you should consider getting one.

## Lesson 1: Revisiting the Friedman Test for Rankings

Interpretation of the statistical technique known as the Friedman test was introduced in the case study in Chapter 2. Because of the relatively common use of performance comparisons through summed rank scores, it allowed a good introduction to analysis of means (ANOM)-type presentation. Some of the statistical issues of that test will now be discussed for practitioners who might be interested.

The summed rank scores were shown in Chapter 2, but Exhibit 7A.1 gives the actual rankings used to calculate the sums for each county, which is needed for the analysis.

As described in a book by Conover,[1] the Friedman test applies the standard two-way analysis of variance (ANOVA) technique on this data (Exhibit 7A.2). The major factor of interest is comparison of performance by county. Each item is considered a separate measure of performance. With 10 measurements, it is like having 10 different snapshots of performance, the sum of which is aggregated into an overall score.

We need to determine if some counties have a consistent tendency toward higher scores and some toward lower scores. In statistical terms, each item is, in essence, a *block* or a *replication*.

**EXHIBIT 7A.2** ◾ **ANOVA for Rank Data**

| Source | DF | SS | MS | F | P |
|---|---|---|---|---|---|
| Item | 9 | 0.00 | 0.00 | 0.00 | 1.000 |
| County | 20 | 1,702.80 | 85.14 | 2.56 | 0.001 |
| Error | 180 | 5,997.20 | 33.32 | | |
| Total | 209 | 7,700.00 | | | |

Source: Davis Balestracci Jr., MS, *Quality Digest,* September 2006. www.qualitydigest.com. Reprinted with permission.

Note the zero sum of squares (SS) for the item source. This is an inherent given because of the nature of each replication perforce having identical data (the numbers 1–21). For statistical interpretation of this table, Conover uses the actual F-test for county (F = 2.56, $p$ = 0.001, which is less than 1 chance in 1,000 of being random). It is obviously significant and there are true differences among the performance scores.

### An Alternative Given in Some Statistical Packages

Conover claims that this interpretation is superior to the more commonly used chi-square statistic given in most computer packages for the Friedman test. This latter test can be approximated from this ANOVA by multiplying SS for county by the factor $12/[T \times (T + 1)]$. T is equal to the number of items being compared, in this case, counties (21).

To interpret this latter analysis, the equivalent $p$-value is found from a chi-square table with (T – 1) degrees of freedom (DF). For this example, the result is a chi-square statistic of $[12/(21 \times 22)] \times 1{,}702.8 = 44.23$ with 20 DF ($p$ = 0.0014).

Technicalities such as this aside, there is little doubt that differences exist among counties, but which ones?

### Finding Differences

For comparisons, how does one determine the standard deviation of each county's score: the sum of the 10 rankings? The analysis was done on the individual scores comprising the summed ranking. So one must use the mean square error ($MS_{error}$) term in the ANOVA along with the fact that 10 items were summed. Statistically, this results in:

$$\sqrt{(10 \times MS\ error)} = \sqrt{(10 \times 33.32)} = 18.25$$

I would then recommend proceeding to construct the ANOM graph using three standard deviations (± ~55) on either side of the average (110), resulting in a lower limit of 55 and upper limit of 165. This confirms the previous analysis (Exhibit 7A.3) of one above-average county and one below-average county.

But some people would insist on looking for differences. How would one proceed in this case? I provide two options, but I hope that it will make you see the wisdom and practicality of ANOM.

### Option 1. Only because the ANOVA gave a significant result, $p$ < 0.05, for county.

Some books espouse using what is statistically called the least significant difference (LSD) to interpret the differences in the summed scores. If nothing else, it is simple and in essence based on using the traditional two-standard-deviations thinking.

EXHIBIT 7A.3 ■ ANOM for 21-County Summed Rank Scores

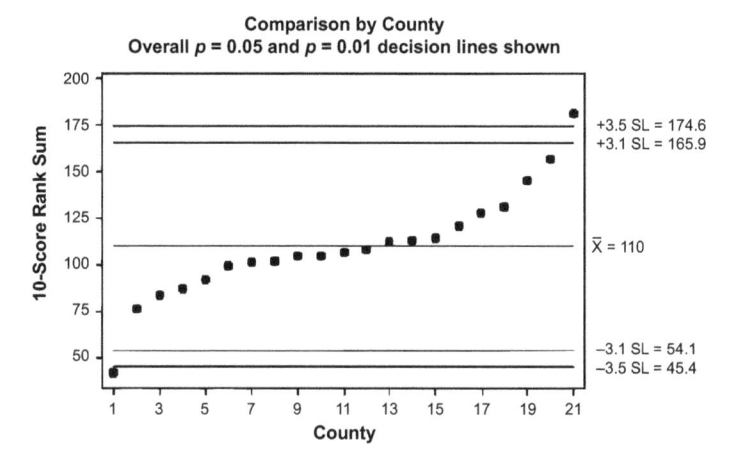

**Comparison by County**
Overall $p = 0.05$ and $p = 0.01$ decision lines shown

+3.5 SL = 174.6
+3.1 SL = 165.9
$\bar{X} = 110$
−3.1 SL = 54.1
−3.5 SL = 45.4

Source: Davis Balestracci Jr., MS, *Quality Digest,* September 2006. www.qualitydigest.com. Reprinted with permission.

Do not forget, one is looking at a *difference*, subtracting *two* numbers *each* with a standard deviation of 18.25. Similar to the preceding equation, the standard deviation of this difference is

$$\sqrt{[2 \times (10 \times \text{MS error})]} = \sqrt{(666.4)} = 25.8$$

So the LSD in this case is $(2 \times 25.8 \approx 52)$.

Note that all significant difference determinations will involve a factor times the standard deviation of an individual average. I have described the best case scenario LSD for this situation; the actual factor (sometimes larger) is affected by the number of DF of the estimate of the standard deviation. Think of it as *approximately* $2 \times \sqrt{2}$, as in this case, $(2 \times \sqrt{2}) \times 18.25 \approx 52$).

**Option 2. The human tendency is to focus arbitrarily on the largest differences.** To account for this prejudice, another possible calculation adds an element of conservatism and balance.

Theoretically, with 21 scores to compare, there are 210 potential pair-wise comparisons. A factor taking this into account, called the *studentized range*, allows one to compare *any* two randomly chosen counties. It is tabulated in most standard statistical texts (my particular favorite is Snedecor and Cochran[2]) and, for this scenario, is 5.01 (note the difference from $(2 \times \sqrt{2}) = 2.82$ for the LSD). Multiplying this factor times the standard deviation of a difference (previous section):

$5.01 \times 18.25 = 91$ (vs. the LSD of 52)

This factor is dependent on how many comparisons are being made and the number of DF in one's estimate of standard deviation.

## Stick with Analysis of Means

Just because I explained it does not mean you have to use these ANOVA alternatives. I am sure these two techniques for looking at differences are helpful. However, I have no doubt that you may be confused (it confused me for years after I got my MS degree in statistics). And, even given this information, there would still be wide human variation in the ultimate interpretation of the table of summed ranks.

Think back to the elegant simplicity, clarity, and intuitive nature resulting from the ANOM: one above-average county, one below-average county, and 19 statistically indistinguishable counties.

What is not intuitive is how to reproduce that analysis using the summary table of rank sums along with the two significant difference values of 52 and 91.

## Lesson 2: Basic Lessons from the Ranking Data — Some Observations about Standard Deviations and Outliers

Using these data once again, I now justify the "three standard deviations is good enough" philosophy of ANOM. This exact ANOM calculation will give many of you sweaty palms. Using three standard deviations with ANOM is probably already giving some of you sweaty palms. So I will also demonstrate a simple alternative technique that can quickly find outliers.

The ANOM graph originally shown in Chapter 2 for this data is reproduced in Exhibit 7A.3. Some of you no doubt notice that the overall $p = 0.05$ and $p = 0.01$ limits of my summed rank scores analysis were approximately 3.1 and 3.5 standard deviations, respectively. You might be wondering how in the world I obtained them. It is a slight twist on what I explained earlier in this chapter, so I demonstrate the calculation and address an additional important point. Generally, given the structure of many data sets, the luxury of calculating exact limits is not an option, so one has to perforce use three, which is usually good enough.

To review the scenario, 10 sets of rankings for each of 21 counties were summed. However, because of the nature of rankings, you do not have 21 independent observations. Once 20 sums are known, the 21st is also known by default. The overall average is always 110 (10 × 11) and is not affected by the individual values. So there are two issues: Statistically, one is making, in essence, only 20 comparisons. Implicitly deleting an observation to test it in relation to the average of the remaining observations is not possible (this means that adjusting the limits via the $\sqrt{(n-1)/n}$ factor discussed earlier in the chapter is unnecessary).

Because we are making 20 simultaneous decisions, what is the probability needed to ensure that, *if there are no outliers*, there is an *overall* risk of 0.05 or 0.01 of creating a false signal? In the current case, if you naively use $p = 0.05$, the probability of at least one data point being a special cause when it is not is $[1 - (0.95)^{20}] = 0.642$, a 64 percent risk.

What level of $p$ makes $(1 - p^{20}) = 0.05$ (and 0.01)? The answers: 0.997439 (and 0.999498), respectively. Further, because these are two-sided tests, I need to redistribute the probability so that half is on each side of the limits, meaning that I need to find the t-values for 0.998719 (and 0.999749), with $[(k - 1) \times (T-1)]$ DF (in this case, 9 × 20 = 180). These t-values are 3.06 (and 3.54).

Thus as explained earlier in this chapter, using three standard deviations is pretty good. In fact, if you remember, I calculated three standard deviation limits for this data in Lesson 1.

EXHIBIT 7A.4 ■ Summary of the 21 Summed Rank Scores, Including Five-Number Summary

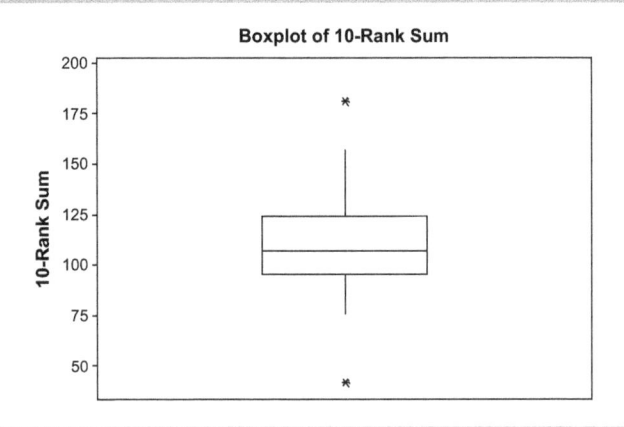

| Variable | N | StDev | Min | Q1 |
|---|---|---|---|---|
| 10-Rank Sum | 21 | 29.18 | 42 | 95.50 |

| Variable | Median | Q3 | Max | |
|---|---|---|---|---|
| 10-Rank Sum | 107.0 | 124.5 | 181 | |

EXHIBIT 7A.5 ■ Box-and-Whisker Plot of 21 Rank Sums

Let's look at a nonparametric robust alternative. Statistically, a *five-number summary* of the 21 rank sums can be constructed (contained in the Exhibit 7A.4 summary): minimum (42), Q1 (first quartile, i.e., ~25th percentile) (95.5), median (107), Q3 (third quartile, i.e., ~75th percentile) (124), and the maximum (181).

A box-and-whisker plot of this data is shown in Exhibit 7A.5. The boxplot is a distribution-free graphic that takes the five-number summary one step further to calculate a criterion to detect potential outliers.

The first and third quartiles form a box containing the middle 50 percent of the data. With the median notated within the box, lines are drawn from the sides of the box to the last actual data values within what is called the *inner fence* (described in the next paragraph). These lines are called the *whiskers*. Actual data values outside of this fence are plotted with an asterisk and are considered possible outliers.

Note the intuitive calculation of the inner fences to determine potential outliers:

1. Find the "interquartile range," that is, (Q3–Q1).
   In this case, 124.5 – 95.5 = 29.
2. Multiply (Q3–Q1) by 1.5: 1.5 × 29 = 43.5.
3. Subtract this quantity from Q1: 95.5 – 43.5 = 52.
4. Add this quantity to Q3: 124.5 + 43.5 = 168.
5. Any number <52 or >168 is a possible outlier (from our data: 44 and 181).

Note that the spread between the inner fence limits, which is (168 – 52) = 116, is very close to the range of 111.8 for the overall 0.05 limits on the ANOM chart.

In this case, it arrives at the same conclusion as the ANOM, and as shown earlier, its range of 52 to 168 is similar to the ANOM's plus or minus three standard deviation limits of 55–165.

(*Note:* As shown in Exhibit 7A.4, the traditional calculation of the standard deviation of all 21 scores yielded 29.2. The inner fence range is (168 − 52 = 113), which converts to 3.97 times this standard deviation or, in other words, plus or minus *two* standard deviations. *Because of the two special cause counties*, this standard deviation calculation is inappropriate. This once again demonstrates that three standard deviations, *calculated correctly*, is a good criterion for declaring outliers.)

## Lesson 3: Deeper Statistical Issues of the Accident and Emergency Continuous Data and Its Analysis Using Analysis of Means

A graphical approximation to ANOM was shown earlier in this chapter for continuous-type data comparing five regions' accident and emergency performance. The separate performances were given the same $y$ scale, making visual comparisons quite easy in this case. Most of the time, this type of presentation will suffice.

I will now demonstrate some deeper analysis that might sometimes be necessary either when things are not as obvious or there are even smaller numbers of observations for each group. To review the situation, a comparative run chart analysis is shown for this data in Exhibit 7A.6. Good judgment helps one discern what I like to call "the most recent stable history." For Regions 1 through 5, this seems to be, respectively, the last 13 observations, all 26 observations, the last 13 observations, all 26 observations, and the last 16 observations of each region's graph.

Generally, one likes to have the luxury of at least 20 observations for a reasonably good estimate of the common cause. For these data, it means that Regions 1, 3, and 5's control charts might benefit from more accuracy. The control charts visually demonstrated the similarity of their common cause ranges to each other and Region 2. Might it be possible to take advantage of that fact to obtain a more accurate overall pooled estimate, and how would one go about doing that?

### *Testing Similarity of Standard Deviations*

An easy first test of the equality of these five regions' standard deviations is to use an S-chart ("S" for "standard deviation"). It is a standard chart and most good statistical software will contain the option to create one.

It is interpreted in a similar way to an ANOM: It takes the standard deviations being compared, assumes they're all the same, calculates the overall standard deviation obtained from pooling all of them together, and then tests whether each individual standard deviation is just statistical variation on that common value. This is pretty much as explained earlier in this chapter for any ANOM comparison. The limits calculated are typically, once again, three standard deviation decision limits.

Exhibit 7A.7 shows the chart comparing the five regions. Region 4's data were subsequently removed from the analysis and calculations (but still plotted), which results in Exhibit 7A.8.

For those of you who might desire a more statistically accurate test *and* have access to a more powerful standard statistical computer package, the two most common are Bartlett's test and Levene's test. The computations are quite complicated, but that is not a problem. The interpretation is relatively simple. One such analysis is shown in Exhibits 7A.9 and

EXHIBIT 7A.6 ■ Comparative Run Charts of Accident and Emergency Performance

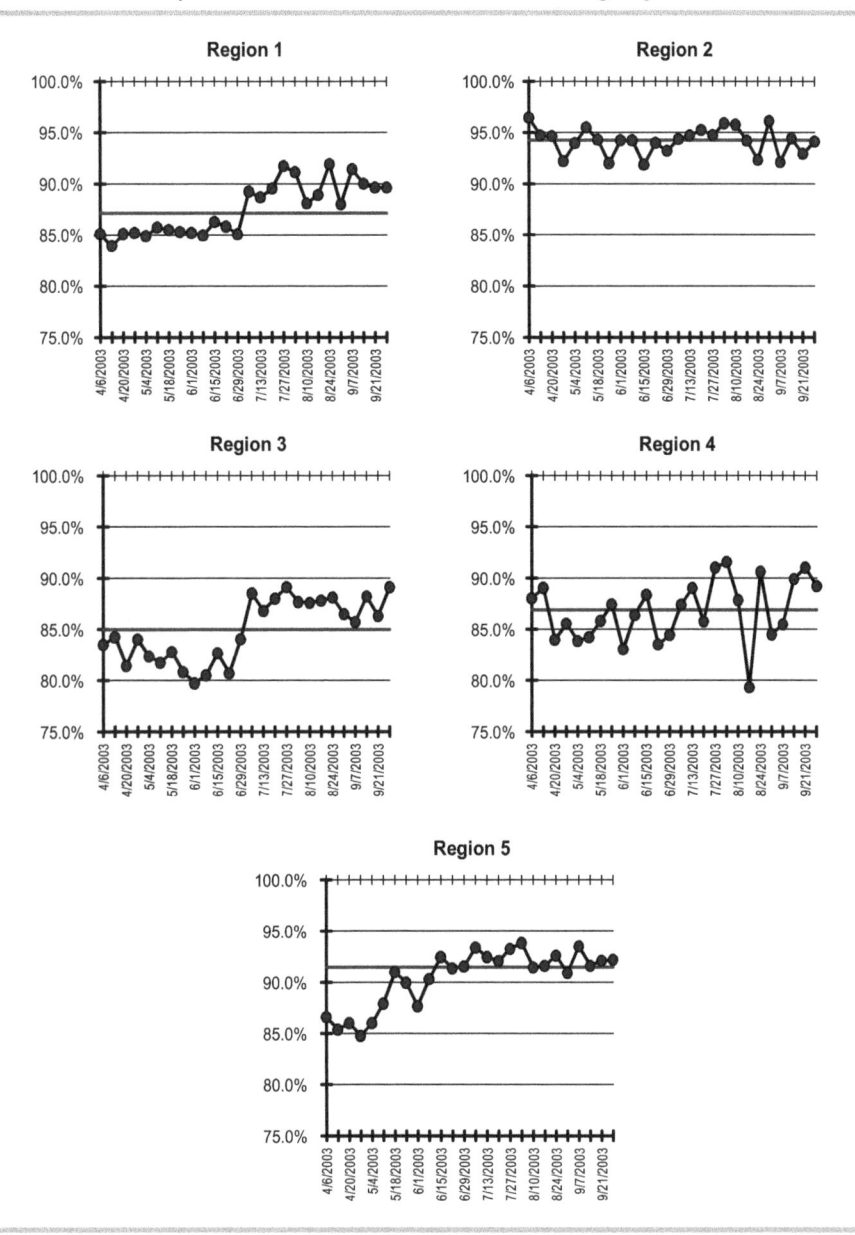

7A.10. It shows the output for both tests simultaneously from the package Minitab with Region 4's data omitted and included, respectively.

Bartlett's test is heavily dependent on the underlying data being normally distributed, while Levene's test is considered robust to departures from normality. If the data are not normally distributed, this is what sometimes causes significance with Bartlett's test; the significance may have nothing to do with testing the equality of the standard deviations.

**EXHIBIT 7A.7** ■ Control Chart Comparison of Five Regions' Deviations Using an S-Chart: Region 4 Data Included in Calculation

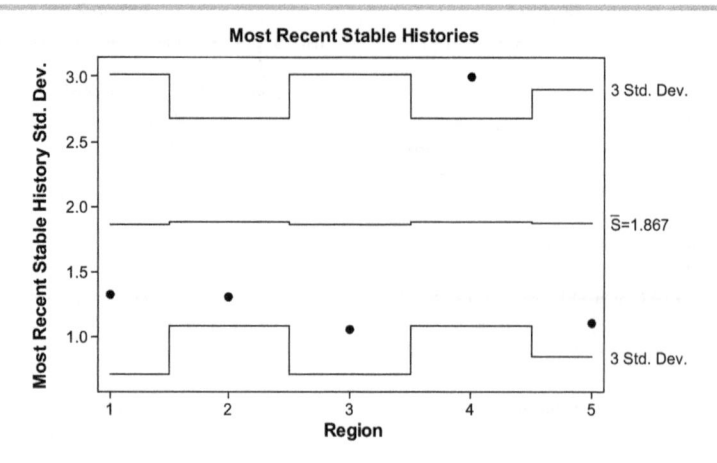

*Note:* Region 4's standard deviation is an obvious outlier.

**EXHIBIT 7A.8** ■ Control Chart Comparison of Five Regions' Deviations Using an S-Chart: Region 4 Data Plotted but Omitted from Calculation

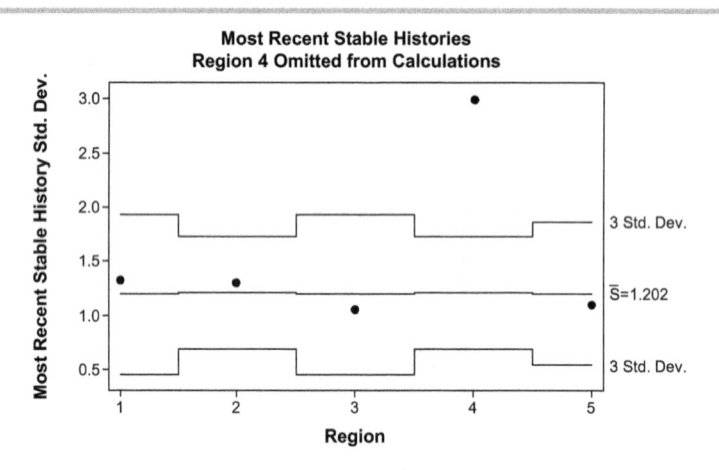

*Note:* Regions 1 through 3 and 5 are all within the limits.

I tested the five regions' most recent stable history for normality and they easily passed. In this case, the results from both tests in Exhibits 7A.9 and 7A.10 can be trusted. They both agree that Region 4 is an outlier (each with $p < 0.001$) and they both agree that the remaining four regions' data seem to have equivalent standard deviations. (Barlett's $p$ = 0.760 and Levene's $p$ = 0.862. This means that declaring the remaining four standard deviations different would run a risk of at least 76 percent of being wrong.)

EXHIBIT 7A.9 ■ Bartlett's Test and Levene's Test for Equality of Standard Deviations: Region 4 Omitted from Calculation

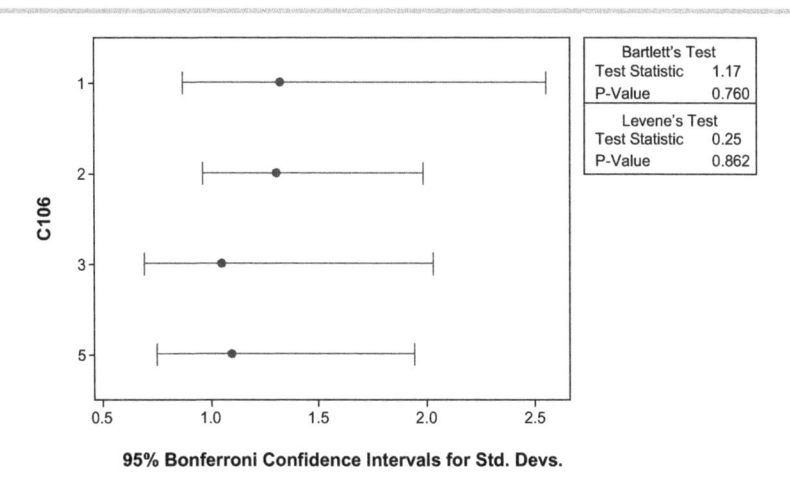

| Bartlett's Test | |
|---|---|
| Test Statistic | 1.17 |
| P-Value | 0.760 |

| Levene's Test | |
|---|---|
| Test Statistic | 0.25 |
| P-Value | 0.862 |

95% Bonferroni Confidence Intervals for Std. Devs.

EXHIBIT 7A.10 ■ Bartlett's Test and Levene's Test for Equality of Standard Deviations: Region 4 Included

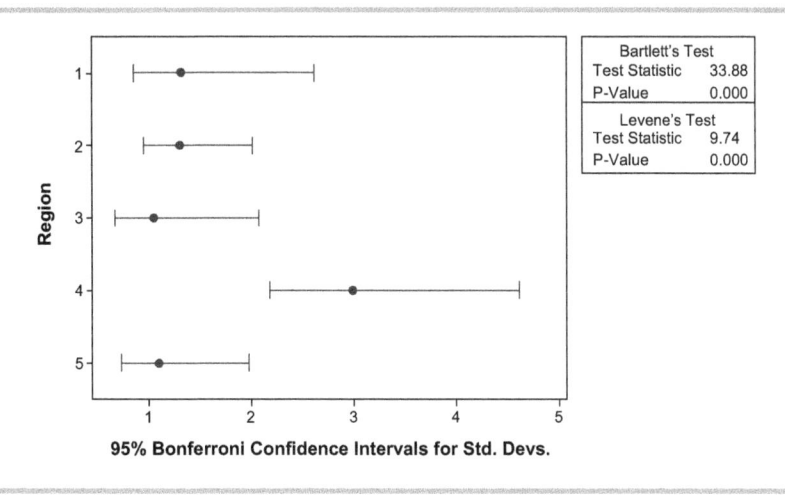

| Bartlett's Test | |
|---|---|
| Test Statistic | 33.88 |
| P-Value | 0.000 |

| Levene's Test | |
|---|---|
| Test Statistic | 9.74 |
| P-Value | 0.000 |

95% Bonferroni Confidence Intervals for Std. Devs.

For those of you who do not have access to a high-power statistical package, trust me: The S-chart (available on any *good* basic statistical process control package, which is what most people reading this book use) will not steer you wrong.

Now that Regions 1, 2, 3, and 5 have similar standard deviations, they can be pooled into their common estimate using traditional one-way ANOVA (in essence, comparing the four regions' performances), which results in Exhibit 7A.11.

To get all the mileage we can out of this exhibit, note that the $p$-value for region is <0.001. Virtually no doubt exists that the performances of the four regions somehow

EXHIBIT 7A.11 ■ ANOVA Table Calculating Pooled Standard Deviation for Regions 1, 2, 3, and 5

One-Way ANOVA: Accident and Emergency Performance vs. Region
(Region 4 omitted)

| Source | DF | SS | MS | F | P |
|---|---|---|---|---|---|
| Region | 3 | 412.21 | 137.40 | 92.66 | 0.000 |
| Error | 64 | 94.90 | 1.48 | | |
| Total | 67 | 507.11 | | | |

Pooled StDev = 1.218

differ. The common standard deviation is obtained from the square root of the MS error (1.48), which is given in the exhibit as pooled standard deviation equaling 1.22.

Now, if you did want to go ahead and calculate the LSD and/or studentized range significant difference (as discussed in Lesson 2), let me vehemently discourage you with something that is more the rule than the exception: Most of the time, *you will be comparing averages with varying numbers of observations.* The example in Lesson 1 had a nice structure where any compared averages had the same number of observations. When they do not (as in this case and as you might be intuiting at this point), it quickly gets messy and confusing.

Further, these data have an additional issue: How does one compare the averages of Regions 1, 2, 3, and 5 to Region 4 with its *different* standard deviation?

Here is what I recommend:

1. Try to compare them via control charts on the same scale.
2. Even though it is slightly different from the exact ANOM calculation, force in the five regions' overall average value of 90.214 as each chart's average.
3. Then force in a standard deviation of 1.22 in Regions' 1, 2, 3, and 5 control charts and let Region 4 use its average (or median) moving range to get its unique common cause.
4. Finally, observe the performance of the data vis-à-vis the forced center line to see whether special cause tests are triggered.

This approach is summarized in Exhibit 7A.12. This approximate analysis still comes to the correct conclusion: Region 1 is average, Regions 2 and 5 are above average, and Regions 3 and 4 are below average. For those interested in the formal ANOM chart, it is shown in Exhibit 7A.13.

In my opinion, this leaves a lot to be desired, and it isn't the easiest graph for the statistical novice to either obtain or interpret. The upper and lower decision limits are set at three standard deviations and each region is being compared to the overall average of 90.2 percent. Note that because of the different sample sizes in each group ($n$ = 13, 26, 13, 26, and 16, respectively), the individual common cause limits vary. And, because of Region 4's larger variation, the limits for its performance are too tight. I think you will agree that this graph is not as intuitive as Exhibit 7A.12, which also handles the issue of interpreting Region 4's performance very well.

**EXHIBIT 7A.12** Approximate ANOM Comparing Five Regions' Accident and Emergency Performance

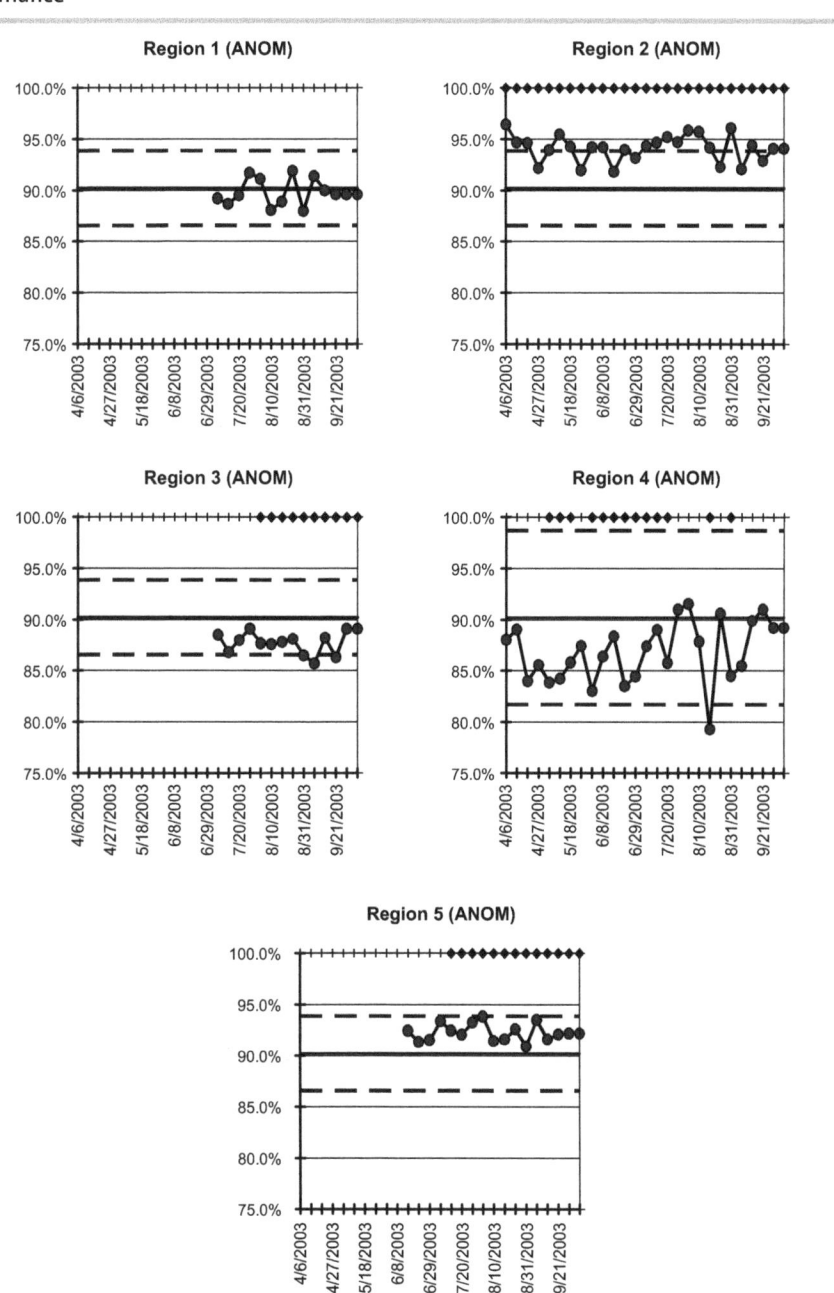

*Note:* Forced common average of 90.214% and common standard deviation (Regions 4's common cause calculated from its own average moving range).

EXHIBIT 7A.13 ■ ANOM Chart Comparing Regional Performance

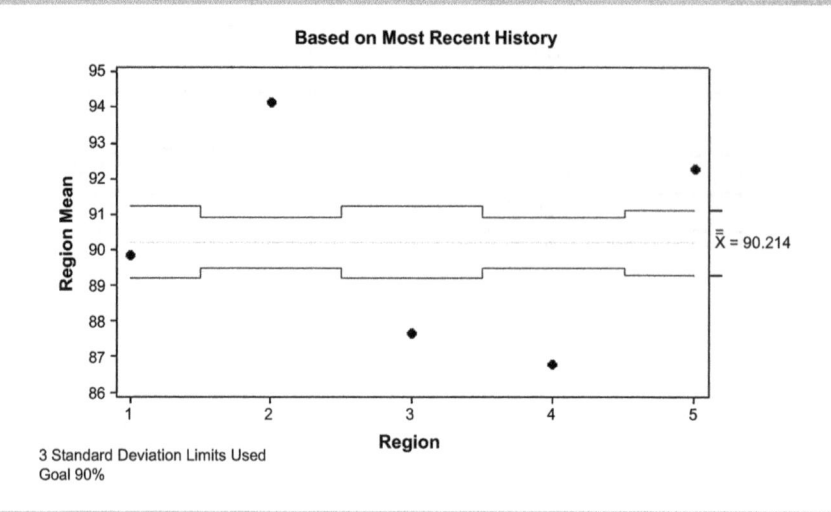

**Based on Most Recent History**

[Chart: Region Mean vs. Region (1–5), with $\bar{\bar{X}} = 90.214$]

3 Standard Deviation Limits Used
Goal 90%

My point with all this detail is a warning: If you are not careful, you can quickly drown in a statistical swamp. And once again, a case is made for using the powerful but elegant simplicity of "just plot the dots."

## Lesson 4: The Empirical Rule

What about normal distribution? Notice that I mentioned it only in this appendix for people who want a little more advanced discourse. It tends to be a robust underlying implicit assumption in a lot of analyses in spite of people not testing it, nor necessarily needing to or having to know about it.

In the greater scheme of things, you have got better things to learn more thoroughly. If you want deeper knowledge about basic statistical theory (distributions, hypothesis tests, etc.), be my guest, but it will not necessarily make you a better practitioner for the types of data and situations you will commonly encounter in *everyday* work. You do not need to teach people statistics; you need to help them solve their problems.

Wheeler developed "The Empirical Rule"[3] to justify using three standard deviation limits on time-ordered control charts. He rarely mentioned the normal distribution in his writings and noticed that *regardless of the distribution* (and assuming the data are from a stable process):

- 60–75 percent of data fall between plus or minus one standard deviation around their average;
- 90–98 percent of data fall between plus or minus two standard deviations around their average; and
- 99–100 percent of data fall between plus or minus three standard deviations around their average.

It is this last point that makes the control chart so useful with its three standard deviation limits and robust to any underlying alleged data distribution. There is nothing

sacrosanct about the statistical platitudes people spew that are based on the normal distribution:
- Two standard deviations is 95 percent confidence;
- Three standard deviations is 99.7 percent confidence;
- Data need to be normally distributed to plot a control chart; and
- A process needs to be in control before you can plot a control chart.

On hearing such nonsense, I advise you to run the other way.

Wheeler and Chambers explain this at length and demonstrate it in their book *Understanding Statistical Process Control* (which I would not recommend to the typical reader of *Data Sanity*). Wheeler also developed more recent publications designed for everyday practitioners. These can be found on his Website, www.spcpress.com. The Website also contains short articles on various topics that might be helpful in many common situations.

As I one time saw Deming *growl* at someone asking a question in one of his seminars about decisions in the context of the normal distribution, "Normal distribution? I've never seen one!" Let's get less obsessed with the normal distribution and more obsessed with solving practical problems practically.

## REFERENCES

1. Conover, W.J. 1980. *Practical Nonparametric Statistics*, 2nd ed., 299–302. New York: John Wiley & Sons.
2. Snedecor, George W., and William C. Cochran. 1967. *Statistical Methods*, 6th ed., 568. Ames: Iowa State University Press.
3. Wheeler, Donald J., and David S. Chambers. 1992. *Understanding Statistical Process Control*, 2nd ed., 61. Knoxville, TN: SPC Press.

## RESOURCES

Arthur, Jay. QIMacros™ www.QIMacros.com.
Balestracci Jr., Davis. 2006. "I Hate Bar Graphs — Part 2: Consider Multiple-Year Data from Another Angle." *Quality Digest* (April). www.qualitydigest.com/april06/departments/spc_guide.shtml.
Balestracci Jr., Davis. 2006. "I Hate Bar Graphs — Part 2 (Cont.): Changing the Conversation, Courtesy of 'Boring' SPC." *Quality Digest* (May). www.qualitydigest.com/may06/departments/spc_guide.shtml.
Executive Learning. 2002. *Handbook for Improvement: A Reference Guide for Tools and Concepts*, 3rd ed. Brentwood, TN: Healthcare Management Directions.
Hoerl, Roger, and Ronald Snee. 2002. *Statistical Thinking: Improving Business Performance*. Pacific Grove, CA: Duxbury.
Neubauer, Dean. 2007. "Pl-Ott the Data!" *Quality Digest* (May). www.qualitydigest.com/may07/articles/05_article.shtml.
Ott, Ellis R., Dean V. Neubauer, and Edward G. Schilling. 2005. *Process Quality Control: Troubleshooting and Interpretation of Data*, 4th ed. Milwaukee, WI: ASQ Quality Press.

QIMacros is an all-purpose statistical process control package designed as an Excel add-in. A 30-day free download is available. Jay Arthur has done a good job of understanding you, the customer. QIMacros works directly off one's current Excel work sheet and costs a little over $200 (most advertised statistical packages are too advanced for the casual user, overly complicated, and cost more than $1,000 per copy). I have tested his calculations, and they are correct (many of the less expensive packages cannot be trusted). Arthur also provides very good customer service and has a lot of information on the Website that puts the package in the context of an organizational quality improvement effort, especially Six Sigma.

The book by Ott and colleagues is probably for the more advanced practitioner. There are no healthcare examples, but much wisdom can be found in this book. Ott invented the analysis of means technique. Neubauer and Schilling were two of his students and they have updated the original material.

Wheeler, Donald J. 1993. *Understanding Variation: The Key to Managing Chaos*. Knoxville, TN: SPC Press.

I highly recommend this book of Wheeler's for all levels of experience.

Wheeler, Donald J. 1997. "Collecting Good Count Data." *Quality Digest* (November). www.qualitydigest.com/nov97/html/spctool.html.

Wheeler, Donald. 2007. "Collecting Good Count Data: Obtaining Good Count Data Is a Mixture of Planning and Common Sense." *Quality Digest* (November). www.qualitydigest.com/nov97/html/spctool.html.

CHAPTER 8

# Beyond Methodology: New Perspectives on Teams, Tools, Data Skills, and Standardization

## KEY IDEAS

Transitioning to implicit quality improvement work teams can be awkward. Many problems in the transition relate to:

- Understanding a situation as an isolated incident rather than an ongoing process breakdown;
- Using inadequate problem definition;
- Implementing known solutions with neither a good baseline estimate of the problem nor piloting a solution with well-designed data collection to assess (and hold) the gains;
- Overusing and improper use of tools;
- Failing to recognize that all change has a cultural consequence, which requires different skills to solve;
- Having variation caused by ad hoc standardization processes that need more formality; and
- Having poor previous cultural experiences because of poor implementation of more formal documentation processes.

## TEAMS AS PART OF LARGER SYSTEMS

"Teams need to be a part of larger contexts and larger systems." This Peter Scholtes comment, taken from his observations on teams (see Chapter 9), is sage advice. It is hoped that the previous chapters as well as suggested resources educate the reader about the theory behind quality improvement (QI). The concepts of process, variation, and data also allow one to get started immediately without making a typical mistake: creation of too many formal project teams working on issues insignificant to the organization's business strategy and future survival. As Chapter 2 made you aware, there are myriad daily opportunities to improve via saner use of data, which will create the time to consider larger scale, more strategic projects anchored in "the world of the solution" (see the "Why Your Customers Lie to You" sidebar in Chapter 10).

QI theory, needed by everyone in the culture, helps to create unified work teams with a common language and sense of purpose. These teams can then recognize *all work* as a measurable process with both internal and external suppliers and customers. This knowledge must become routinely used by frontline work teams to be truly effective. An efficient use of data, awareness of variation, and proper reaction to both creates a strong foundation in which project teams can thrive in the larger organizational context.

Replacing a cultural tendency to blame people by recognizing processes as the sources of most problems will increase morale and reduce fear. Dysfunctional behavior related to confrontation and blame of lower-level workers can be minimized when organizational management sets expectations of zero tolerance for this. People will finally be able to recognize that what they previously perceived to be individual, unique problems (*special causes of variation*) were really the same few problems repeated in various guises (*common causes*).

Routine process thinking exposes the true, hidden opportunities in the lack of daily processes as well as existing hidden time and data inventories. Part of the hidden opportunity for management is the realization that special causes of variation (i.e., problems) at a local level may actually be symptoms of *common causes of variation at a much higher level*. Examples of those higher levels include organizational purchasing, technical training, communication skills training, maintenance, promotion, and hiring processes.

Brian Joiner provides an excellent example of this when one company lost a major contract proposal. The company treated it, as always, as a special cause, but further investigation showed it to be the first time that the bad processes lurking within their *overall organizational proposal process* (common causes) *randomly* came together to sabotage a potential contract. If it had not happened on this contract, it was waiting to happen on a future one. To paraphrase Joiner regarding typical special cause reactions, "fire the guilty, blame the customer, or do nothing."

Once again, the issue is transformation, not merely improvement. Transforming current managerial behavior through these skills will cause profound improvement of an organization and its culture. However, once the organization is aligned, additional issues and questions (beyond the scope of this book) remain. I can recommend no better resource than *The TEAM Handbook* by Scholtes, Joiner, and Streibel to answer these questions of sound project methodology and logistics (see Resources).

Consider the following: Will mere improvement keep you in business 5 to 10 years from now? What processes will help the organization face and deal with unexpected changes in the outside culture? What processes will help you innovate? Do these processes formally exist today?

## Transformation through Projects

The previous editions of *Quality Improvement: Practical Applications for Medical Group Practice* (see Resources) were written when continuous quality improvement (CQI) was the dominant improvement philosophy in healthcare. This resulted in organizations creating myriad project teams under a new administrative arm known as *quality improvement*, which generally existed side by side with the traditional, more hardwired clinical quality assurance. Clinical and administrative projects were considered distinctly different from one another. Lots of activity resulted, especially tools training, but most organizations failed to reap all of the promised benefits, creating increasing executive and middle management cynicism.

In the early 1990s, Rummler and Brache developed a unique methodology to integrate process improvement into an overall framework and saw seven deadly sins of process improvement, to which many CQI programs at the time succumbed:[1]

1. Process improvement was not tied to strategic issues.
2. Process improvement did not involve the right people, especially top management, in the right way.
3. Process improvement teams were neither given clear direction nor held accountable.
4. Reengineering was considered the only way to make significant improvements.
5. There was no consideration of how changes would affect the people who had to work in the new process.
6. The focus was more on redesign than on implementation.
7. There was consistent failure to leave behind a measurement system and other parts of the infrastructure that were necessary for holding any improvement gains.

As previously stated, projects are necessary, but they are not sufficient to transform the status quo. That said, a disciplined approach to any improvement is necessary to get to root causes and hold any gains. This chapter will concentrate on good project methodology and logistics regardless of the type of project chosen. It contains information needed to guide you through any project from beginning to end in terms of both sequencing and diagnostic tools needed.

The QI climate has evolved over the years. Many projects increasingly deal with issues of clinical guideline implementation and work standardization. These issues have their own unique problems and are discussed separately later in the chapter. In fact, as Lean enterprise and Toyota Production System become more prominent as organizational improvement approaches, standardization is actually at their core.

## SOME WISDOM FROM JURAN

Juran's writings have been influential on my thinking. He believed the approach to improvement to be project based with each project consisting of two separate journeys: a *diagnostic journey* from symptom to cause followed by a *remedial journey* from cause to remedy:

$$\text{Symptom} \rightarrow \text{Cause} \rightarrow \text{Remedy}$$

$$\underbrace{\phantom{\text{Symptom} \rightarrow \text{Cause}}}_{\text{Diagnostic Journey}} \underbrace{\phantom{\text{Cause} \rightarrow \text{Remedy}}}_{\text{Remedial Journey}}$$

Ongoing undesirable variation indicates an underlying problem or opportunity. To find its root causes, the diagnostic journey requires asking many different questions to understand the hidden sources of variation. A team of diverse staff with varying experiences, knowledge, and skills is necessary.

As described in Chapter 5, data collection within the context of the diagnostic journey helps to identify the significant improvement opportunities within the observed process (demonstrated in the three examples in Appendix 8A). This requires theories about the root causes, study of work in progress, and analysis. The diagnostic journey includes uncertainty and depends largely on technical expertise about the process to identify a root problem cause.

At the end of the diagnostic journey, a potentially viable solution is developed. This solution is usually tested and evaluated on a pilot scale. If deemed unfeasible, the solution is discarded or revised, and the diagnostic journey continues. Exhibit 8.1 outlines the diagnostic journey.

After obtaining a viable solution, the remedial journey begins. There are not as many technical unknowns and questions in this journey as compared to the diagnostic journey. The solution is now known, and the appropriate areas can be targeted for change. The remedial journey's focus is more specific.

As you've seen from the extensive discussion in Chapter 3, the issues surrounding the remedial journey involve more psychology than technology. The new solution must overcome people's natural resistance to change. Once the change is made, the QI process requires standardization of the new work process and proof that the theorized gains are made and held. The issue then becomes hardwiring the solution into the culture. Exhibit 8.2 outlines the remedial journey.

**EXHIBIT 8.1 ■ Diagnostic Journey — A Breakthrough in Knowledge**

- Choose a problem.
- Understand the process.
- Fix obvious problems I.
- Establish stability and baselines.
- Fix obvious problems II.
- Generate theories for causation.
- Localize a major opportunity.
- Identify proposed solution.
- Pilot and evaluate proposed solution.

**EXHIBIT 8.2 ■ Remedial Journey — A Breakthrough in Behavior**

- Overcome resistance to change.
- Bring about standardization.
- Hold gains.

The diagnostic and remedial journeys are different in purpose, skills, and people involved. Juran deemed their sequence a universal, natural progression for proper QI.

It is useful to look at a specific process improvement as going through this natural progression for two reasons. First, there can be a tendency to jump from symptom directly to remedy. This could add complexity to a process if the remedy does not address the true root causes. Second, most project teams underestimate, if not totally ignore, the implications of the remedial journey. As you are aware from the discussion in Chapter 3, planning the remedial journey is not trivial. Often, minimal consideration is given to its key aspects. *A solution's impact on the work culture should always be evaluated prior to its implementation.*

Data from a well-designed pilot is a start for providing objective proof, but they do not necessarily address the sometimes mysterious reasons for resistance (stated reasons vs. real reasons). Now that you have an overview of the entire project journey, I will discuss the individual journeys separately.

### Become an Organizational Change Agent

As improvement professionals, part of our learning curve is the experience of facilitating project teams that fail miserably. Despite the necessary lessons learned, there still remain some real dangers lurking in any project, but it goes beyond organizing and facilitating a team. We need to avoid the project trap: too many projects that are too vague and will have minimal impact.

In the postmortem, if indeed there even is a postmortem, the question that inevitably arises for projects that didn't get close to desired results is, "Why was this project chosen in the first place?" With a collective shoulder shrug, the consensus many times seems to be, "It seemed like a good idea at the time."

Here are five project evaluation criteria by Matthew E. May,[2] an expert on innovation (see Resources). He suggests scanning the current organizational project portfolio and evaluating your role by giving each project a star rating: one star for each criterion. Ask yourself, *"What percentage of my work is five-star projects?"*

1. **Passion** (Personal passion for your project is a good indicator of potential engagement.)
   - Does it call on your key talents and strengths? Does it require you to stretch them, so that you'll learn and grow?
   - If it's a team project, are the talents and values of your project team aligned to the project? Does your project team believe in the purpose of the work?

2. **Impact**
   - Will there be big, noticeable, positive change and walloping impact for your intended audience?
   - Who is on the receiving end of whatever it is you're going to deliver?
   - Who is truly interested in the outcome of your project?

3. **Rave**
   - Will your project create raving fans — people whom you will wow with expectations, needs, or requirements that are exceeded? (In today's social media world, it's much easier for a raving fan to broadcast your project's virtues.)
   - Will these results be strong enough to not only create followers and zealots, but also motivate them to tell others, who will tell others, and so forth? (It's important to create critical mass.)
   - Will it make that 25–30 percent critical mass of leaders you've worked hard to create look good?

4. **Breakthrough**
   - Does your project represent a breakthrough, revolutionary improvement, or innovation; that is, does it require your best creative thinking and problem-solving ability?
   - Will it deliver something distinctly better in terms of greater value, not merely just new or different?

5. **Visibility**
   - Ensure that you have a high-profile, high-stakes project that will attract resources (i.e., people and money).
   - Recognition plus resources equals a higher probability of success.
   - If you've worked the first four criteria well, this shouldn't be a problem. But if visibility is a problem, are you fully leveraging them to sell it?

As you can see, there are business, human, and practical issues to consider when choosing a project or situation to study. Remember, the goal is to transform daily work life so that QI is imbedded in all aspects of the culture. If you can use this wisdom during steps 1 and 2 of the road map of major steps to transformation (Exhibit 1.2), especially with the evolving critical mass, you will ensure a successful start for your organizational transformation. This will also be thoroughly discussed in Chapter 9.

In previous chapters, I suggested "safety" as a good place to start your transformation, which dovetails with another recent movement in healthcare. Many health insurance companies are formally refusing to pay for unavoidable and unanticipated events that "shouldn't" have happened.

What if you could bring some sanity to the root cause analysis subindustry? You can turn an undesirable situation into a major educational moment when executives put away their wishful thinking (and tantrums about accountability) and realize that organization might be *perfectly designed* to have things happen that shouldn't happen (e.g., complaints, falls, pressure sores, central-line infections, hospital-acquired infections), which would be a major breakthrough in thinking.

## A PROCESS FOR IMPROVEMENT

*The TEAM Handbook* is an outstanding resource for guiding you in the facilitation of project teams. It brings a process-oriented framework to a situation and uses it within the context of the "seven sources of problems with a process." A guiding road map that integrates this context and Juran's data strategies is shown in Exhibit 8.3.

Exhibit 8.4 shows the improvement process from the perspective of a service or administrative work culture. It also includes improvement activities. This excellent framework was developed by Joiner Associates as "The Seven Step Method." The minutiae are not important, but the overall context and theory are virtually identical for *any* good improvement model.

### Don't Standardize Just to Standardize

Just as there is no such thing as improvement in general, there is no such thing as standardization in general. If you want to see full-fledged resistance (and stonewalling), make the following general grand announcement: "Because of our commitment to [CQI, Six Sigma, Lean, etc.], we need to develop standard work processes."

Of course you need to develop a standard work process, and ultimately, you will, after process language is ingrained in your organizational culture (a three-to-five-year transition). Remember, if you currently do not have standard processes, it is because you are not designed to have them. This includes clinical *and* administrative processes. Some questions that need to be asked are:

- Because of a lack of standard processes, what kinds of problems are observed in the work culture? Which of these are the most serious barriers to desired strategy and values?
- What are the 20 percent of the processes causing 80 percent of the problems?
- Which clinical guidelines would most benefit patients?
- What are the 20 percent of the clinical issues that cause 80 percent of your costs? Are there hidden opportunities for simultaneous cost reduction and better clinical outcomes through standardization?
- What level should be worked on first? Should we start small or big?
- Whom should they involve?
- Exactly what needs to be standardized?
- How does one ensure people use standards once they are in place?

## EXHIBIT 8.3 ■ A General Five-Stage Plan for Improvement

| Stage 1 Understand the Process | Stage 2 Eliminate Errors | Stage 3 Remove Slack | Stage 4 Reduce Variation | Stage 5 Plan for Continuous Improvement |
|---|---|---|---|---|
| • Describe the process | • Error-proof the process | • Streamline the process | • Further operationally define key customer variables | • PLAN for Monitoring Changes |
| • Identify customer needs and concerns and operationally defined measures of them | 3. Errors and mistakes in executing procedures? | 5. Unnecessary steps, inventories, wasting time, wasteful data collection? | • Expose hidden special causes | • DO the Monitoring |
|  | 4. Can preventive measures be designed into the process? |  | • Reduce variation in the process | • CHECK the Results |
| • Develop a standard process |  | *Study the current process* | • Assess process capability | • ACT to Make Improvements Continuous |
| 1. How does the process currently work? | *Study the current process* |  | 6. Variation in inputs and outputs? | • Document and Standardize Improvements |
| 2. How should the process work? |  |  | *Cut new windows* | • Collect Data to Hold Gains |
| *Exhaust in-house data* |  |  |  | *Designed experimentation* |

◄──────── Fix obvious problems at any time ────────►

Source: Adapted from Peter R. Scholtes, Brian L. Joiner, and Barbara J. Streibel. 2003. *The TEAM Handbook*, 3rd ed., 5-9. Madison, WI: Oriel. Used with permission.

- Where in a chosen process are the high-leverage points that must be standardized because variable methods (or poor handoffs) are seriously hindering the ability to provide consistently high-value service?

The workforce needs to know why it is developing standards beyond merely documenting what they are currently doing. If done on a vital organizational process (clinical or administrative), this will result in the ultimate reduction in confusion, conflict, complexity, and chaos. Employees will then begin to understand how different facets of their work affect the products and services delivered to customers. They will also know which elements are most critical to producing high-quality output with minimal waste and see the need to perform those tasks consistently.

Standards must not:

- Stifle creativity and lead to stagnation;
- Interfere with a customer focus;
- Add bureaucracy and red tape;
- Make work inflexible or boring, especially at low-leverage process points;

EXHIBIT 8.4 ■ The Joiner Seven-Step Method (with emphasis on administrative processes)

### 1. Project

**Goal:** *To define the project's purpose and scope.*

Questions to be answered:
- What problem or "gap" are you addressing?
- What impact will closing this gap have on customers?
- What other reasons exist for addressing this gap?
- How will you know if things are better?
- What is your plan for this project?
  - Define the boundaries.
  - Develop measures.
  - Identify all the players, their needs, and concerns.

### 2. Current Situation

**Goal:** *To further focus the improvement effort by gathering data on the current situation. Can one isolate the 20% of the process causing 80% of the problem?*

Questions to be answered:
- What is the history?
- Can you study the current process?
  - What are the key process indicators?
  - Is data available to get a baseline that quantifies the extent of the problem?
- Can the problem or situation be depicted in a high-level sketch or flowchart as it really works?
- Are there obvious problems that can be fixed immediately?
- What happens now when the problem appears? What are the symptoms?
  - Where do symptoms appear? Where don't they appear?
  - When do symptoms appear? When don't they appear?
  - Who is involved? Who isn't?
- Analyze the data: Common cause or special cause strategy needed? Do you need to regroup?

### 3. Cause Analysis

**Goal:** *To identify and verify deep causes with data; to pave the way for effective solutions.*

Questions to be answered:
- Have you isolated the 20% of the process causing 80% of the problem?
- From studying the current process, what are the possible causes of the symptoms? Which of these are verified with data?
- What are possible deeper causes of the verified causes?
  - Construct a cause-and-effect diagram.
  - Ask "Why?" five times.
  - Do you need to further dissect the process and get data?
- How does the verification of causes affect decisions about who should be working on this effort?

### 4. Solutions

**Goal:** *To develop, try out, and implement solutions that address deep causes.*

Questions to be answered:
- Generate a variety of solutions.
  - What solutions could address the deep causes?
  - What criteria are useful for comparing potential solutions?

(Continues)

## EXHIBIT 8.4 (Continued)

- What are the pros and cons of each solution? How do they relate to the gaps and causes?
- Which solutions seem best? Which will you select for testing?
- How will you try them on a small scale?
  - What data will you collect?
    - What lurks to compromise your data process?
    - Did you use the eight questions of data collection?
  - What are the cultural barriers to the solution?
- Which trial solution turned out to be most effective?
- What are the plans for implementing it full scale? Can you use successive plan-do-study-act cycles?

### 5. Results

**Goal:** *To evaluate both the solutions and the plans used to implement them.*

Questions to be answered:
- How well do results meet the targets?
- How well was the plan executed? *What can this tell you about planning for future improvements?*

### 6. Standardization

**Goal:** *To maintain the gains by standardizing work methods or products.*

Questions to be answered:
- What is the new standard method or product?
  - Has it been formally documented?
  - Has it been error-proofed?
- How will all employees who do this work be trained?
- What's in place to ensure the process is hardwired?
- Is there simple data monitoring that will demonstrate that gains are being maintained and will detect and prevent backsliding?
- How will anyone know if things are working the way they should work?
- What means are in place to foster ongoing improvement?

### 7. Future Plans

**Goal:** *To anticipate future improvements and to preserve the lessons from this effort.*

Questions to be answered:
- Is it time to bring the project to closure?
- What remaining needs were not addressed by this project?
- What are your recommendations for investigating these remaining needs?
- How will the documentation be completed? What happens to it when it's finished?
- What did you learn from this project?
  - How can these lessons be communicated so that future projects can benefit from a better improvement process?

Source: Adapted from Peter R. Scholtes, Brian L. Joiner, and Barbara J. Streibel. 2003. *The TEAM Handbook*, 3rd ed., 5-15–5-17. Madison, WI: Oriel. Used with permission.

- Only describe the minimal acceptable output;
- Be developed and not used;
- Be etched in granite forever;
- Be imposed from the outside; or
- Waste time.

Standards should:
- Make progress more visible and make it easier to track that progress over time;
- Capture and share lessons;
- Evaluate points of consistent weakness in the process;
- Evaluate how and by how much new initiatives helped to improve quality;
- Help workers communicate more effectively with other functional areas;
- Help workers communicate more effectively among themselves;
- Be treated as living, breathing guidelines than can and *must be* constantly improved;
- Focus on the few things in a process that truly make a difference, and
- Provide a *foundation* for improvement.

Many people in Institute for Healthcare Improvement (IHI) hospital-based initiatives are stating that one of their values in IHI initiatives is patient safety, which is a wonderful platform for introducing the accompanying care bundles. However — and I still cannot emphasize this enough — you will still have to audit your current culture's current performance vs. its gap with your new desired performance. You need to study the current situation, understand how it got that way, and identify the vested interests in keeping it that way.

Because of variation between organizations, you will need to discover the 20 percent of the guideline that accounts for 80 percent of *your* culture's potential opportunity and realize this 20 percent will probably be different for each individual hospital. If you do not start there, the whole guideline will seem overwhelming to the culture (stated reason). It might be better to begin by getting data on current performance to identify your cultural issues before making any grand announcement about care bundle implementation.

The process in Exhibit 8.5 might be helpful. It is an adaptation of the plan-do-study-act (PDSA) cycle made famous by W. Edwards Deming called *plan-do-check-act* (PDCA). It is used specifically for standardization and subsequent auditing. However, should there be a theory that the standard process could be improved, then it would be tested using PDSA.

### Training Issues of Standardization: Train and Retrain

After the best-known methods have been developed and documented, you need to know how to make sure they are used. Education and training play a key role, but whom does one train? New employees and new managers are obvious. But what about experienced employees who seem to have a tendency to naturally, and many times conveniently, forget? It is these experienced employees who are usually the first to tell new employees, "I know you're taught that, but you don't need do it that way." This is an example of cultural initiation and a stated reason. The real reason is more to the effect of "If you do it that way, then I'm going to get hassled about not doing it that way, and I will make your life

**EXHIBIT 8.5** ■ A Process for Understanding Standardization at a Local Level

**Questions to be answered at the beginning:**
- Are the current documented standards best?
- How do they compare with the methods the people are actually using?
- What about new ideas being recommended?
- Can we eliminate certain steps or inventory or inspection, or are they there for a reason?

**Check: Understand the current process.**
- Make sure you understand *why* the work is being done. See if this purpose is clearly documented and is compatible with the project's purpose.
- Locate any existing documentation of methods. Compare actual practice with the documented methods.
- If there are no documented standards, compare different practices among the people doing the work.
- Compare how the effectiveness of the work is supposed to be checked with how it is actually checked.

**Act: Establish a consistent framework upon which improvements can be built.**
- Reconcile the actual practices and the documentation, changing whichever of the two needs to change (i.e., change the actual practices to match the documentation, or change the documentation to match the actual practice).
- Do this for both how the work is supposed to be done and how it is supposed to be checked.
- If no standard methods are in place and no one can show with data which methods are really best known, a practical alternative at this stage is simply to agree on a method they all will use.

**Plan: Make the documentation more useful.**
- Develop a plan for upgrading the documentation.
- Develop a plan for encouraging the use of the documented standard.
- Determine how to detect flaws and potential improvements in the standard.

**Do: Train to the new documented standard. Use the new standard.**

**Check: Once again compare actual practice with documented standards.**
- Determine inconsistencies.
- Investigate those inconsistencies.
- If the standards are not being followed, for example:
  - Is it because the documentation is too difficult to use?
  - Because people don't appreciate the need for using the standard?
  - Because the standard doesn't allow people to keep up, or prevents them from doing quality work?
  - Because people have found a better way?

**Act: Again, reconcile the actual practice with the documentation, changing whichever data shows needed change.**

miserable as a result." In considering some tolerated cultural elements that have allowed barriers to standardized processes to proliferate, ask:

- Has work ever been checked to monitor performance? If so, was the purpose to police the employees or to deliver the consistent best process to the customer?
- What are the plans for a feedback system?

A high degree of standardization is needed to make effective training possible.

- Without standardization, training is cumbersome, inefficient, ad hoc, and generally ineffective.
- Without effective training, any standard is soon lost.

### Employees Will Resist

Be prepared for these stated reasons for employee resistance:

- "Management doesn't know how to do my job."
- "Sharing my knowledge will make me vulnerable."
- "Rules are going to be enforced for rules' sake, not considering the customer."
- "I'm experienced. I don't need documentation."

Therefore, given the many dysfunctional beliefs people have accumulated from past experiences with standardization efforts, how does one let people experience the benefits, which are less waste, less rework, higher customer satisfaction, and saner lives for themselves? One strategy is to involve the people actually doing the work in the current situation process, once again using PDCA.

- Facilitate creation of a **plan** for how the work will be done and know how to measure whether it is effective.
  - Make sure employees understand (internal and external) customer needs.
  - Involve specialists or other knowledgeable people as partners who understand how the process does or should work; these are people who can teach employees about the underlying theory or principles that guide the work.
  - Be aware of major blocks that because of current culture may be virtually immovable, and treat them as givens. Change only those that promise major benefits.
  - Preserve the components of the existing process. Localize or focus the changes and minimize the disruption employees incur in their daily work.
- **Do** the work according to the plan.
- **Check** how well the work is going, using indicators employees helped to create.
- **Take action** to put in place immediate remedies. Participate in developing ways to prevent problems from recurring.
- **Designate an owner** who will be responsible for keeping visible the documentation, for updating the standard and its documentation as improvements are identified, and for ensuring that newcomers and others are trained. If a process is not updated with an improved version at least every three months, that's sometimes a signal that no one is using the standard.

## Some Proven Realities of Teams

In addition to his sage advice about project choice, May also shares some seemingly unshakable truths about projects, even well-chosen ones.[3] Can you develop the skills to recognize and deal with these very normal traps that most cultures are perfectly designed to have occur?

- A major project is never completed on time, within budget, or with the original team, and it never does exactly what it was supposed to.
- Projects progress quickly until they become 85 percent complete. Then they remain 85 percent complete forever — sort of like a home improvement project.
- When things appear to be going well, you've overlooked something. When things can't get worse, they will.
- Project teams hate weekly progress reports because they so vividly manifest the lack of progress.
- A carelessly planned project will take three times longer to complete than expected. A carefully planned project will only take twice as long as expected. Also, 10 estimators will estimate the same work in 10 different ways. And one estimator will estimate 10 different ways at 10 different times.
- The greater the project's technical complexity, the less you need a technician to manage it.
- If you have too few people on a project, they can't solve the problems. If you have too many, they create more problems than they can solve.

As your role expands, be careful and take care of yourself. Being human and passionate about improvement, it is easy to (1) have delusions of success and a bias for optimism, (2) take on more than one should, (3) routinely exaggerate the benefits, and (4) discount the costs.

As I see all the time in conference presentations, people exaggerate their abilities as well as the degree of control they had over events, tending to take credit for success and blaming failure on external events. To cover themselves and justify the existence of their role, there can be a tendency to overscope, overscale, and oversell while simultaneously underestimating, under-resourcing, and underplanning.

*Any* size project will become complex and challenging. Competing interests and conflict *will* occur, and individual members' performances *will* vary widely. Besides these human factors, there are the inevitable, continual shifts in direction and frequent stalls that slow momentum and demand constant planning, adjustment, and improvisation.

I hope I have made the case to avoid a flurry of project teams unless leaders have at least the step 1 understanding (see Exhibit 1.2 and Chapter 9) to apply process thinking, problem-solving tools, statistical thinking, and the "accountable question" in responding to cultural victim behavior (Chapter 3) as the new concepts are being practiced. The best strategy for educating leaders is to expose everyday opportunities to use data sanity to solve high-level problems and get results that make them look good. Well-chosen projects using May's criteria can be used to help develop the crucial 25–30 percent critical mass of leaders who will passionately commit to excellence.

The approach I am giving you is robust to any improvement philosophy. If your organization is forcing a formal structure such as Lean Six Sigma or Toyota Production System on an environment whose leadership behaviors telegraph commitment to the status quo and getting better by evolution, I'm willing to bet that some of you are frustrated.

Although this topic is beyond the scope of this book, I offer a few brief articles in the list of Resources.

## Standardization before Tools

The successful improvement approaches are increasingly emphasizing and nearly demanding the need for process standardization as a prelude to the inevitable whirlwind of activity. Because of the impression made on me by Mark Hamel (see Resources), I believe that understanding standardization as a process is more important than statistical tools and their mechanics. Leadership needs to respect and empower frontline workers and their processes as a necessary prelude. Tools are important, but I find myself using fewer of them and finding myself in awe of what can be done with critical thinking questions, new conversations motivated by a run and/or control chart, and, when appropriate, understanding a situation as common cause.

### Be Careful

A hot topic at the moment, especially in healthcare, is rapid-cycle PDSA. In many cases, I'm seeing it presented as a process for the ordinary employee to test good ideas in routine work as a way to circumvent sluggish management.

PDSA requires the improvement practitioner to grasp the situation. The plan portion of PDSA calls for understanding and comparison of what is happening vs. what should be happening and what people know vs. what they don't know. In other words, we should not willfully further process ignorance.

This means that PDSA can take time. Unfortunately, the all-too-common rallying cry is: "What can we do now? By next week? By tomorrow?" This has led to the invention of rapid-cycle PDSA:

- Test on a really small scale. For example, start with one patient or one clinician at one afternoon clinic and increase the numbers as you refine the ideas.
- Test the proposed change with people who believe in the improvement. Don't try to convert people into accepting the change at this stage.
- Implement the idea only when you're confident you have considered and tested all the possible ways of achieving the change.

There are many cultural, human landmines that work against this simple concept. The original intent of small tests of change was to enable learning how a particular intervention works in a particular setting. The goal was not to test a hypothesis but to gain insight into the workings of a system and improve that system. It is culture specific. I am seeing signs that the emphasis on "rapid" has unintentionally morphed this methodology to a platform to test ideas that come more out of intuition than critical thinking. If not careful, "plan" can easily become "come up with a good idea to champion," which, if it works, then needs to be forced on a resistant culture and shared with the healthcare community at large to copy.

Critical thinking does not necessarily result from using a practitioner's toolbox framed within a formal improvement structure such as Six Sigma, Lean enterprise, Lean Six Sigma, or the Toyota Production System. It's easy to be seduced by all the fancy tools, acronyms, Japanese terminology, and promises.

Even with the best planning, many of us have discovered that rapid-cycle PDSA can easily become a complex tangle of a network whose application involves frequent false starts, misfires, plateaus, regroupings, backsliding, feedback, and overlapping scenarios

EXHIBIT 8.6 ■ If Only It Were This Simple

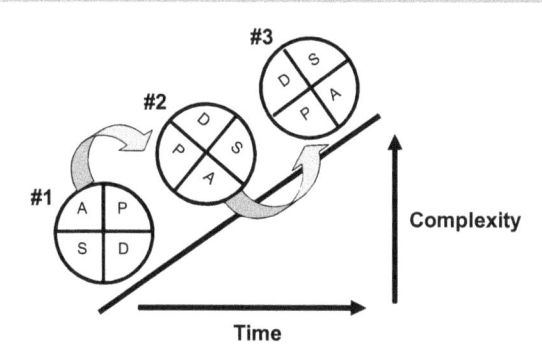

within any one cycle (hardly like the ubiquitous graphic of perfect PDSA circles rolling up an incline shown in Exhibit 8.6).

Despite the messy reality, *proper* execution of PDSA cycles as a strong, reliable methodology for improvement remains fundamental. Its intuitive nature provides the discipline necessary for good critical thinking and appropriate formality in the midst of inevitable variation present everywhere, including the variation in variation experienced among similar facilities.

My approach prefers far fewer tools in conjunction with critical thinking to understand variation in one's native language. That said, all improvement practitioners should read my 2014 article "PDSA...or Rock of Sisyphus?" (see under the "Rapid-Cycle PDSA and Its Lurking Traps" section in Resources), which applies critical thinking to the rapid-cycle PDSA process and lays out the raw reality, and *The Improvement Guide* by Langley and colleagues (see Resources).

## WHAT ABOUT THE TOOLS?

Tools and their mechanics are secondary to the statistical thinking behind their use. The overall motivation in QI is to understand the variation in a situation and reduce the inappropriate and unintended variation, which is to have the process move along the correct path as close to 100 percent of the time as possible. Putting tools in this perspective, the emphasis should be on:

- Process-oriented thinking through **flowcharts**;
- Proper planning of data collection through appropriate **data aggressiveness** and design of **check sheets** or **data sheets** using the eight questions of data collection (see Chapter 5);
- Initial assessment of stability of processes in time and their capability (desired vs. actual performance) through **run charts and control charts** (see Chapter 6); and
- Identification of possible sources of variation and special causes in inputs to a process through **stratification (Pareto analysis, stratified histogram)**, an **Ishikawa (fishbone) diagram** of a *significant isolated* special cause of variation (i.e., 20 percent of the process causing 80 percent of the problem), and **scatterplots** to establish possible causal relationships.

EXHIBIT 8.7 ■ Pareto Diagrams of Accident Data by Department and Accident Category

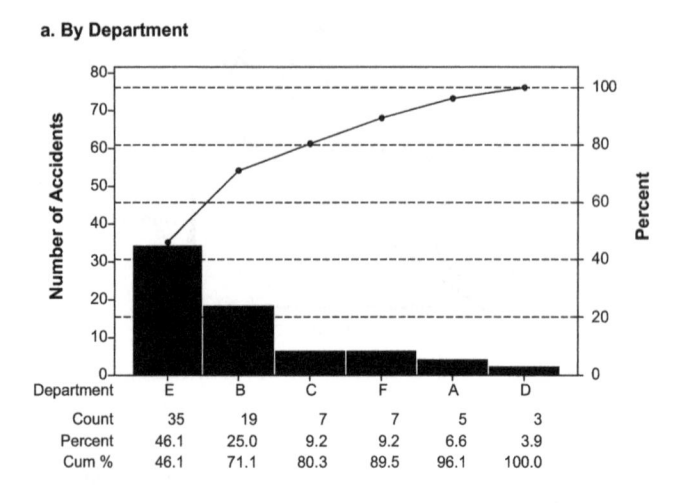

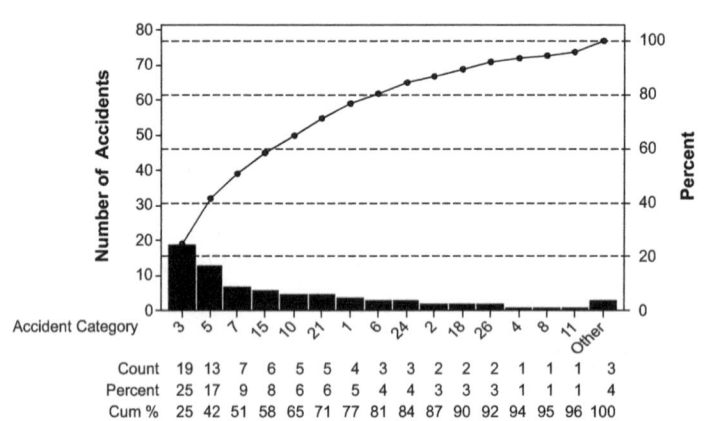

**a. By Department**

| Department | E | B | C | F | A | D |
|---|---|---|---|---|---|---|
| Count | 35 | 19 | 7 | 7 | 5 | 3 |
| Percent | 46.1 | 25.0 | 9.2 | 9.2 | 6.6 | 3.9 |
| Cum % | 46.1 | 71.1 | 80.3 | 89.5 | 96.1 | 100.0 |

**b. By Accident Category**

| Accident Category | 3 | 5 | 7 | 15 | 10 | 21 | 1 | 6 | 24 | 2 | 18 | 26 | 4 | 8 | 11 | Other |
|---|---|---|---|---|---|---|---|---|---|---|---|---|---|---|---|---|
| Count | 19 | 13 | 7 | 6 | 5 | 5 | 4 | 3 | 3 | 2 | 2 | 2 | 1 | 1 | 1 | 3 |
| Percent | 25 | 17 | 9 | 8 | 6 | 6 | 5 | 4 | 4 | 3 | 3 | 3 | 1 | 1 | 1 | 4 |
| Cum % | 25 | 42 | 51 | 58 | 65 | 71 | 77 | 81 | 84 | 87 | 90 | 92 | 94 | 95 | 96 | 100 |

Good data are crucial throughout this process, and well-designed check sheets (see Exhibit 5.12) will ensure a robust data process (but you still will not be able to anticipate everything those darn humans will unintentionally do to sabotage it).

The **Pareto principle** was demonstrated in the accident safety data example in Chapters 2 and 5. To turn a stratified data collection into a Pareto diagram bar graph, plot the bars in descending order, show the individual percent contribution of each, and plot a line graph above the bar graphs to show the cumulative percentage of the preceding bars. Exhibit 8.7 contains two Pareto diagrams of the tabulated accident data stratified by department and accident type. However, as you remember in this particular case, it told a much different story when presented in its matrix form. Regardless, it is initially useful to brainstorm possible categories of stratification when studying the current process (see Chapter 5).

## EXHIBIT 8.8  Pareto Diagram of Reasons for Delays in Discharge

*Note:* There are 14 categories of delayed discharge, but the first 4 account for 80 percent. The first reason alone (physician related) accounts for 35 percent.

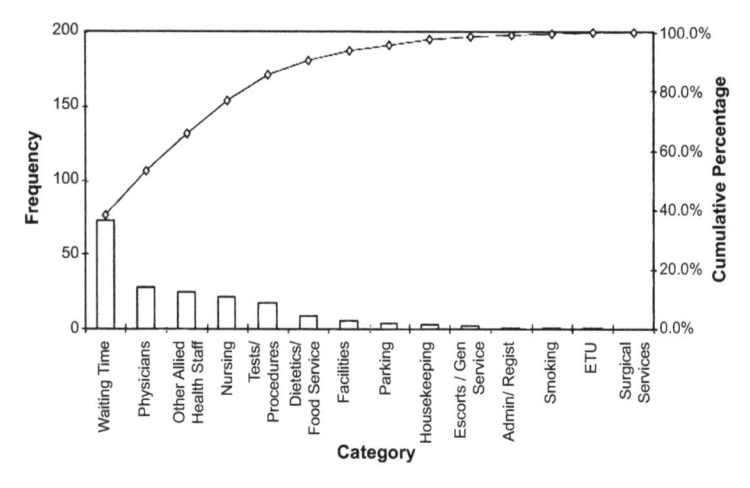

## EXHIBIT 8.9  Pareto Diagram of Patient Complaints from Comment Cards

*Note:* Once again, 14 categories of complaints, but the first 4 account for 80 percent.

It's not so much Pareto diagrams, but using Pareto analysis to isolate and focus on a major opportunity within a vague situation that is so important. Exhibits 8.8 and 8.9 show analyses of reasons for delay in discharge and patient complaints, respectively.

Sometimes, it is not only helpful to tally the incidents, but also to convert the tally to the actual cost to the organization. Exhibit 8.10 shows a Pareto analysis of both reasons and cost for discarded surgical items.

**EXHIBIT 8.10** ■ Pareto Analysis Contrasting Frequency vs. Cost

a. Surgical Items Discarded (by volume)

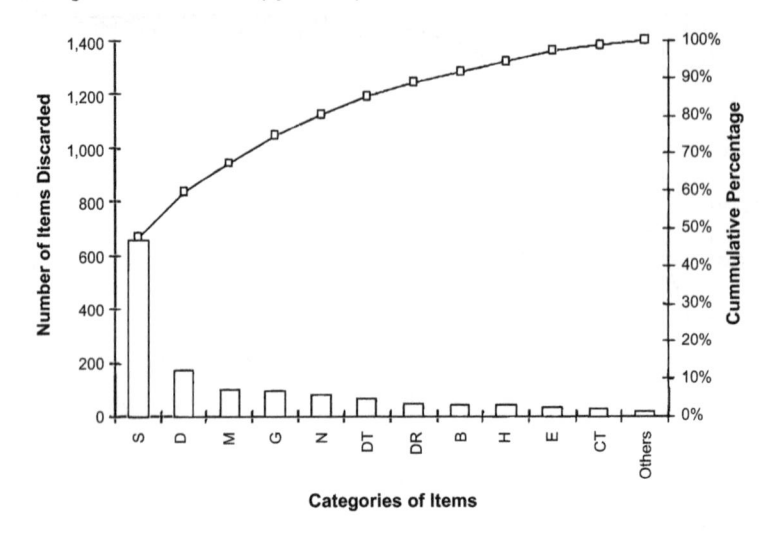

b. Surgical Items Discarded (by total cost)

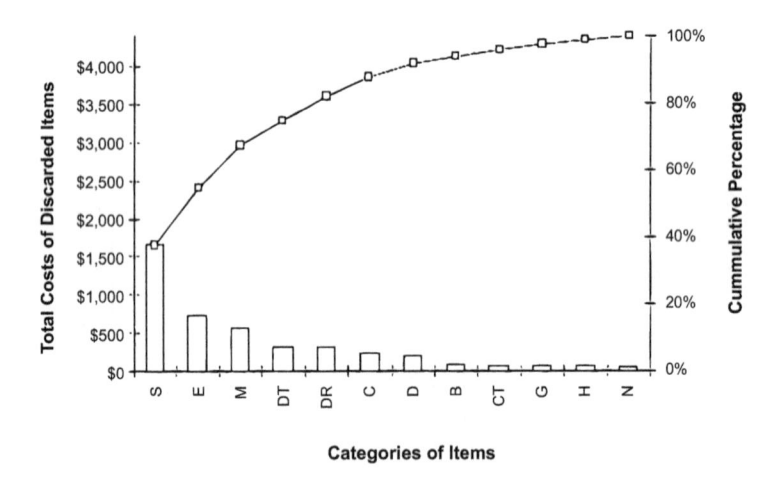

**Ishikawa (fishbone) diagrams** help organize brainstormed ideas about causes of undesirable variation. They are developed by the project team working on the process and represent the relationship of a problem to its major inputs: people, methods, machines, materials, measurements, and environment. They should be used sparingly, usually after proper flowcharting and stratification or Pareto analysis have localized a major opportunity. Otherwise, they commonly and quickly become unwieldy, as shown in Exhibit 8.11. It is sometimes used in conjunction with the tool of "asking 'Why?' five times" (Exhibit 8.12) with the resulting causes put on the appropriate bone of the diagram.

EXHIBIT 8.11  Fishbone (Ishikawa) Cause-and-Effect Diagram: Vague vs. Localized

**Localized Problem**

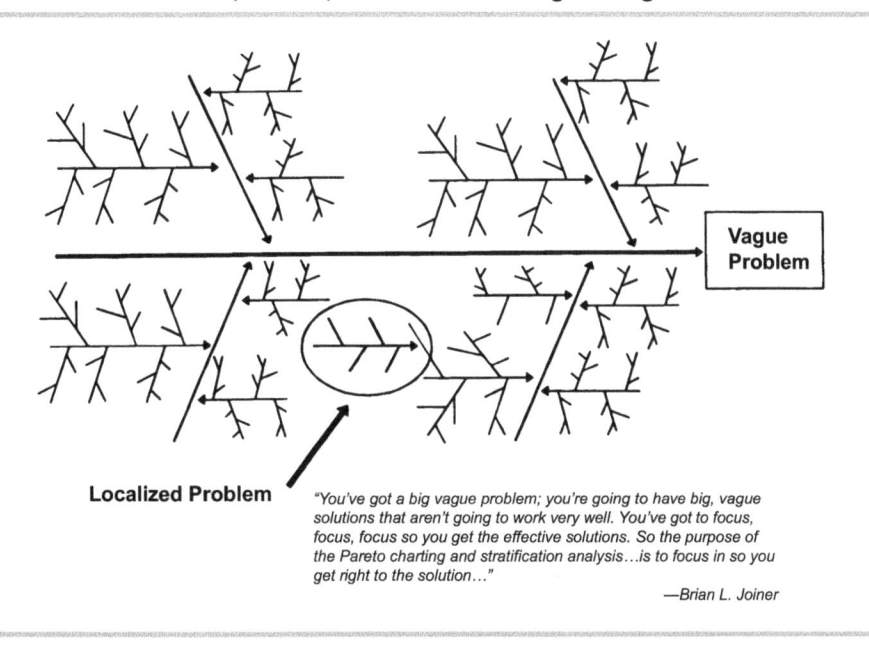

*"You've got a big vague problem; you're going to have big, vague solutions that aren't going to work very well. You've got to focus, focus, focus so you get the effective solutions. So the purpose of the Pareto charting and stratification analysis…is to focus in so you get right to the solution…"*

—Brian L. Joiner

EXHIBIT 8.12  "Ask 'Why?' Five Times" Analysis as a Prelude to a Fishbone Diagram

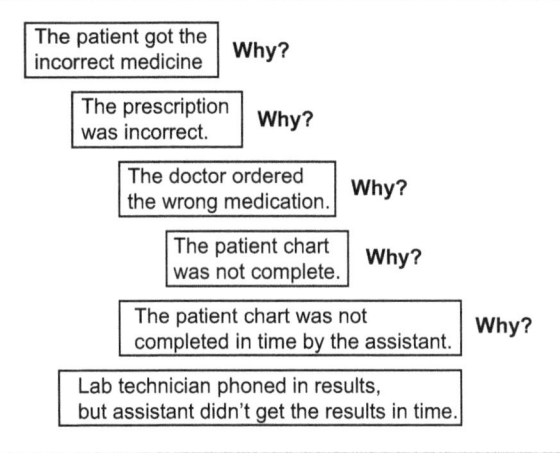

- The patient got the incorrect medicine — Why?
- The prescription was incorrect. — Why?
- The doctor ordered the wrong medication. — Why?
- The patient chart was not complete. — Why?
- The patient chart was not completed in time by the assistant. — Why?
- Lab technician phoned in results, but assistant didn't get the results in time.

A **scatterplot** graphically tests a simple theory about whether an input affects a process output. By plotting the output on the vertical axis and the theorized input on the horizontal axis, you usually observe one of three patterns: a positive relationship (output increases as the input increases), a negative relationship (output decreases as the input increases), or no relationship (the data appear as a shotgun pattern; see Exhibit 8A.16). Exhibit 8.13 contains a scatterplot of charges vs. length of stay. The plot shows that as the length of stay increases, the charges rise as well.

EXHIBIT 8.13 ▪ Scatterplot of Charges vs. Length of Stay

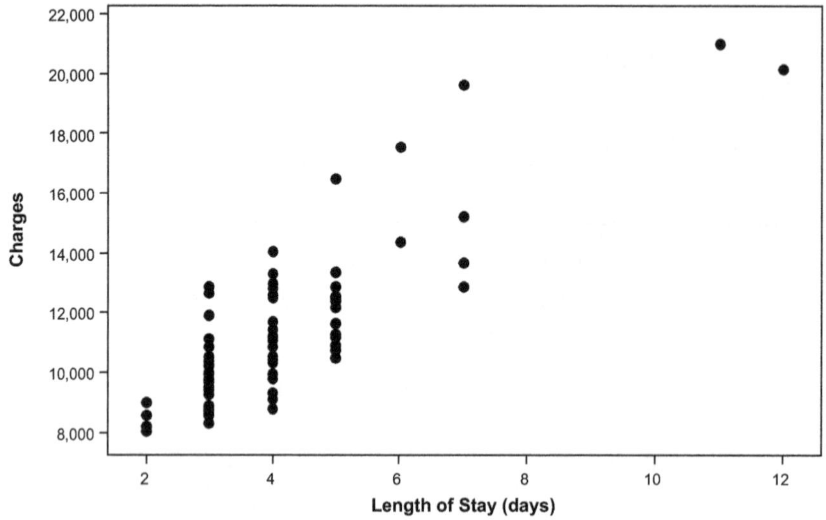

*Note:* This scatterplot shows a positive association between length of stay and total charges.

Scatterplots can be useful when exhausting in-house data and studying the current process. Many times, a formal statistical linear regression is performed on these types of data. Actually, the graph provides much more information than a linear regression analysis, even a statistically significant one, because again, *such an analysis may not be appropriate*: "A picture is worth a thousand numbers."

Regression analysis without plots may also fail even when a relationship exists. If the relationship is not linear, regression analysis could show either misleading significance or no significance. An isolated outlier can also create false statistical significance. Additional danger lurks when a tenuous linear relationship is extrapolated for future prediction beyond the range of the current data. Exhibit 8.14 is a famous example where the four totally different scatterplots yield the identical statistical regression analysis in every number.

The two graphs in Exhibit 8.15 illustrate the association between state performance (there are 50 data points) and two important indicators. There does seem to be some association, but does it need to be expressed mathematically as shown? Visually, it seems to have more merit in Exhibit 8.15a, but what about the performance of Montana (MT) in the upper left quadrant? Using these graphs will lead to much better discussion as opposed to an equation with statistical significance.

It is important to remember that just because an input and an output show a pattern on a scatterplot does not necessarily guarantee a cause-and-effect relationship. For example, ice cream sales and the murder rate show a positive relationship on a scatterplot. Does this mean that ice cream causes murder? A more likely explanation is a third variable, which is temperature, whose increase causes both ice cream sales and the murder rate to rise.

A **stratified histogram** is another method used as a common cause strategy. Unlike a Pareto chart, which uses tallied *counts* of the number of times an event has occurred,

EXHIBIT 8.14 ■ The Potential Deceptiveness of Linear Regression: Plot the Dots!

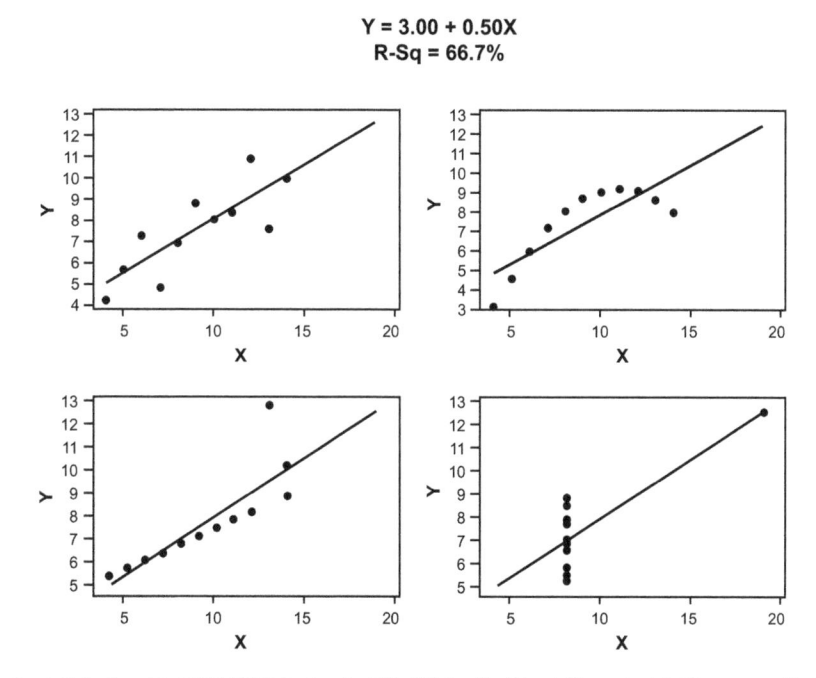

$$Y = 3.00 + 0.50X$$
$$R\text{-}Sq = 66.7\%$$

Source: Davis Balestracci Jr. 2007. "SPC for the Real World." *Quality Digest* (November) 2007. www.qualitydigest.com. Reprinted with permission.

a stratified histogram is its analog for *continuous* data. If a run or control chart displays common cause, theories are generated to possibly explain the process's tendencies toward either high or low values. One can either somehow code the plot for these factors (as in the laboratory data in the "Real Common Cause" example in Chapter 6) or create separate histograms on the same scale (Exhibit 8.16; see also Exhibit 8A.15). In this case, one looks for distinct shifts of one category vis-à-vis others.

*The TEAM Handbook*, *Statistical Thinking*, and *Handbook for Improvement* (see Scholtes and colleagues in Resources) contain extended explanations of these tools with capsule summaries and examples, including healthcare examples. Do not get bogged down in the mechanics and minutiae of the tools. Their purpose is to understand variation.

Exhibits 8.17 and 8.18 relate various tools to the improvement process. Exhibit 8.17 lists the steps of Joiner's Seven-Step Method (see Exhibit 8.4) and some questions and activities that are part of each step. Exhibit 8.18 is a chart showing which tools go with which steps. Following the data thought process as outlined will help you decide when it is appropriate to use a particular tool.

Appendix 8A demonstrates simple, powerful, practical use of several of these tools through three actual everyday scenarios from my consulting. People approached me with vague anecdotes that were not formal organizational projects. I helped them plan a data collection to study their current process. Any work environment is teeming with these

**EXHIBIT 8.15** ▪ Scatterplots That Show Some Relationship (But Do They Need to Be Quantified?)

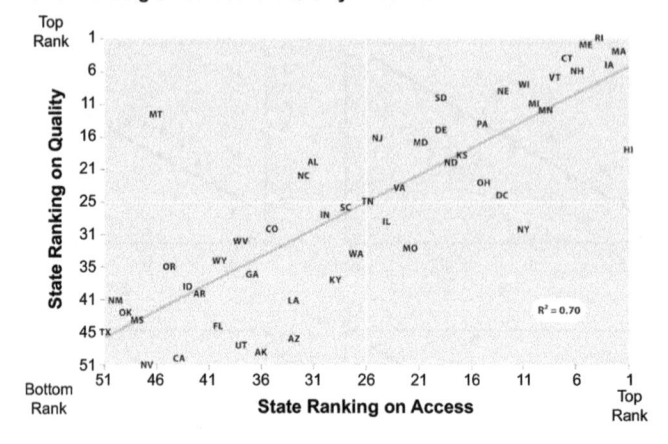

**a. State Ranking on Access and Quality Dimensions**

$R^2 = 0.70$

Avoidable Hospital Use and Costs

**b. Medicare Reimbursement and 30-Day Readmissions by the State, 2003**

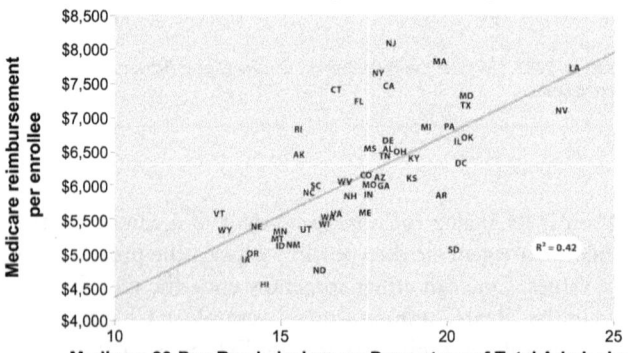

$R^2 = 0.42$

Data: Medicare reimbursement—2003 Dartmouth Atlas Health Care;
Medicare readmissions—2003 Medicare SAF 5% Inpatient Data

Source: The Commonwealth Fund. www.commonwealthfund.org.

kinds of opportunities, as well as heaving with meetings that are well-meaning everyday attempts to improve them without using this process.

The intent of these examples is to show how a simple data collection can be used, with very little data and effort, to move from a vague situation described anecdotally to profound process understanding with intelligent follow-up. Of course, plotting the dots is a big part of it. There is a simple, practical *thinking process* that will yield profound results regardless of whether used on formal projects or more informally in everyday work.

Many projects or improvement opportunities fail because of vague missions, too much premature detailed flowcharting, no baseline estimate of the extent of the problem,

**EXHIBIT 8.16** ■ Examples of Stratified Histograms

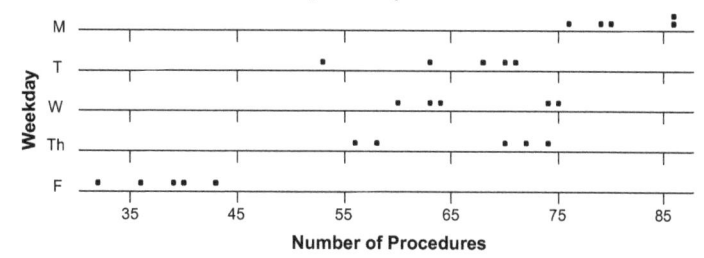

a. Number of Procedures Stratified by Weekday

b. Histogram Comparison of Cardiac Mortality Performance

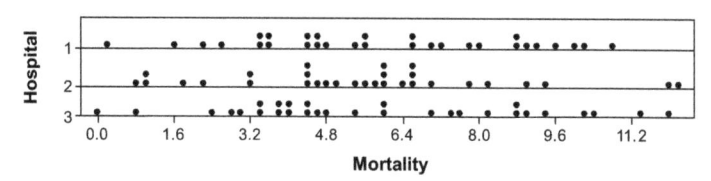

c. Histogram of Recent Stable Behavior

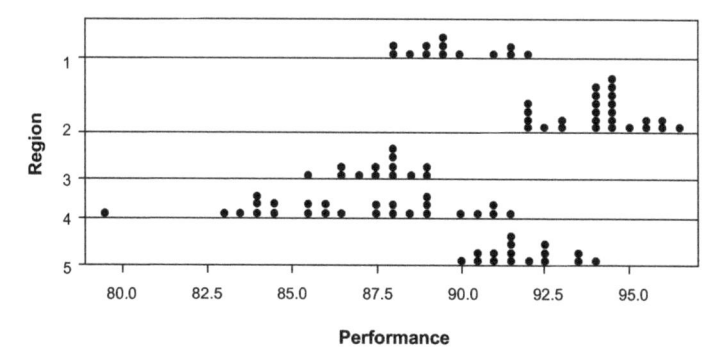

Source a and b: Davis Balestracci Jr. 2005. "Real Common Cause." *Quality Digest* (August); source c: Davis Balestracci Jr. 2007. "A Blinding Flash of the Obvious." *Quality Digest* (July). www.qualitydigest.com. Reprinted with permission.

and failure to understand the current situation (Step 2 in Joiner's Seven-Step Method in Exhibit 8.4). *Being able to focus a situation is one of the most crucial skills a quality practitioner needs to learn and develop*, as well as learning to recognize that most opportunities will be dealing with common cause.

## NO MORE TOOLS — IT'S TIME FOR THE REMEDIAL JOURNEY

Once a solution is found or a process is standardized, Juran's remedial journey begins, which involves different skills to bring a project to closure and hardwire results into the culture. This is summarized in Exhibit 8.19. Many of these are inherent in the previously

EXHIBIT 8.17 ■ Process Improvement: Questions and Activities

1. Situation selection
2. Current situation assessment
    - How does the process work?
    - How should it work?
    - What data are already available?
    - Is there a historical baseline?
3. Cause analysis
    - Are there errors and mistakes? Do they contain special causes or are they common cause?
    - Can we localize a major opportunity?
      - Should we study the current process? (stratification)
      - Should we cut new windows? (disaggregation)
    - Is the current process capable vis-à-vis desired performance?
    - Does the process need to be redesigned? (designed experimentation)
4. Solutions
    - Technically, what will solve the problem?
    - How will this solution affect the work culture?
    - Where should we pilot the solution on a small scale?
    - How will we know if the solution works?
5. Results
    - Is the problem basically solved?
    - Can additional waste be eliminated from the process?
    - Were there any unexpected side effects?
    - Have we sufficiently integrated dealing with cultural resistance into the solution?
6. Standardization
    - Has everyone been properly trained?
    - Are there any cultural side effects?
    - Is the proper data collection in place to hold gains?
7. Future plans

Source: Adapted from Peter R. Scholtes, Brian L. Joiner, and Barbara J. Streibel. 2003. *The TEAM Handbook*, 3rd ed., 5-15–5-17. Madison, WI: Oriel. Adapted with permission.

described improvement processes, but because many project solutions will involve frontline personnel directly, the psychology of cultural resistance to change will again be reviewed and discussed.

## Change Would Be Easy If It Weren't for All the People

Many QI projects come to excellent solutions only to have the same problems mysteriously return six months later. An obvious beneficial remedy to a situation should create no problems. However, an unexpected backlash of delaying tactics or outright rejection of the remedy often occurs. These come from various sources: a manager, the workforce, an external customer, or a union. The reasons given for resistance may seem puzzling, senseless, or even illogical to the advocates of the change. Many times resistance comes from the very people who will benefit from the change.

EXHIBIT 8.18 ■ Grid of Process Improvement Steps and Process Improvement Tools

**Process Improvement Tool**

| Process Improvement Setup | Flowchart | Cause-and-Effect Diagram (Ishikawa) | Pareto Chart / Stratification Analysis | Scatterplot | Stratified Histogram | Run Chart/ Control Chart | Operational Definitions | Check Sheet |
|---|---|---|---|---|---|---|---|---|
| 1. Situation Selection | x | | x | | | x | | |
| 2. Current Situation | x | x | x | | x | x | x | x |
| 3. Cause Analysis | x | x | x | x | x | x | | |
| 4. Solutions | x | x | | | | | | |
| 5. Results | | | x | | x | x | | |
| 6. Standardization | x | | | | | x | | |
| 7. Future Plans | x | x | x | | x | | | |

EXHIBIT 8.19 ■ The Needed Tasks of the Remedial Journey

**Standardization**
- Overcome cultural resistance to change.
- Use Juran's "Rules of the Road."
- Provide ongoing training.
- Provide formal documentation.

**Hold gains**
- Use data collection to assess ongoing current state of process.

Because improvement means change, resistance to change must be considered in each improvement plan to bring about effective, lasting improvement. As I discussed thoroughly in Chapter 3, Juran extensively studied the resistance phenomenon and named it *cultural resistance to change*. This discussion will focus more on this phenomenon as it relates to specific project implementation.

There are two elements common to all change:

1. The change itself (usually technological); and
2. A social consequence of the change.

The social consequence of change is usually the source of resistance because it is an uninvited guest in the culture. It is critical to understand and plan for the nature of the social consequence of any change.

## Juran's Rules of the Road

As an organization grows and matures, its culture develops patterns. Change is difficult when these patterns are disrupted. Society is defined as a continuing body of human beings engaged in common purposes. Without exception, all human societies display cultural patterns — habits, status, beliefs, traditions, practices. These patterns stem from real needs of law and order: to defend the society against danger, to explain mysterious phenomena, and to continue the perpetuation of the society itself. Once a pattern is established, all members are taught the accepted pattern of behavior, and new members must conform to this pattern or face unpleasant consequences.

The cultural pattern is a stabilizer and reinforces existing emotional boundaries. People count on the pattern's predictability for comfort. *Any* change is perceived as a threat to this predictability and must be examined in light of what threat it poses to the culture. As previously discussed in Chapter 3, one many times needs to look beyond the stated reasons to intuit the real reasons.

Stated reasons for resistance may include:

- Specific points of a change;
- Concern for another person; and/or
- Issues about safety or quality.

These are all legitimate considerations. However, the real reasons may be concerns about the individual's status, security, respect, and stress level. Many times he or she might say, "I just haven't thought this through yet." A complicating factor is that the mixture of stated and real reasons applies to both the advocates of change as well as the members of the work culture whom that change will affect.

Any team proposing a solution should consider whom the solution will affect, how they will be affected, and how they are likely to react. Which habits, whose status, and what beliefs are threatened? To understand, ask yourself:

- Are people being asked to perform new, unfamiliar tasks?
- Are they losing face by having to accept the fact they were doing things "wrong?"
- Are they being asked to work harder, do someone else's job, or take on additional (or fewer) levels of responsibility?
- Are they losing autonomy?
- Will employees lose contact with long-time associates and/or need to interact with new people?
- Will daily work schedules and activities, including lunch and break times, need to change?
- Will past resentments reappear because of perceived power issues?

Depending on the proposed solution, reactions can include fear, hostility, overt resistance, passive resistance, and stress.

If strong reactions are anticipated, Faith Ralston's conversational model (see Exhibit 3.1) can also be used here because of the strong emphasis on identifying and acknowledging personal feelings and business needs. Although individuals may perceive a conflict between the two, *if business needs are separated from personal needs, and facts are separated from feelings*, the chance of success is significantly greater.

Juran also provided some refreshing practicality and clarity on these points. He studied the recommendations of several anthropologists and developed guidelines for implementation of a solution. These "Rules of the Road"[4] are quite simple, relevant to any improvement effort, and can have a profound effect on improvement planning, piloting, and implementation.

### *Provide Participation*

At one time or another, everyone has been a victim of NIH (not invented here). Resistance often results when key participants in a process are not meaningfully involved in both the change planning and implementation. Soliciting ideas from participants throughout the improvement process helps them develop ownership in the change and facilitate its eventual acceptance. Providing participation during data collections and sharing results make the project goings-on less of a surprise. If the solution can be kept at a general enough level, the participants (the culture) should help design its details because they know the actual situation the best. This ensures a smoother and more successful pilot.

Juran pointed out that at the outset, participation serves mainly to flush out the objections that are bound to appear. This could be advantageous while proposals are still in a somewhat fluid state. It could also be advantageous to involve a third party with no vested interest in either the change or the status quo to supply balance and objectivity. This is especially important with clinical leaders who are often mistakenly left out of administrative improvements. One coding project site found that when physician leadership was actively involved, the team was able to successfully implement change, while a similar team working on the same process without physician leadership was not.

### Provide Sufficient Time

Change cannot be rushed. People need mental preparation time. They must evaluate the merits of the change in relation to their habits, status, and beliefs. There is always the additional perceived need to develop or negotiate an accommodation with the proposed change.

### Start Small

Always pilot a proposed change on a small scale. This reduces risk and facilitates acceptance by proponents of both the new and old ways. Pilots have the additional benefit of exposing unforeseen bugs in the process as well as unintended consequences that would cause untold damage to the project if rolled out and experienced on a larger scale. They also provide another opportunity for the culture to evaluate and accept the change and expose potential saboteurs.

### Avoid Surprises

Cultures thrive on predictability and continuity. Sudden surprises are shocking and disturb the peace. Maintain constant communication at all levels and allow appropriate time for adequate planning.

### Choose the Appropriate Time for Change

Are too many other changes going on? Is there negative fallout from previous QI efforts? Will current relations with management sabotage this effort before it is even begun? All these questions are vital in choosing the appropriate time for change.

### Keep Solutions Free of Excess Baggage

Solutions should address deep, root causes. People can only absorb so much change at one time. A typical resistance strategy is to distract from the major issue by focusing on the baggage, not the proposal's basic merits. Acknowledge that many issues will be addressed during the improvement process, but continually redirect attention and energy toward the root cause.

### Work with the Recognized Informal Leadership of the Culture

Which frontline workers have earned the respect of their colleagues? It's important to work with the recognized informal leadership of the culture.

### Treat People with Dignity and Understand Their Position

Try to see the change through the culture's belief system. Listen actively, ask for input, respond seriously and directly to input provided. Sometimes, a little bit of attention is all it takes.

### Name the Resistance for What It Is, and Deal Directly with It

Demonstrate flexibility and change specific objectives that can either benefit or have a neutral effect on the solution. It's vital to deal directly with resistance.

### Offer a Quid Pro Quo

In exchange for their support, offer those affected something in trade that they value. The trade does not have to be related to the change.

### Forget It

If all else fails, abandon the effort. Some battles, ultimately, are just not worth fighting. If the issue turns into a vicious power struggle, the culture will virtually always win. Some things to keep in mind:

- Keep the change in the context of the situation;
- Communicate clearly and often;
- Let commitment grow and don't ask for an immediate pledge of allegiance;
- Let people air past resentments, but keep them looking and moving forward;
- Define expectations and results *clearly* and *give feedback*;
- Reward achievement and effort;
- Show your commitment to the change by providing appropriate resources; and
- Whenever possible, maintain current social structures.

## SUMMARY

Projects are important and necessary, but not sufficient, to achieve true organizational transformation. Even when projects are well chosen, the logistics of running a team are key to success or failure. All good team processes come out of the same theory, and I have chosen to summarize the excellent framework given in *The TEAM Handbook* and *Fourth Generation Management*. The dynamics among team members is another issue and beyond the scope of this book. However, some of Chapter 3 might be helpful, and *The TEAM Handbook* covers these issues very well.

Juran's wisdom has shown that any problem has two journeys to traverse: (1) a diagnostic journey from symptom to cause (*analytical skills*); and (2) a remedial journey from cause to remedy (*logistical and psychological skills*).

These journeys have completely different purposes and require totally different skills that go far beyond the usual training emphasis on quality tools. Juran's practical synthesis of "resistance to change" is still the most realistic context for considering a project result's implementation, and his Rules of the Road are most helpful.

The need for good clinical guidelines in a healthcare culture is becoming more critical. Yet, these too need to be tied to an organization's mission, vision, and values. Most

healthcare organizational cultures are not designed to have open attitudes toward standardization. They have the following cultural realities, which add increased variation:
- Management has never effectively emphasized the use of documented standards.
- Few employees have experienced the benefits of effective standardization. Many have been subject to rigid implementation of arbitrary rules.
- Virtually no one sees the need for standards.
- Most employees receive little training on how to do their jobs. Instead, the majority are left to learn by watching a more-experienced employee.
- Most employees have developed their own unique versions of any general procedures they witnessed or were taught. There is a tendency to think, "My way is the best way."
- Changes to procedures happen haphazardly; individuals constantly change details to counteract problems that arise or in hopes of discovering a better method.

Standardization has to be considered a process, and unfortunately past experiences have created many individual cultural beliefs that will need to be overcome, especially with regard to status and autonomy. The paradox is that standardization does *not* stifle creativity:
- Standardization frees the mind to put its energy on improving the process and not constantly reacting to variation, which results in mental exhaustion and only working around the process; and
- Any standardized process can be improved and has a higher probability of being improved.

A documentation process will need to become part of the overall standardization process:
- If process documentations are not constantly being updated, it is evidence they are not being used.
- It does not need to be cumbersome. There are many easy-to-use flowchart software packages.

The purpose of standards is to create exceptional service with maximum efficiency. Standardization focuses on methods of getting work done to answer the questions:
- "What will we do differently to achieve new, consistently higher levels of performance, prevent occurrences of common problems, and maintain the gains discovered and made?" or
- "Should we improve what we have or start over from scratch, with a clean sheet of paper?"

And, regardless, I hope the discussion on resistance to change has shown that:
- Redesigning a process on paper is easy; implementation is another matter.
- Hassle and chaos may be greater than additional benefit.
- *All* change is social change; minor matters to one party are radical changes to someone else.

Doesn't most improvement boil down to these two simple questions?
1. Why does routine care delivery (or product quality) fall short of standards we know we can achieve?
2. How can we close the gap between what we know can be achieved and what occurs in practice?

## APPENDIX 8A: SIMPLE DATA ISSUES AND STUDYING THE CURRENT PROCESS

The following three examples, increasing in complexity, demonstrate the elegant simplicity and necessity of studying the current process to gain an understanding of it (a vital part of Joiner's Step 2 of his Seven-Step Method in Exhibit 8.4). I have explained the analyses in detail to help review and solidify the concepts of Chapters 5, 6, and 7, and plotting the dots will be a big part of it. This will increase your skill in the ability to focus a vague situation, especially helping people resist the urge to jump to process dissection (Juran's "cutting new windows") before stratification. Helping people avoid collecting too much data too soon will help get you results sooner as well as gain increased respect for your role and the quality improvement process in the culture.

### Example 1: The Adverse Drug Event Data

A hospital joined a major initiative for reducing adverse drug events (ADEs). Because it was well known that these errors were underreported, there was a substantial education effort early in the project to increase awareness of such errors, reduce fear of punitive consequences, and set up a reliable process for reporting errors. It was believed that with this support an honest assessment of the current state of the process would be obtained.

The data in Exhibit 8A.1 were collected after the initial expected dramatic rise was observed on a run chart. Plotting the dots as an initial understanding of the new ADE reporting process results in the run chart in Exhibit 8A.2 in which we see that there are no trends.

The next step is to check for eight in a row either all consecutively above or below the median. The longest run is length 12, from February 26 through March 10. Even though this covers 14 days, two of them had values of 4, that is, the median. These are not included in the count of the run length, but, regardless, this is evidence of a special cause. Note that there is another long run (length 9) from April 11 through April 19.

Looking at the run chart, the process average decreased over this time period. At this point it could either indicate an improved process with fewer errors or a backslide into underreporting. A good question to ask initially might be, "Was there a system in place to hold any gains (in reporting)?"

The most recent stable history of this data period appears to begin March 17. The run chart and analysis (Exhibit 8A.3) show that there are no trends.

The runs analysis shows the longest run is length 7, from April 11 through April 19. Even though this covers nine days, two of them had values of 3, that is, the median. (They are not included in the count of the run length.)

The same is true for a run covering April 22 through April 28. There are only 5 nonmedian values, so the run is of length 5, not 7. This is not enough to declare a special cause although we have some provocative observations: There is an interesting run of length 7 from April 11–19, which looks somewhat like a "needle bump" as of April 20, and April 22's result looks high.

With this in mind and given that there were no special causes indicated by the run chart, I created a c-chart of all this data (Exhibit 8A.4); these are incidents and the average is less than 5.

There are several outliers and things now get interesting. Looking at the high data points (March 20 and 27, April 3 and 10), whether outside the upper limit or not, they all occur on a Wednesday. Regarding the high value of 12 on April 22, on investigation,

EXHIBIT 8A.1  ADE Data

| Date | ADE | Date | ADE |
|---|---|---|---|
| 2/26 | 11 | 3/29 | 6 |
| 2/27 | 11 | 3/30 | 0 |
| 2/28 | 6 | 3/31 | 3 |
| 2/29 | 10 | 4/1 | 1 |
| 3/1 | 6 | 4/2 | 4 |
| 3/2 | 4 | 4/3 | 10 |
| 3/3 | 11 | 4/4 | 3 |
| 3/4 | 8 | 4/5 | 2 |
| 3/5 | 6 | 4/6 | 3 |
| 3/6 | 6 | 4/7 | 0 |
| 3/7 | 4 | 4/8 | 3 |
| 3/8 | 9 | 4/9 | 4 |
| 3/9 | 5 | 4/10 | 6 |
| 3/10 | 8 | 4/11 | 2 |
| 3/11 | 2 | 4/12 | 0 |
| 3/12 | 6 | 4/13 | 0 |
| 3/13 | 11 | 4/14 | 2 |
| 3/14 | 5 | 4/15 | 3 |
| 3/15 | 6 | 4/16 | 3 |
| 3/16 | 8 | 4/17 | 2 |
| 3/17 | 3 | 4/18 | 1 |
| 3/18 | 3 | 4/19 | 1 |
| 3/19 | 1 | 4/20 | 5 |
| 3/20 | 8 | 4/21 | 2 |
| 3/21 | 3 | 4/22 | 12 |
| 3/22 | 5 | 4/23 | 4 |
| 3/23 | 0 | 4/24 | 3 |
| 3/24 | 1 | 4/25 | 5 |
| 3/25 | 3 | 4/26 | 6 |
| 3/26 | 4 | 4/27 | 3 |
| 3/27 | 9 | 4/28 | 8 |
| 3/28 | 4 | 4/29 | 1 |

it was found this was caused by a new fax machine that was set to the wrong paper size, which resulted in an atypically large number of errors. Eliminating those four results yields the c-chart in Exhibit 8A.5.

To summarize, it appears to be a stable time period averaging close to three error reports per day (typical daily range of 0–8: Note that the upper limit, if rounded, was attained on one day).

It was still believed that the number of errors was underreported, so there was another major education effort (data shown in Exhibit 8A.6). This data for the subsequent month was added to *the most recent stable history* of the previous graph. The run chart in Exhibit 8A.7 thus begins at March 17 and contains 75 observations. There are no trends and no runs of length 8 or greater.

**EXHIBIT 8A.2** ADE Run Chart of Initial Data

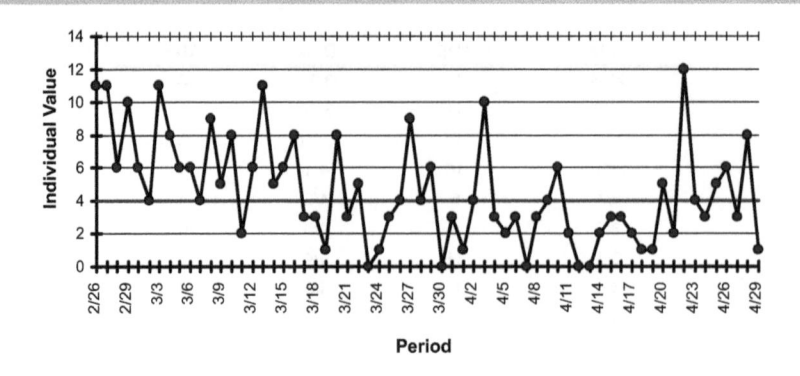

**EXHIBIT 8A.3** Most Recent Stable System Run Chart

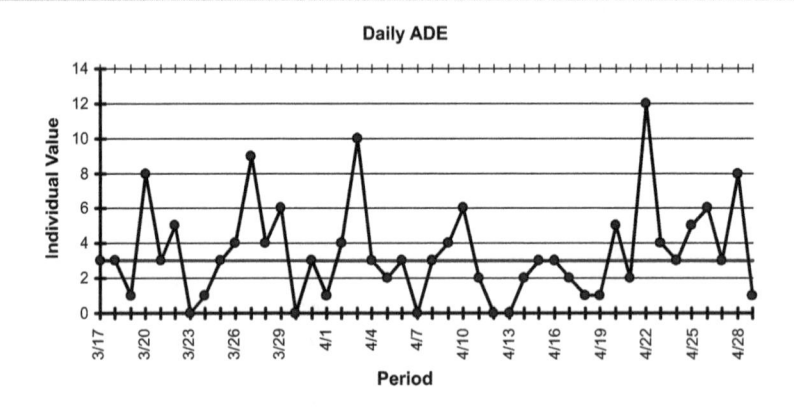

Daily ADE

**EXHIBIT 8A.4** Stable System ADE C-Chart: March 17–April 29 (all data used)

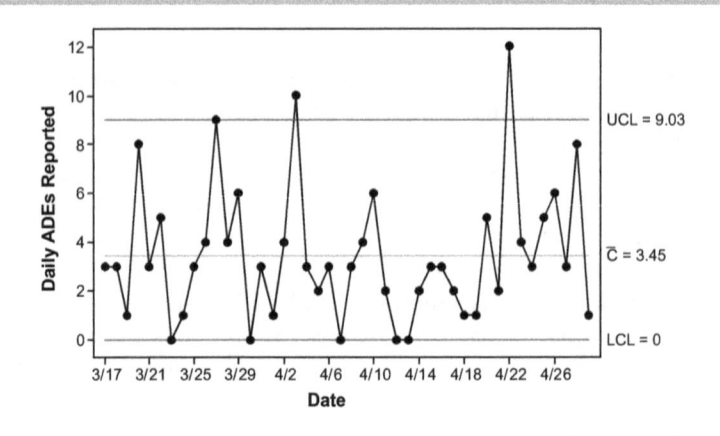

UCL = 9.03
$\bar{C}$ = 3.45
LCL = 0

EXHIBIT 8A.5 ■ Stable System ADE Data C-Chart: March 17–April 29 (outliers deleted)

[Control chart: Sample Count vs dates 3/17 to 4/26; UCL = 7.713, $\bar{C}$ = 2.744, LCL = 0]

Note: 3/20, 3/27, 4/3, 4/10, and 4/22 results omitted from analysis.

EXHIBIT 8A.6 ■ Data after Educational Intervention

| Day | ADE | Day | ADE |
|---|---|---|---|
| 5/1 | 7 | 5/17 | 2 |
| 5/2 | 5 | 5/18 | 0 |
| 5/3 | 4 | 5/19 | 0 |
| 5/4 | 3 | 5/20 | 3 |
| 5/5 | 6 | 5/21 | 8 |
| 5/6 | 10 | 5/22 | 4 |
| 5/7 | 7 | 5/23 | 12 |
| 5/8 | 1 | 5/24 | 1 |
| 5/9 | 1 | 5/25 | 14 |
| 5/10 | 1 | 5/26 | 4 |
| 5/11 | 5 | 5/27 | 1 |
| 5/12 | 4 | 5/28 | 3 |
| 5/13 | 5 | 5/29 | 10 |
| 5/14 | 5 | 5/30 | 5 |
| 5/15 | 7 | 5/31 | 2 |
| 5/16 | 5 | | |

Using a test not covered in this book (see my 2008 article in Resources, "An Underrated Test for Run Charts"), there was a special cause: a special cause *that one desired to create*. The education had some effect. The question is whether the effect could be maintained.

A control chart for the stable period (outliers deleted) and the intervention data (change shown) is given in Exhibit 8A.8.

A stable reporting process is needed for meaningful aggregation via a common cause strategy. Note that it is still not back to the level that resulted from the initial education. Could this possibly be because definitions of errors are clearer and people are being more

**EXHIBIT 8A.7** ■ Baseline Run Chart with Post-Education Performance

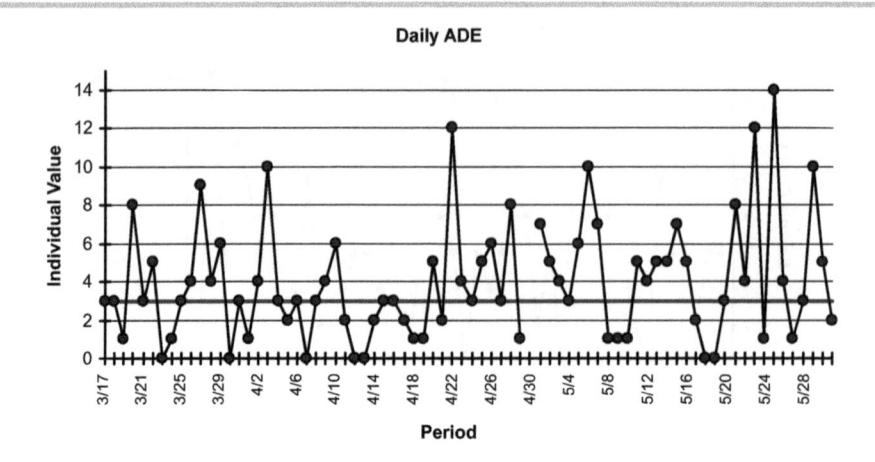

**Daily ADE**

*Note:* You might ask what the effect of the education was.

**EXHIBIT 8A.8** ■ Stable System and May 1 Intervention ADE Data C-Chart

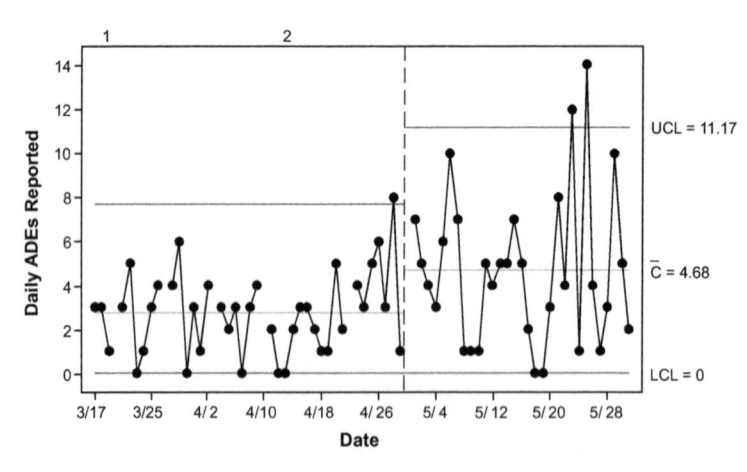

UCL = 11.17
$\bar{C}$ = 4.68
LCL = 0

*Note:* 3/20, 3/27, 4/3, 4/10, and 4/22 results omitted from analysis.

careful only because of the attention being given ADEs? And now there are also those two special causes on May 23 and May 25.

Now that the process has somewhat stabilized, a Pareto matrix aggregating the errors from the most recent stable history (probably not including May 23 and May 25) or comparing it to a Pareto matrix of the aggregated stable history before the current one to see exactly what factors in the process were affected by the intervention could be quite enlightening. In other words, were specific underlying factors or errors affected or was it just the total number of errors reported that was affected proportionately?

EXHIBIT 8A.9 ■ Patient Transfer Times

| Patient (Time Order) | Transfer Time | Patient (Time Order) | Transfer Time |
|---|---|---|---|
| 1 | 22 | 32 | 55 |
| 2 | 27 | 33 | 28 |
| 3 | 12 | 34 | 39 |
| 4 | −4 | 35 | 75 |
| 5 | 30 | 36 | 16 |
| 6 | 24 | 37 | 28 |
| 7 | 22 | 38 | 8 |
| 8 | −12 | 39 | 13 |
| 9 | 56 | 40 | 6 |
| 10 | 38 | 41 | 46 |
| 11 | 306 | 42 | 38 |
| 12 | 0 | 43 | −3 |
| 13 | 39 | 44 | 2 |
| 14 | 293 | 45 | 38 |
| 15 | −21 | 46 | 7 |
| 16 | 38 | 47 | 47 |
| 17 | 117 | 48 | −3 |
| 18 | 150 | 49 | −15 |
| 19 | 230 | 50 | 76 |
| 20 | 17 | 51 | 90 |
| 21 | 28 | 52 | 18 |
| 22 | 29 | 53 | 54 |
| 23 | 23 | 54 | −58 |
| 24 | 0 | 55 | 67 |
| 25 | 3 | 56 | 56 |
| 26 | −4 | 57 | 123 |
| 27 | 80 | 58 | 180 |
| 28 | 26 | 59 | 26 |
| 29 | 70 | 60 | 43 |
| 30 | −6 | 61 | 30 |
| 31 | 28 | 62 | −3 |

This is an example of studying the current process while simultaneously getting a baseline with which to measure improvement efforts, yielding more questions to get to deeper process answers.

## Example 2: The Patient Transfer Time Data

A multidisciplinary team at a hospital wanted to improve the process of transferring patients from the intensive care units (ICUs) to noncritical care units. A measurement was obtained by subtracting the time the patient left the unit from the time the data were transferred in the computer system. Sixty-two patients were transferred in one week. The data are shown in their time order in Exhibit 8A.9, and the resulting run chart is shown in Exhibit 8A.10, which reveals that the median is 28; there are no trends; and there are no runs of eight in a row all above or below the median. So far, it shows common cause.

EXHIBIT 8A.10 ■ Transfer Times Run Chart — All Data

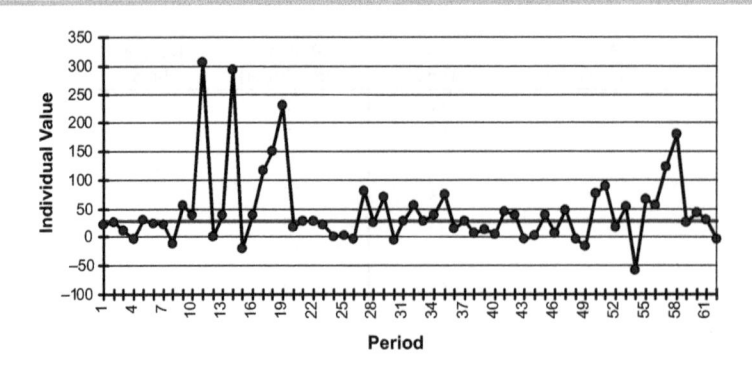

Some of the observations (11 and 14) look quite high. Some of the times are also negative. On inquiry, it was not unusual for the data to arrive at the noncritical care unit before the patient left the ICU.

The median moving range of the 62 observations is 34. From this, it is easy to calculate the maximum expected moving range due to common cause: $MR_{Max} = 3.865 \times 34 = 131.4$.

Note that both moving ranges involving observation 11 (values of 268 and 306) and observation 14 (values of 254 and 314) far exceed 131, which is usually an indication of being an outlier.

The moving ranges from observation 19 to 20 (value of 213) and observation 58 to 59 (value of 154) are also special causes, but the interpretation is not so clear. Looking at the sequence of lower values immediately after 19 and 59, it might suggest whether the transfer point was "batching," that is, accumulating several records, then transferring them all as a batch at the same time, maybe even in the reverse order from which they were received.

The resulting control chart is shown in Exhibit 8A.11. There are no surprises: Observations 11, 14, 19, and 58 (probably 18 as well) are special causes. The average of this chart is a mixture of extremes and not a useful number. In trying to characterize the typical process for the typical patient, omitting those five observations results in Exhibit 8A.12.

With the outliers deleted, the average went from 45 minutes to 28.6 minutes. It also looks like there might two more outliers (observations 17 and 57), but they are not affecting the analysis very much. (Deleting them brings the average down to 28 and barely changes the common cause.)

Therefore, on the average, patients' records typically arrive about 30 minutes after they leave the ICU, plus or minus about 100 minutes. There are various things to consider here:

1. It might be nice to understand more deeply how the data transfer time is operationally defined and whether it is useful as is.
2. When everything that can go wrong does go wrong, it may take well over two hours to get an individual record transferred. If that were to happen (and it will), would that compromise patient care?
3. Meanwhile, what about those five excessive special cause times? From the moving range analysis and looking at the chart, is batching an issue that could eventually contribute to an undesirable event?

**EXHIBIT 8A.11** Transfer Times Control Chart — All Data (median moving range used to calculate limits)

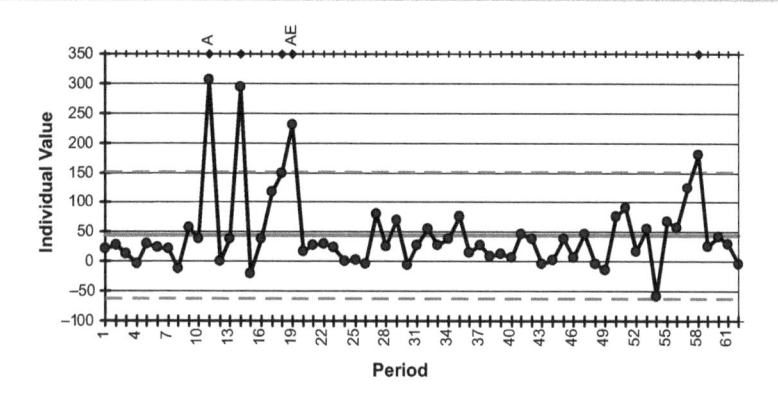

**EXHIBIT 8A.12** Time to Transfer Patient Data — Special Causes Deleted (average moving range used to calculate limits)

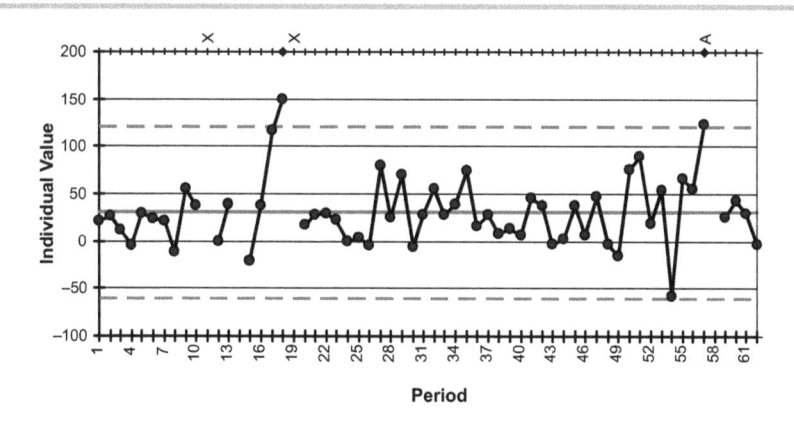

4. The only data I had were the times. Other easily taken additional information was not recorded. Might aggregating the common cause times of this chart, then doing a stratified histogram by *time of day when transferred* (hourly, 2-hour, or 4-hour blocks) show that certain times of the day have higher transfer times than others? Might other stratifications be by noncritical care location or diagnosis?

5. Does the system inherently have an ongoing *approximate* 5/62 = 8 percent occurrence of excessive data transfer time? Are there commonalities to the five excessive times that might allow one to predict when they are going to happen, such as a particular type of patient or during the lunch hour?

6. If 30 minutes is acceptable, what are the process factors that might cause the large variation (e.g., batching, lunch breaks)?

7. Some more general questions are: Is this a high priority with the ICU staff? Is it easy to transfer the data? Is the location to which the data should be sent obvious for all patients?

After further stratification to isolate a major opportunity, one can get more data-aggressive and cut new windows, if appropriate, to dissect the various components making up the total time. The desire is a focused effort on the 20 percent of the process causing 80 percent of what is deemed (if there is a goal) "excessive" times.

Wouldn't you say that's a good start from 62 data points?

## Example 3: The Emergency Department Lytic Data

An emergency department supervisor was receiving vague anecdotal comments about problems with the process of mixing thrombolytic drugs. He decided to study the process by which patients with a suspected heart attack obtained these crucial drugs. The supervisor collected data on the next 55 patients treated for such a condition (i.e., studied the current process). He recorded the number of minutes it took from the time the patient came through the door until the patient received the drug. These times are given in Exhibit 8A.13 and are sorted in the order in which the patients were treated.

This supervisor had some potential theories in mind regarding the variation in the process. Thus he recorded which shift was on duty. He listed these as: Shift = 1

**EXHIBIT 8A.13** ▪ Emergency Department Lytic Data

| Order | Time | Shift | RN | Order | Time | Shift | RN |
|---|---|---|---|---|---|---|---|
| 1 | 9 | 1 | 2 | 30 | 40 | 1 | 2 |
| 2 | 20 | 2 | 2 | 31 | 50 | 1 | 2 |
| 3 | 20 | 1 | 3 | 32 | 30 | 2 | 2 |
| 4 | 20 | 1 | 2 | 33 | 58 | 1 | 2 |
| 5 | 37 | 2 | 2 | 34 | 43 | 2 | 2 |
| 6 | 55 | 1 | 2 | 35 | 20 | 1 | 2 |
| 7 | 37 | 2 | 2 | 36 | 18 | 2 | 2 |
| 8 | 20 | 2 | 2 | 37 | 28 | 2 | 2 |
| 9 | 37 | 2 | 1 | 38 | 16 | 1 | 2 |
| 10 | 29 | 2 | 2 | 39 | 20 | 1 | 2 |
| 11 | 33 | 2 | 2 | 40 | 58 | 2 | 2 |
| 12 | 33 | 2 | 2 | 41 | 32 | 2 | 2 |
| 13 | 6 | 2 | 2 | 42 | 16 | 2 | 2 |
| 14 | 100 | 2 | 2 | 43 | 35 | 1 | 2 |
| 15 | 98 | 1 | 2 | 44 | 40 | 2 | 2 |
| 16 | 20 | 2 | 2 | 45 | 16 | 1 | 2 |
| 17 | 73 | 1 | 2 | 46 | 16 | 1 | 2 |
| 18 | 14 | 2 | 2 | 47 | 18 | 1 | 2 |
| 19 | 50 | 1 | 1 | 48 | 22 | 2 | 1 |
| 20 | 25 | 1 | 2 | 49 | 22 | 1 | 2 |
| 21 | 40 | 1 | 2 | 50 | 55 | 1 | 2 |
| 22 | 120 | 1 | 2 | 51 | 31 | 1 | 1 |
| 23 | 18 | 2 | 2 | 52 | 20 | 2 | 2 |
| 24 | 44 | 2 | 2 | 53 | 15 | 2 | 2 |
| 25 | 24 | 1 | 1 | 54 | 21 | 2 | 2 |
| 26 | 10 | 1 | 2 | 55 | 55 | 1 | 1 |
| 27 | 106 | 2 | 2 | | | | |
| 28 | 22 | 1 | 2 | | | | |
| 29 | 15 | 2 | 3 | | | | |

EXHIBIT 8A.14 ■ Run Chart of All Data in Time Order

**Time to Receive Drug — All Shifts**

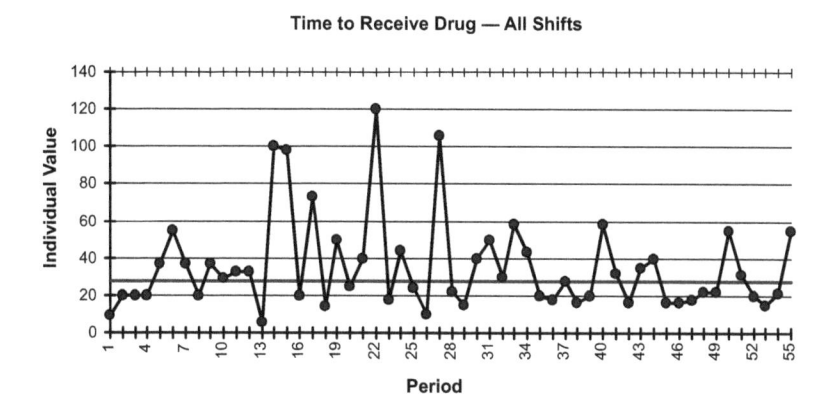

EXHIBIT 8A.15 ■ Stratified Histogram by Shift

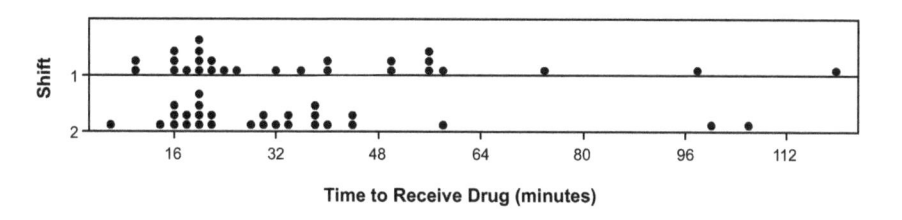

(7 a.m.–3 p.m.) or Shift = 2 (any other time, i.e., 3 p.m.–7 a.m.). He also thought that it was important to know how many registered nurses (RNs) were on duty at the time. These additional pieces of information will be considered after we begin by plotting the dots via a run chart. Exhibit 8A.14 shows that there are no trends and there are no runs of eight in a row all above or below the median.

The supervisor thought there might be a difference by shift. Given that the run chart showed common cause, one can now do a stratified histogram by shift (Exhibit 8A.15) to see whether one shift has a tendency toward higher or lower values.

There seems to be no noticeable difference between performances of the two shifts. The supervisor also thought the time to receive the drug was inversely proportional to the number of nurses on duty, that is, the more nurses, the shorter the time.

If you feel that two things are related, a simple scatterplot of one variable vs. the other is powerful for visual evidence of a trend (or other relationship). Exhibit 8A.16 shows this plot for the data.

There is no indication of a strong relationship between performance and number of RNs on duty. Because there was enough data available for each shift (27 observations for Shift 1 and 28 for Shift 2), it is also possible to do the simple visual analysis of simultaneous run charts putting each shift's data on the same scale (Exhibit 8A.17).

**EXHIBIT 8A.16** ■ Scatterplot of Time to Receive Drug vs. Number of Nurses on Duty

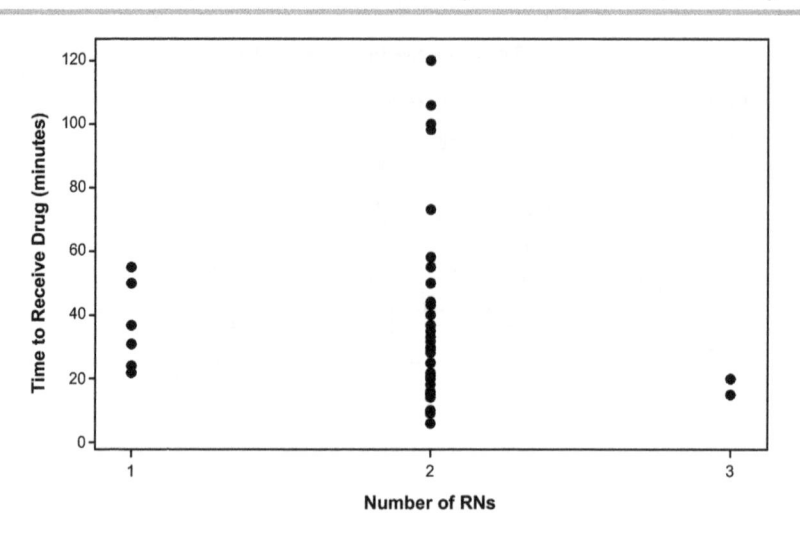

**EXHIBIT 8A.17** ■ Run Chart Comparison by Shift (same scale)

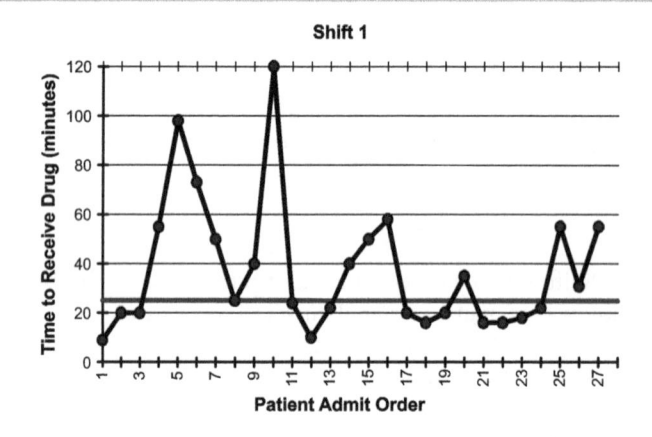

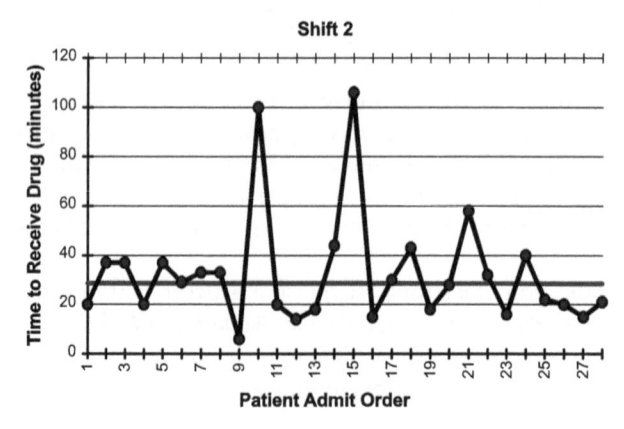

EXHIBIT 8A.18 ■ Initial Analysis of Means via I-Charts to Compare Time to Receive Drug by Shift (forced: overall average of all data used)

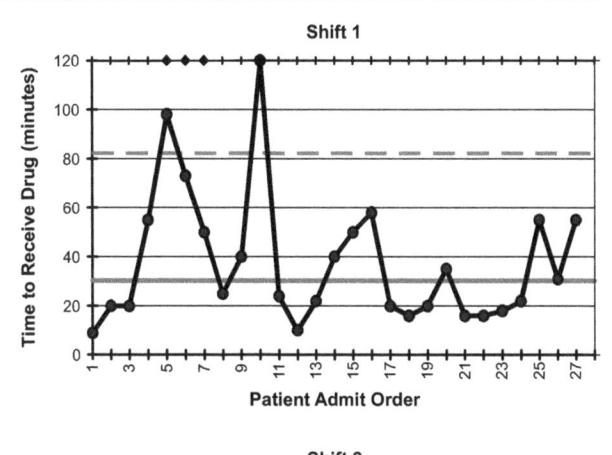

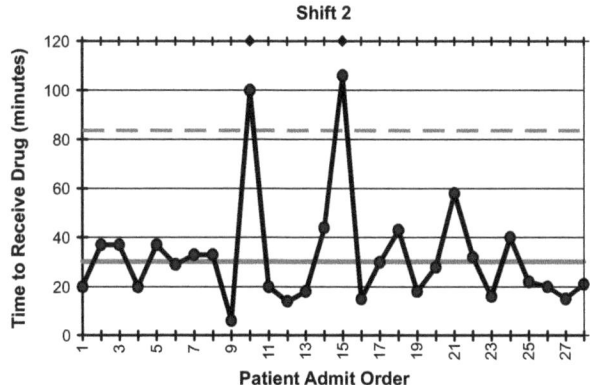

**Shift 1**

[I-chart: Time to Receive Drug (minutes) vs. Patient Admit Order (1–27)]

**Shift 2**

[I-chart: Time to Receive Drug (minutes) vs. Patient Admit Order (1–27)]

The performances look similar and are virtually indistinguishable. To demonstrate just how similar the performances are, Exhibit 8A.18 contains Exhibit 8A.17 converted to two control charts on the same scale.

Note that the common cause was calculated individually, yet they are similar. The typical range encountered by a patient is anywhere from virtually immediate treatment to as long as 80 minutes. This latter value occurs if everything that can go wrong does go wrong, which cannot be predicted because the treatment time seems related neither to the shift nor how many RNs are on duty.

Both shifts contain two outliers each (special causes), which will most probably benefit from separate investigation — individually and as a group because an interesting question arises: "Is there a *certain stable percentage* of patients who *will* have a longer waiting time than 'average?'" And, if so, can this type of patient be *predicted* when he or she comes through the door (special cause strategy)?

So far, this is very little data but might suggest a theory that this percentage could be as high as 4-out-of-55 or 7.3 percent.

Because of the outliers, the median moving range was used for each shift's common cause calculation.

**EXHIBIT 8A.19** ■ Analysis of Means via I-Charts Comparison by Shift of Time to Receive Drug (outliers deleted — forced common average)

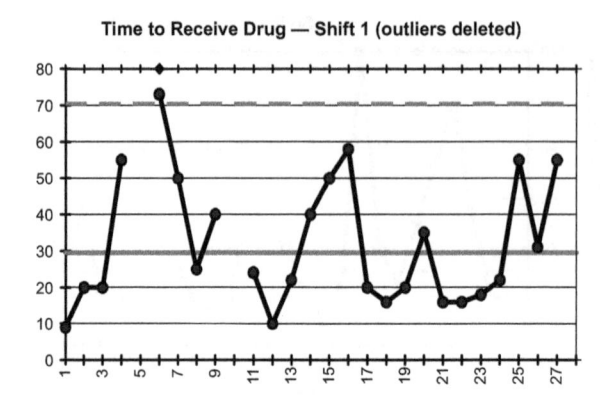

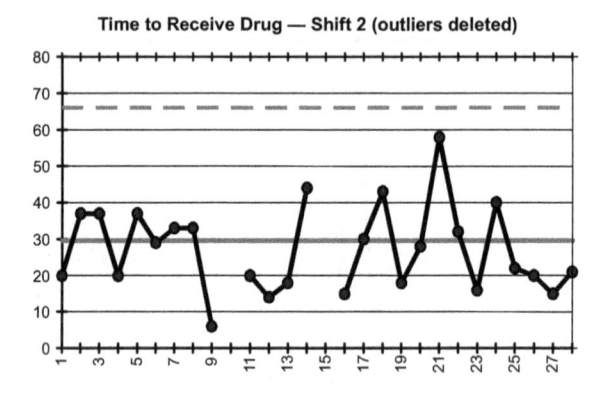

*Time to Receive Drug — Shift 1 (outliers deleted)*

*Time to Receive Drug — Shift 2 (outliers deleted)*

Finally, the two outliers from each shift are deleted from the analysis (but not from future consideration), and the I-charts approximating the analysis of means process are replotted to see whether the "typical" performance of Shifts 1 and 2 differ (Exhibit 8A.19).

Even with the outliers deleted, the performances are virtually identical in both average and variation (average moving range used for each shift's individual calculation of common cause; with outliers deleted, it actually yielded tighter limits than using the median moving range).

There is quite a bit of variation. In quickly assessing a situation and testing simple theories, some theories tested were shown not to apply. Does there need to be more study of the current situation?

## REFERENCES

1. Rummler, Geary A., and Alan P. Brache. 1995. *Improving Performance*, 2nd ed., 126–133. San Francisco: Jossey-Bass.
2. May, Matthew E. 2013. "How to Pick a Project." *Just a Thought* (blog). (August 9). http://matthewemay.com/how-to-pick-a-project.

3. May, Matthew E. 2013. "The Seven Truths of Projects: It's Up to the Project Team to Prove Them False." *Quality Digest* (August 22). www.qualitydigest.com/inside/quality-insider-column/seven-truths-projects.html.
4. Juran, Joseph M. 1964. *Managerial Breakthrough,* 152–157. New York: McGraw-Hill.

## RESOURCES

Balestracci Jr., Davis. 1996. *Quality Improvement: Practical Applications for Medical Group Practice,* 2nd ed. Englewood, CO: Center for Research in Ambulatory Health Care Administration of Medical Group Management Association. First edition published 1994.

Balestracci Jr., Davis. 2008. "An Underrated Test for Run Charts: The Total Number of Runs Above and Below the Median Proves Revealing." *Quality Digest* (October). www.qualitydigest.com/magazine/2008/oct/department/underrated-test-run-charts.html.

Balestracci Jr., Davis. 2013. "Activity Is Not Necessarily Impact: Focus!" *Quality Digest* (September 24). www.qualitydigest.com/inside/quality-insider-column/activity-not-necessarily-impact.html.

Executive Learning. 2002. *Handbook for Improvement: A Reference Guide for Tools and Concepts,* 3rd ed. Brentwood, TN: Healthcare Management Directions.

Hamel, Mark R. 2009. *Kaizen Event Fieldbook: Foundation, Framework, and Standard Work for Effective Events.* Dearborn, MI: Society of Manufacturing Engineers.

Hamel, Mark R. 2014. "Balancing Two Types of Knowledge for Lean Transformation." *Gemba Tales* (blog). http://gembatales.com/.

Hoerl, Roger, and Ronald Snee. 2002. *Statistical Thinking: Improving Business Performance.* Pacific Grove, CA: Duxbury

Joiner, Brian L. 1994. *Fourth Generation Management.* New York: McGraw-Hill.

Langley, Gerald J., Kevin M. Nolan, Clifford L. Norman, and Lloyd P. Provost. 2009. *The Improvement Guide: A Practical Approach to Enhancing Organizational Performance,* 2nd ed. San Francisco: Jossey-Bass.

This is the absolute best reference on how to properly use the plan-do-study-act (PDSA) cycle.

May, Matthew E. 2012. "*Healthcare Kaizen*: Five Questions with Mark Graban." *Quality Digest* (November 30). www.qualitydigest.com/inside/health-care-column/healthcare-kaizen-five-questions-mark-graban.html.

May, Matthew E. n.d. [Article archive]. *Quality Digest.* www.qualitydigest.com/read/content_by_author/29064.

May writes extensively about innovation. If you need a timeout for a bit of professional fresh air, read some or all of this articles in the *Quality Digest* archive.

Scholtes, Peter R., Brian L. Joiner, and Barbara J. Streibel. 2003. *The TEAM Handbook,* 3rd ed. Madison, WI: Joiner/Oriel Inc.

## RAPID-CYCLE PDSA AND ITS LURKING TRAPS

Balestracci Jr., Davis. 2014. "From Davis Balestracci — Things Are the Way They Are Because They Got That Way…" *Harmony Consulting, LLC Newsletter* (January 27). http://archive.aweber.com/davis-newslettr/4.OHn/h/From_Davis_Balestracci_.htm.

Balestracci Jr., Davis. 2014. "'Just Do It!' Still Won't Do It." *Quality Digest* (January 29). www.qualitydigest.com/inside/quality-insider-column/just-do-it-still-won-t-do-it.html.

Balestracci Jr., Davis. 2014. "From Davis Balestracci — How About Applying Critical Thinking to the Process of Using Rapid Cycle PDSA?" *Harmony Consulting, LLC Newsletter* (April 7). http://archive.aweber.com/davis-newslettr/76Wtr/h/From_Davis_Balestracci_.htm.

Balestracci Jr., Davis. 2014. "PDSA…or Rock of Sisyphus? PDSA Is a Messy, Ugly, Nonlinear Process…That You Absolutely Need." *Quality Digest* (April 16). www.qualitydigest.com/inside/quality-insider-column/pdsa-or-rock-sisyphus.html.

## PROJECTS AND PROJECT TEAMS

I recommend the following brief articles whose content is beyond the scope of this book. They also make a very strong case for leadership "walking the talk" and process standardization, *which remains one of the most resisted and counterintuitive concepts of a large-scale improvement effort*. It is also one of the most crucial if an organization is to succeed.

Balestracci Jr., Davis. 2014. "From Davis Balestracci — Before Your Management Says, 'Next!'" *Harmony Consulting, LLC Newsletter* (January 13). http://archive.aweber.com/davis-newslettr/JlHcH/h/From_Davis_Balestracci_.htm.

Hamel, Mark R. 2013. "Respect the Process: And It Will Respect You." *Quality Digest (October 2)*. www.qualitydigest.com/inside/quality-insider-column/respect-process.html.

Hamel, Mark R. 2013. "Build the Lean Management System, and the Behaviors Will Come: Not Exactly." *Quality Digest* (December 5). www.qualitydigest.com/inside/quality-insider-column/build-lean-management-system-and-behaviors-will-come.html.

I trust Mark's work the most of any Lean practitioner. See previous page for his excellent book *Kaizen Event Fieldbook*.

CHAPTER 9

# Cultural Education and Learning as a Process

## KEY IDEAS

- Quality education is not about skills, but rather about changing thinking.
- Learning is a process, and translating adult learning into behavior change is a complex process.
- It is an unrealistic expectation for any education or training within a short time frame to result in self-sufficiency in what is taught.
- One seminar will not change behavior, especially if delivered as an "information dump."
- Do not expect a flurry of multiple simultaneous projects to create improvement.
- Creative curricula with continuous daily reinforcements and subsequent actions connected directly to well-chosen $R_2$ results could be the best way for educating a culture in needed $B_2$ beliefs.
- Physicians have different immediate needs than administrative personnel, even though many long-term needs are the same.
- A deeply entrenched physician belief system of individual accountability taken to an extreme, resulting from medical training and experiences, is unintentional and a serious barrier that must be overcome for success.
- Both clinical and administrative staff must be meaningfully involved from the beginning for an improvement effort to be successful. False distinctions between clinical and administrative projects can create confusion and waste because of inherent interactions.
- Resist the temptation of using a parallel universe of clinical outcome improvement projects to create physician buy-in.
- There are core concepts that need to be taught to create a common organizational language of "process" in the entire culture.

## A FRIENDLY WARNING

Adam Walinsky said, "If there are twelve clowns in a ring, you can jump in the middle and start reciting Shakespeare, but to the audience, you'll just be the thirteenth clown."[1] This Walinsky quote sheds some insight as to why it's so difficult to get work cultures to take quality improvement (QI) as seriously as we do. Thinking back to Exhibit 1.1, if you have been forced to retrofit QI into such a culture, what do you expect? And what are you going to do about it to get the respect you deserve?

Robert Middleton offers, "If you make excuses for not doing something, you're just lying to yourself. It's as simple and as painful as that. The question is, do you want results more than the comfort of avoiding results?"[2]

Do you spend a lot of time delivering internal education and training seminars? Does your leadership team demand to know what the payback is for all the training? Do they threaten it with the first cutbacks when cost-cutting season arises? And how is it all contributing to a "big dot" in the boardroom?

The following material is probably going to make many people with formal QI responsibility uncomfortable. Take a deep breath and remember that your strong reactions are never for the reasons you think (see Chapter 3). Like me, you have put much effort into your organizational QI endeavors and education. After years of good seminar reviews with nothing subsequently changing, I took Middleton's challenge and decided I wanted results more than the comfort of avoiding results. It remains an ongoing challenge.

I want to motivate a new $B_2$ belief system in you about organizational training and education and their delivery. Recall the classic definition of *insanity*: doing things the way you have always done them and expecting different results. Many of your current $B_1$ beliefs are going to be severely challenged. In the context of a new organizational $B_2$, QI is a "learning and growth" sub-business of the organization as well as the strategy for the organization accomplishing its strategy and $R_2$ results.

## IMPLICATIONS FOR ORGANIZATIONAL EDUCATION

Many QI education efforts do not have clear goals other than nebulous "quality training." There is no denying their good intentions. People work hard and intuitively do their best. However, truly objective analysis would show that many training programs are not necessarily designed with the customer or workforce in mind. Courses can typically overwhelm participants with too much conceptual knowledge and jargon in a lecture format and passive participation through unrealistic, patronizing, rote exercises ("Let's flowchart the process of making coffee."). The focus tends to be on skills, skills, and more skills in a compressed time frame, and results are reported in terms of the number of people trained, not the ultimate results of the training.

The typical mixed audience training session, as administered through a human resource or QI department, is just not conducive to problem solving. Most are offered in more of a mini-university rather than a team atmosphere. The focus becomes the activity and not the ultimate impact. Even training courses targeted to specific departments tend to be ineffective because of the overly formal structure and lack of focus on real problems. Motivation to learn and use tools and skills is often lost by bogging down in their minutiae.

Many times both the instructors and participants assume an objective of self-sufficiency, resulting in courses that are too long. Implicit in this assumption is that the participants will be left to decide how and when to apply the methods. When people have not been shown how to use information properly, they will generally misapply it, if they even feel motivated to try to apply it.

From the model in Chapter 3, which will be reviewed here, one can only hope to create some awareness and breakthrough in knowledge to motivate the beginning of a breakthrough in thinking. Going beyond that, with lack of a meaningful application, is a waste of time. A goal of complete self-sufficiency in methods and skills through a course or series of short courses is unrealistic. So stop designing courses that imply or expect self-sufficiency as an objective.

## Don't Forget the 85/15 Rule

There is a widely held belief that an organization would have few, if any, problems if only workers would do their jobs correctly. In fact, the potential to eliminate mistakes and errors lies mostly in improving the systems through which work is done, not in changing the workers.

In spite of the 85/15 rule, frontline workers are often the ones mandated to take in-depth training while executives and management get enough abbreviated training to "know what's going on." Although hiring the best people and putting them through quality training may be a good policy, even the best people are up against 85 to 15 odds (see Chapter 1). At best, they have direct control over only 15 percent of their work problems ("Put a good person in a bad process and the process wins *every* time"). The 15 percent may certainly need attention, but, even then, they are usually not issues vital to business survival. However, in the case of demotivators, as discussed in Chapter 4, they may be important for employee morale.

The 85/15 rule is also manifested when employees are trained and subsequently empowered to choose a project. Unfortunately, the problems chosen and presented directly to managers usually tend to be obvious, related to the 15 percent, and do not represent deep fixes. As has been emphasized repeatedly, *the important problems are the opportunities that no one is aware of.* In essence, management has charged 85 percent of the workforce to provide less than optimal (but well-meaning) solutions for 15 percent of available improvement opportunities. This does not seem to be a sensible deployment of resources.

## The Lack of Value in Training the Trainer

Many a disaster has also occurred as a result of "train the trainer" programs. These are programs in which outside resources are used to train a select few, who then train the organization, including other trainers. My experience has been that these courses are too long, too heavy on teaching tools, and try to teach too much in too short a time frame. The participants, many of whom may not even truly understand why they are there, are overwhelmed (usually after the first two hours) and are eventually expected to do this in their spare time. People do not need to teach tools, they need to teach people to solve their problems.

In addition, unintentional $B_1$ filtering takes place as knowledge is passed from one set of trainers to the next set of trainers. Eventually, any resemblance between what the "trained" trainers teach and what was originally taught is purely coincidental. Mastering aspects of a tool is much different from effective application of a tool. I can know how to use a hammer to drive a nail, a saw to cut a piece of wood, and a level to make sure things are even, but if the whole purpose is to ultimately build a house, I am in big trouble.

Once again, unintended human variation becomes the enemy of the quality of education and training; teaching tools as ends in themselves can easily become an end in itself. People need to understand the world of the QI process.

Mark Silver, in "Why Your Customers Lie to You" (see Chapter 10 sidebar), explains a context of understanding "the world of the solution." Most customers do not. To them, the world of the solution is what works in *their* unique world.

Seminar participants could be considered internal customers of your organizational education process. And, if they do not understand the world of the solution (and the people teaching them do not understand it), teaching them things such as "creativity" is a total waste of time as well (see Carnell and Gregerman in Resources).

The key to successful training is not to teach methods and skills, but to teach people how to use these skills — how to solve their problems and the problems that are barriers to the organization's $R_2$ results. Any conceptual knowledge should support a problem-solving process and be immediately applied.

## Changing Adult Behavior

Even if the correct knowledge is taught, there is still a process by which people understand and assimilate new information. This process was discussed in Chapter 3 and involves the following four phases, only the latter two of which can create true, competent self-sufficiency based in the proper context of the world of the solution:

- Phase 1: Having awareness;
- Phase 2: Achieving a breakthrough in knowledge;
- Phase 3: Choosing a breakthrough in thinking; and
- Phase 4: Demonstrating a breakthrough in behavior.

Each of these four phases is part of the human psychological process. Each has its unique, deliberate pace and challenges. All learning launches participants on a journey through these phases. The human change process takes time. Any training that goes beyond an individual's current phase is wasted and could actually be counterproductive by creating unneeded psychological frustration. Given the behavior model from Chapter 3, unless the seminar participants (and instructor) are clear about the $B_2$ belief context in which the tool is used, they will filter information through their current $B_1$, virtually guaranteeing limited comprehension and ineffective application.

One of the biggest disappointments in a QI effort occurs when concepts learned in a course do not translate into action. Human nature being what it is, logic is not always persuasive (see Chapter 3). Formidable barriers are erected by people's natural resistance to change, such as the link between statistical thinking and methods to the common $B_1$ math anxiety and a job that is already perceived to take up more than 100 percent of their time. The impact of these barriers is virtually impossible to overestimate.

Unique problems are encountered when teaching adult learners. A partial list includes participants' perceived lack of immediate applicability; inappropriate material being taught; people's natural resistance to change (even though they acknowledge the need for change); courses quickly getting ahead of what people are capable of realistically absorbing; and, probably most important, the inertia caused by the company's need to stay in business. The current way is the only known way and absorbs the total organizational "digestive capacity." Thus new knowledge is not immediately applied and is soon forgotten, if indeed it was learned properly in the first place.

Jim Clemmer[3] recommends the following as important considerations in teaching adults:

- Understand why the skill is important;
- Discuss the specific behaviors involved in the skill;
- Watch a demonstration of the skill;
- Practice the skill;

- Receive constructive feedback; and
- Identify opportunities for using the skill.

If the goal is awareness, keep the time frame appropriate to creating awareness. Further damage occurs when, despite a multitude of classes taught, management discovers no overall organizational financial benefit and laments the loss of productivity due to time demands, and QI resources are the first to suffer in budget cuts. When the leadership team neither participates in training nor models the appropriate skills, negative cultural consequences also result.

*No course or instructor can change people.* People must choose to change themselves. Unless the delivery of the education is designed to address this issue and spark individual internal motivation, *it has no value.* Long-held $B_1$ cultural beliefs (about both the material and internal training) must be challenged in such a way that people accept the challenge and become excited about being led into the future.

## Beyond Awareness

Proper education puts training in perspective. (Think of it this way: Would you rather your children or grandchildren have sex "education" or sex "training"?) Awareness and the resulting breakthrough in knowledge need to be seen as the potential beginning of an ultimate journey toward breakthroughs in thinking and behavior, the final phase of understanding and assimilating knowledge. However, as you remember from Chapter 3, there is another phase that must take place before the education can translate into truly meaningful action. The education and awareness phase's breakthrough in knowledge must be processed via a necessary but awkward painful transition phase: struggling with the needed changes in a belief system to create the breakthrough in thinking.

This phase is extremely difficult to impose on a culture for reasons discussed previously, and it is naive to believe that one or even a series of short, intense courses geared toward self-sufficiency can change a lifetime of ingrained habits. A flurry of teaching activity should not be confused with impact.

It is not realistic to expect an immediate or even a necessarily correct application of material recently learned. In fact, part of the breakthrough-in-thinking phase will involve learning from *mis*applications of skills through the filter of old habits and real-time constructive feedback. "Thinking statistically" in terms of processes and properly identifying and understanding variation are many times — and especially initially — overwhelming and counterintuitive.

People are being pushed out of their comfort zones, and they must have time to acclimate as well as see proof that the culture values this change. If management demonstrates the desired behaviors, acts as teachers and coaches, rewards use of the behaviors, and allows people to take pride in their everyday work resulting from application, the pace of training results will still be deliberate, but it will accelerate and have a chance of succeeding.

## KEEP THE PROJECTS HIGH LEVEL

Do not overdo projects on allegedly obvious problems expecting improvement in general. The reality of designating continuous QI as an organizational goal by itself is necessary, but not sufficient for improvement. At first QI will be perceived as pulling energy away from normal daily tasks that already take up more than 100 percent of everyone's time. Whereas myriad uncoordinated QI projects can become an energy drain, seeing QI as a transformational strategy has the potential to pull the energy inward to create an organizational synergy through a common strategy and desired results, with the data sanity of Chapter 2 as a key catalyst. Teams are a necessary part of it, but there are things an organization must do in parallel with the teams' efforts to complement them and create the aforementioned synergy.

A resource I consider indispensable for any QI facilitator is *The TEAM Handbook*, now in its third edition (see Scholtes and colleagues in Resources). To quote the late Peter Scholtes, a major contributor to the first edition in 1988 and author of the foreword for the second edition:

> The importance and popularity of teams have escalated dramatically in the last several years. As someone who perhaps helped to contribute a bit to that trend, I feel a need to offer a caution: teams are not a panacea. Teams are one vehicle for getting work done. Teams will not always be the best vehicle. A given team may not be able to deal with the causes of the problem or the needs of the system. There is no substitute for leadership, good planning, well-functioning systems, excellent services, well-designed and executed products, and an environment of trust and collaboration. Some managers seem to want to proliferate teams, the more the better. But teams need to be a part of larger contexts and larger systems: systems that select priorities, systems and processes for providing goods and services to the customers, systems for training and educating the workforce. Without purpose…there can be no system. And without purpose and systems, there can be no team. Leaders, therefore, must focus on their organization's mission, purpose, and the systems needed to successfully accomplish that mission and purpose.[4]

As many organizations have learned, committing to a QI framework is at best an awkward adolescence that can neither be created by establishing a QI department in the organization nor attempting to implement part of the QI philosophy in bolt-on fashion without embracing the entire concept of organizational transformation.

It is much easier to begin than to keep going. Experience shows that the initial enthusiasm, which can almost border on intoxicating, is often followed by a nasty hangover. As I and many others have learned, an initial flurry of training and team creation generates a lot of heat, but probably not much light, and improvements do not necessarily last long after project completion, if projects even come to completion.

Management must resist acting on the initial outburst of enthusiasm to create projects on long-standing organizational problems with scopes that are too wide and vague. There is also a tendency to populate the teams with frontline people so that they will feel empowered. Trust me, they will not thank you.

People perceive their jobs as already taking up all of their time. Now, in addition to performing their daily job responsibilities, staff members are trying to improve their work processes using new concepts and tools that have been poured into their heads, generally in a stimulus-response short-course format. People are out of their normal comfort zones.

At any time for justification purposes, it is easy and tempting to report how many people have been through how many courses and what percentage of people have participated on a team. Yet the leadership teams become impatient waiting for the promised big payoff to appear. Yes, for QI to succeed, everyone must use at least basic QI skills as a common language in their jobs. However, best intentions and training do not necessarily

EXHIBIT 9.1 ■ Quality Improvement vs. Transformation

| Quality Improvement (QI) | Transformation |
|---|---|
| "One-shot" skills training via courses | Routine, continuous education through daily work |
| Many teams of key personnel focused on routine daily operational issues | Few top management-led teams focused on key strategic issues |
| Heavy emphasis on tools | Entire work culture educated in QI theory |
| Obvious, current problems (3–15% of opportunity)<br>▪ Formal problem identification<br>▪ Problem-solving tools<br>▪ Management guidance teams<br>▪ Formal team reviews<br>▪ Storyboards<br>▪ QI coordinator and formal quality structure | Hidden problems (85–97% of opportunity)<br>▪ Appreciation of systems<br>▪ Psychology<br>▪ Variation<br>▪ Use of data to test improvement theories<br>▪ Continuous establishment and documentation of routine processes important to customers |
| Team facilitators with QI tool skills | Change agents with formal cultural change skills |
| Arbitrary numerical goals | Understanding variation, process capability, integrated measurement system via balanced scorecard |
| Management behavior<br>▪ Manage status quo<br>▪ Solve problems<br>▪ Reactive response to variation (treat as unique, special causes)<br>▪ Choose projects, review progress<br>▪ Send people to "courses" | Management behavior<br>▪ Understand and improve processes<br>▪ Facilitate problem solving and remove cultural barriers<br>▪ Proactive response to variation (Asks: common or special cause?)<br>▪ Exhibit QI skills through behavior<br>▪ Teach QI through routine daily work and meetings |
| Quality "certain percent" of the job and explicit | Quality 100% of the job and implicit |

translate to expected behaviors, especially with adult learners. Quality is more than just training, teams, and projects.

The QI coordination function is necessary, but its role must be one of directing a transformation of organizational behavior, with accountability for facilitating key organizational $R_2$ results. A comparison of a typical QI approach with that of transformation is contrasted in Exhibit 9.1.

What this implies in terms of needed everyday managerial behaviors is summarized in Exhibit 9.2. These skills need to become routine in any organization.

## AN INNOVATIVE APPROACH TO ORGANIZATIONAL EDUCATION

It's time to admit the lessons still not learned. According to Clemmer, "Too often, companies rely on lectures ('spray and pray'), inspirational speeches or videos, discussion groups and simulation exercises. While these methods may get high marks from participants, research (ignored by many training professionals) shows they rarely change behavior on the job. Knowing isn't the same as doing; good intentions are too easily crushed by old habits. Theoretical or inspirational training approaches are where the rubber meets the sky."[5]

## EXHIBIT 9.2 ■ Summary of Skills to Be Routine in All Organizations

**Understand Your Process**
- Convert anecdotes via process language.
- Understand internal and external customer relationships and their true needs; interconnectedness of processes.
- React with questions, not necessarily action.
- Prepare a flowchart to reduce human variation in perception.
- Always consider seven sources of problems with a process (see Chapter 1).
- Plot data and obtain a baseline to establish the extent of a problem.

**Ensure Data Quality**
- Apply the Pareto principle to organizational data: What are the 20 percent of the numbers that account for 80 percent of leadership attention and actions?
- Eliminate wasteful data (no objectives, vaguely defined process outputs) (see Chapter 5).
- Avoid unnecessary, vague, written surveys (see Chapter 10).
- Convert anecdotes (define and tabulate occurrences).
- Conduct simple, efficient collections at the appropriate level of aggressiveness (see Chapter 5).
- Remember that the data collection process itself is not trivial (see Exhibit 5.12 ).
- Use data as a basis for *action*.

**Localize Problems**
- Operationally define fuzzy outputs.
- Stratify by process input to expose special causes.

**Assess Efforts to Improve and Hold Any Gains**
- Use run charts and control charts.

**Plot "Hot" Numbers, That Is, the Numbers That "Make You Sweat"**
- Remember: Losses due to tampering are incalculable.

**"When You Don't Know, You Don't Know"**
- Ask questions.
- Allow observed variation to drive questions you ask.

**Beware of Arbitrary Numerical Goals**
- Ask, "Is the process capable of achieving that goal?" and "Is the variation from the desired goal due to a common or special cause?"

According to Snee,[6] despite the steep learning curve of the last 30 years, the following six common mistakes continue to be made:

1. Focusing on training rather than improvement;
2. Failing to design improvement approaches that require the active involvement of top management;
3. Failing to use top talent to conduct improvement initiatives;
4. Failing to build the supporting infrastructure, including personnel skilled in improvement and management systems, to guide improvement;
5. Failing to work on the right projects, which are those that deliver significant bottom-line results; and
6. Failing to plan for sustaining the improvements at the beginning of the initiative.

Isn't it time for improvement professionals to stop bemoaning these issues and do something about them? No one is better poised than you, but you must also develop the talents to broaden your job responsibilities to deal with the mistakes listed.

## Create Awareness

Initially create awareness for your leaders by connecting the dots for them and solving their problems. The 10 Lessons in Chapter 2 suggest a wealth of opportunity for simple, effective applications.

- Can you attempt to forge a partnership with your leadership team using data sanity to *translate data into intelligent action at the appropriate level?*
- Can you eliminate some routine meetings mired in data insanity (treating common cause as special cause) through effective use of statistical thinking to *solve everyday* problems?
- Can you use everyday data and meetings to help your leadership team learn and apply statistical thinking to their work and free up *significant* time for them in the process?
- Can you cut through their initial resistance by quietly solving a significant longstanding organizational issue to make your case?

## A Guide for Education

Using "A Road Map: Major Steps to Transformation" (see Exhibit 1.2) as a guide, establish awareness and education for your leadership team and build critical mass. These are the two major steps to transformation. And the summary of key basic concepts described in Appendix 9A should be a vital part of education design to create a universal improvement language for its desired resulting behaviors.

### Step 1

The onus is on you to lead top management toward breakthroughs in thinking and behavior through awareness and education. Your objective is to learn and apply the following in everyday work:

- Use process thinking and begin to eradicate blame.
- Introduce statistical thinking and the value of plotting data over time to change the conversations in the boardroom and on the leadership team. Have them experience agreeing on a situation within seconds, resulting in changed, more productive conversations that *solve* issues.
- Be aware of common and special causes of variation and how to deal with each. Be careful of treating all variation as special cause. Use the existence and power of common cause strategies for improvement and be wary of loosely using terms such as *above* or *below average*, *top* or *bottom quartile*, or top or *bottom 10 percent* **without plotting the dots.**

### Be Innovative

From reading the first eight chapters of this book, you know that you are swimming in opportunity to create change in your organization's culture. You can do this by demonstrating to both leadership and staff how the routine use of statistical thinking will free up major chunks of time for them and eradicate dreaded meetings rife with data insanity. The usual leadership team 20-minute overview will not do it. Don't bore leaders to death with W. Edwards Deming's "red beads" or a quincunx. *Solve real problems* by changing conversations; for example, solve a major longstanding problem affecting a number that makes leaders perspire. Safety could be a great start (see the section "Educating a Culture on Improvement" under Resources). As an added result you will gain the respect you deserve and much more interesting work.

The purpose is to gain the support of leadership and align the organization in its improvement work. As a quality professional, you should now take on the duty of recognizing and stopping the siloed, frenetic, no-yield activity that comes from treating common causes of variation as if they were special causes (*especially excessive root cause analyses*) and people confusing hard work with impact.

### Step 2

Build critical mass by continuing your education behaviors in Step 1. The goal is to get 25–30 percent of leadership to *demonstrate* commitment to quality in everyday work, *that is, display visibly changed behaviors.* In other words, create $A_2$ that might help change the cultural $B_1$ to $B_2$, which will in turn drive work behaviors ($C_2$) to obtain desired organizational $R_2$.

You will know that critical mass is taking place when you observe the beginnings of cultural data sanity. Are bar graphs, trend lines, tabular data reports, and traffic light reports slowly disappearing, as well as the meetings that previously used them, and people don't miss them? Run charts will start to be used at board meetings, and leaders will deal with resistance by being insistent and showing results.

You will notice that elements of "universal improvement language" (see Appendix 9A) are being routinely used in the culture, such as process, variation, common cause, special cause, "count to eight," and plot the dots. You will hear people ask if we are perfectly designed for an issue or if the issue is a common or special cause.

Are there fewer meetings accounting for performances as compared against arbitrary numerical goals? Do you see a process focus as opposed to the previous meeting-the-goal focus? Are improvement initiatives based on moving "big dots" and are they beginning to get higher or top priority at meetings?

When you see common cause strategies being routinely used for solving significant problems, you will know that critical mass is taking place. And you will witness a cultural process focus developing *zero* tolerance for blame and victim behavior, and benevolent, routine use of the question-behind-the-question (QBQ) to create true cultural empowerment. What do your organization's schedules, budgets, and meeting agendas telegraph as to values and priorities?

You will see the critical mass leaders using the freed-up time to walk around, seek feedback, and gently coach. And the beginnings of frontline teaching done via solving problems or using Exhibit 5.3 to understand their work as a process will develop. Finally, you will see that promotions are now based on demonstrating commitment to quality and the expectation of leaders to generate their own run charts and control charts on important numbers, then intelligently present and discuss them. (These are the people to whom you devote a lot of mentoring time. Allow them to look good and *let them have all the credit* for any outstanding results.)

At this point you should see:

- Only 20–30 percent of the organization needs to be educated in quality philosophy.
- Only 10–20 percent of the organization needs to be trained in basic tools for QI.
- Only 1–2 percent of the organization needs to be trained in advanced tools.
- In everyday conversations, you begin to hear frontline stirrings that "something feels different around here."

You will now be set up for true success in creating the culture conducive to the success of the third and fourth steps of transformation, as described in Exhibit 1.2. Appendix 9A also provides the educational road map for one of the third step's most important tasks: "All employees are educated in basic QI tools and philosophy."

You will also see thinking and belief systems begin to evolve towards ultimately creating the culture inherent in Step 5, where improvement will be built in to your organizational DNA.

## WHAT ABOUT THE PHYSICIANS?

My experience has been that the typical frontline physician has neither the time, patience, nor interest to sit through formal in-house seminars. This is especially true if their compensation depends on productivity. Quite frankly, it is a poor short-term strategy to try to convince physicians of the importance of QI skills and to teach skills to such an actively resistant culture. Physicians have their own ideas about this "QI stuff" and their medical training has unfortunately entrenched a self-defeating belief in many of them of absolute individual accountability if *anything* goes wrong as well as a clinical trial belief system about statistics (see the appendix at the end of this book).

However, chief medical officers and various department heads need the same education as executives and middle management. It will take the same critical mass of 25–30 percent of them actively demonstrating commitment to improvement principles to begin to align *both* their physicians and nonphysician employees into embracing this style of leadership.

Openness to learning and practicing improvement-based leadership behaviors should be a requirement for promotion to such positions.

In my presentation experience, the most enthusiastic participants have consistently been chief medical officers. The refreshing practicality of the data sanity approach resonates with their frustration with poor data presentations in the many meetings they attend. Physicians have a strong peer connection, and many of these presentations unintentionally malign their colleagues inappropriately regarding practice patterns, utilization, clinical outcomes, undesirable incident occurrences, and peer rankings. They somehow knew that clinical trial statistics didn't apply but didn't know an alternative, and now they have one in the elegant simplicity of data sanity. Being an advocate for stopping the "name and shame" tactics would be a major quid pro quo conduit to encourage physician buy-in to commit to a culture of true excellence.

### The False Barrier between Clinical and Administrative Issues

Illustrating one source of this division from the physician perspective, Berwick states:

> For many physicians, the central notion of "process, not people" as the most powerful cause of both quality and flaws contradicts long-standing assumptions about individual responsibility and the shouldering of blame in medical care. Process thinking challenges strongly held views — enshrined in medical rituals and lore — that the quality of care rests fundamentally on the shoulders of the individual physician.
>
> Of course, that challenge is illusory; QI counsels not an abandonment of individual responsibility, but rather that individuals, through systematic methods, take on even deeper responsibility to help develop and improve the interdependent processes of the work in which they are inextricably bound.

Teamwork and individual responsibility are not opposites; indeed, the former implies the latter.[7]

Identical processes and thinking are used for both clinical and administrative improvement. Very few processes are purely clinical, that is, involving only doctors and patients, or purely administrative, that is, not involving doctors at all. Almost all important healthcare processes touch physicians as either customers, suppliers, or processors.

Physicians in formal administrative roles and informal physician opinion leaders must be involved from the beginning in efforts to use QI as a strategy. But do not fall into the seductive trap of involving physicians through creating a parallel universe of clinical improvement teams on best practices.

## Core Knowledge for Physician Buy-In

All healthcare improvement efforts eventually reach a point where physicians' lack of knowledge and misperceptions about QI will present a roadblock to organizational transformation. The many rapid changes in healthcare have added to the sense of lost control experienced by many physicians. It is no surprise that one social consequence of QI is resistance. Physicians perceive it as someone else "looking over their shoulder" — they feel accused.

A consequential issue to consider is what core knowledge and format would increase the probability of the critical mass effect among physicians. With this in mind, self-sufficiency in QI skills is not an objective but rather the awareness of QI's power by operationalizing data sanity via the concepts shown in Chapter 2 to the routine data used to judge physician performance.

To deal with some of their stated reasons for resistance, you can use material from the appendix at the back of the book as needed to put some of their biases about QI to rest. Contrasting clinical trial thinking vs. QI thinking is one major issue. Physicians will get nervous when you talk about QI being used for "reducing variation"; instead *always* say "reduce inappropriate and unintended variation."

The main objective is to overcome misconceptions and make physicians aware of their place in a system designed for a core process of delivering healthcare. Presentations of data on routine daily work can provide the convincing that physicians typically need to change behavior by showing that QI is merely an extension of their deeply held sacred belief in the scientific method, but in this case, applied to the *delivery* of healthcare in addition to strictly clinical outcomes. Usually data sets similar to the cesarean-section and pharmacy utilization scenarios of Chapters 6 and 7 are enough to get a QI agenda in "through the back door" to daily work.

The key learning objectives are to:

- Distinguish between traditional quality assurance and continuous improvement;
- Apply concepts of *process*, *customer*, and *variation* to everyday work;
- Construct run charts and control charts to understand and improve their work processes; and
- Understand the danger of suboptimizing a process at the expense of the whole system.

To create an organizational common language, they need to be aware of the concepts in Appendix 9A. A leadership development course for potential department heads using Joiner's *Fourth Generation Management* as a text and taught by the chief medical officer and executives could be a powerful cultural signal.

## SUMMARY

When it comes to changing to the thinking required to transform to a QI mind-set, traditional models of organizational training and education have become obsolete. How does one teach "integrity," "listening skills," or "creativity," or measure, as a result of education, "level of caring and quality," which go deeper than being conceptually understood and practiced?

People must discover these *for themselves, within themselves* and break through to new levels of understanding. Unlike many opportunities in the past, education is no longer a simple replication process. QI demands that people look at their jobs through a new lens to motivate different actions on their part, and the delivery of the education will need to motivate the new desired belief system in participants.

In early QI efforts, many organizations used a parallel universe of project teams in addition to the everyday required work (and, in some cases, created yet another parallel universe of clinical improvement project teams), expecting that the activity, in addition to "spray and pray" in-house QI training, would yield unprecedented quality results. Unfortunately, time has shown this belief system to be naive.

Projects may be necessary, but they are not sufficient. Initially, keep them to a few, limited in scope, high level, and related to strategic issues on key $R_2$ results.

Besides the project activity, everyday use of data must transform through a common language of process-oriented thinking and use of process plots with the goal of reducing inappropriate and unintended variation. These are key concepts that *everyone* in the culture needs to learn, not just a chosen few or "belts" (á la Six Sigma).

Past issues of entrenched physician attitudes of individual accountability and "me, my, mine" can no longer be ignored, and integration of physicians into any QI effort remains a consequential and necessary task.

## APPENDIX 9A: KEY QUALITY IMPROVEMENT CONCEPTS NEEDED BY THE ENTIRE CULTURE TO CREATE A "UNIVERSAL IMPROVEMENT LANGUAGE"

### Part 1: Concepts

#### Processes and Systems

Thinking in terms of processes is perhaps the most profound change that comes with adopting a quality management approach.

- A *process* is a sequence of tasks directed at accomplishing a particular outcome.
- Better processes mean better quality, which means greater productivity.

Thinking in terms of processes allows us to:

- Focus on customers;
- Better understand our jobs;
- Define the starting and ending points of work under our control;
- Identify errors, waste, and other problems; and
- Figure out what data will help us improve the effectiveness of our processes.

If a series of related tasks can be called a process, a group of related processes can then be seen as a *system*. Selling a product or delivering a service, for example, are systems that involve thousands of interrelated processes. If a project team feels overwhelmed by its assignment, perhaps it is being asked to study a system, not a process.

Six sources of problems with a process are:
1. Inadequate knowledge of how a process does work;
2. Inadequate knowledge of how a process should work;
3. Errors and mistakes in executing the procedures;
4. Current practices that fail to recognize the need for preventive measures;
5. Unnecessary steps, inventory buffers (time), wasteful measures/data; and
6. Variation in inputs and outputs.

### Customers and Suppliers

Think about the processes you work with daily: The people or organizations whose output you receive are your suppliers, and those who use your product or service are customers. Suppliers inside your organization are referred to as *internal*; those outside your organization are referred to as *external*.

In the new view of organizations, you will start to see yourself as a customer of preceding workers, and start to identify your customers, the people to whom you pass on your work.

### Quality

Quality in the new business world has two aspects.
1. **Quality of target values and features: doing the right things.** Are you delighting customers? Are customers getting the products or services they need, precisely when and how they need them? *High quality* means choosing target features based on the needs, wants, and capabilities of intended customers.
2. **Quality of execution: doing things right.** How efficient are the processes used to design, manufacture, deliver, and provide maintenance for your products? How well do you plan and provide services to your customers?

### The 85/15 Rule

As discussed earlier in the chapter, systems as currently designed create the majority of problems. The initial tendency to blame individual workers for problems must stop. Front-line workers must recognize this as well and instead need to be taught to ask which system needs improvement, then seek out and find the true source of a problem.

Two good examples are related to purchasing: a production line worker cannot do a top-quality job when working with faulty tools or parts, and a surgical nurse cannot do a good job with gloves that do not fit. And there is a deeper issue that is often overlooked: even when it does appear that an individual is doing something wrong, often the trouble lies in how that worker was trained, which, if not consistent, is a system problem.

### Pareto Principle

The Pareto principle is sometimes called the 80/20 rule: 80 percent of the trouble comes from 20 percent of the problems. Though named for turn-of-the-century economist Vilfredo Pareto, it was Juran who applied the idea to management and advises us to concentrate on the "vital few" sources of problems and not be distracted by those of lesser importance.

### Teams and Teamwork

A single person using quality improvement practices can make a big difference in an organization. But rarely does a single person have enough knowledge or experience to understand everything that goes on in a process. Therefore, major gains in quality and productivity most often result from teams — a group of people pooling their skills, talents, and knowledge. With proper training, teams can often tackle complex and chronic problems and come up with effective, permanent solutions. Teams have another distinct advantage over solo efforts: the mutual support that arises between team members.

### Scientific Approach

A scientific approach is nothing more than a systematic way for individuals and teams to learn about processes. It means agreeing to make decisions based on data rather than hunches, to look for root causes of problems rather than react to superficial symptoms, to seek permanent solutions rather than rely on quick fixes. It means paying attention to *methods* of getting things done as well as results.

A scientific approach need not involve using sophisticated statistics, formulas, and experiments — in most cases, simple tools are all you need.

### Complexity

Many times the root causes of problems are buried deep in procedures and processes. They surface only as *complexity* that was generated in working around the problem. Complexity is a general term for unnecessary work — anything that makes a process more complicated without adding value to a product or service.

Complexity arises when people repeatedly try to improve a process without any systematic plan. They try to solve one piece by adding or rearranging steps, not realizing that they are distorting other parts of the process. As the problems resulting from the distortion start to surface, more and more steps are added to compensate.

Complexity is everywhere and often is the first type of problem that project teams identify. There are at least four sources of complexity:

1. Mistakes and defects;
2. Breakdowns and delays;
3. Inefficiencies; and
4. Variation.

Each of these factors causes rework: handling products more often than is necessary, fixing an existing product, redelivering a service.

### Variation

The three key ideas to remember about variation are:
1. **All processes have variation.** With all the factors that affect the output of a process — some of which we can control, others of which we cannot — it is inevitable that there will be differences in products or services.
2. **It is helpful to classify variation into two categories: common cause variation and special cause variation.** Common cause variation arises from the many

**EXHIBIT 9A.1** ■ The Fundamentals of Variation

1. Good data collection requires planning, which is equally as important as the data themselves.
   - The first question must be, "What is the objective?"
2. Good data analysis requires knowing how the data were collected or will be collected. The analysis must be appropriate for the method of collection.
   - Raw data say little.
   - Graphical methods are the first methods of choice.
   - Trend lines are generally worthless.
   - Bar graphs plotted over time have no meaning. (They are only appropriate for stratification and Pareto analysis.)
   - The proposed analysis should be clear before one piece of data is collected.
3. All data result from a measurement process.
   - Is the measurement process agreed on and reliable?
   - Have vague terms been operationally defined for data consistency?
   - Do the people actually collecting the data understand the data's purpose and the processes of how to measure and collect them?
4. Variation exists in all things, but may be hidden by:
   - Excessive round off of the measurement;
   - Excessive aggregation; and
   - Using "rolling" or "moving" averages.
5. All data occur as an output from some process and contain variation. This variation is caused and has sources that can be better identified through proper data collection.
6. There are sources of variation due to inputs to a process (people, methods, machines, materials, measurements, and environment) and variation in time of these individual inputs as well as their aggregate. Both are reflected in the output characteristic being measured.
7. All data occur in time.
   - Any process must first be assessed by plotting its performance in time order.
   - Neglect of the time element may lead to invalid statistical conclusions.
8. The stability (over time) of the process producing the data is of great importance for knowing how to take proper action or predict future performance.
9. Any source of variation can be classified as either a common cause or a special cause. It is important to distinguish one from the other to take appropriate action.
   - If something doesn't "go right," as in the occurrence of an undesirable incident, then that is also variation. Even though it "shouldn't" have happened, it could be due to either common or special cause. If it is common cause, root cause analysis (treating it as a special cause) will not be fruitful.
   - The presence of special causes of variation may invalidate the use of certain statistical techniques.
   - Any and all data analyses must be based in sound theory and help to interpret the observed variation meaningfully in terms of identifying common and special causes.
   - Any good analysis will motivate additional questions that can be investigated with further data collection.
10. There is variation (uncertainty) even when an object or situation is measured only once.

EXHIBIT 9A.2 ▪ Eight Common Statistical Traps

**Trap 1:  Treating all observed variation in a time series data sequence as special cause**

- The most common form of tampering — treating common cause as special cause.

  This is frequently seen in traditional monthly reports: month-to-month comparisons, year-over-year plotting and comparisons, variance reporting, comparisons to arbitrary numerical goals.

**Trap 2:  Fitting inappropriate "trend" lines to a time series data sequence**

- Another form of tampering — attributing a specific type of special cause (linear trend) to a set of data that:

  - Contains only common cause; or
  - Contains a different kind of special cause, usually, a "step" change(s) in the process average.

- Risk or severity adjustments of data through linear regression is a subtle manifestation of this trap.

**Trap 3:  Unnecessary obsession with and incorrect application of the normal distribution**

- Ignoring the time element in a data set and inappropriately applying enumerative techniques based on the normal distribution

  This can cause misleading estimates and inappropriate predictions of process outputs (aggregated averages, standard deviations, year-to-date summaries). This is a case of "reverse" tampering — treating special cause as if it is common cause.

*A data summary should not mislead the user into taking any action that the user would not take if the data were presented in a time series.*

- Inappropriate routine testing of all data sets for normality

- Misapplying normal distribution theory and enumerative calculations to binomial data (percentages based on ratios of occurrences of individual events relative to the number of possible opportunities), or Poisson distributed data (counts of events where the number of possibilities of occurrence are infinite), or Poisson counts turned into rates

**Trap 4:  Incorrect calculation of standard deviation and sigma limits**

- Grossly overestimating (inflating) the true standard deviation by using the "traditional" calculation taught in most courses

  - Because of this inflation, people tend to arbitrarily change decision limits to two (or even one) standard deviations from the average or "standard." The three standard deviations criterion with the correctly calculated value of sigma gives an overall statistical error risk of approximately 0.05.

  - The two best estimates of standard deviation for a given situation are obtained from the time sequence of the data:

    - The **median** moving range divided by 0.954, which is robust to outliers (i.e., the analysis is largely unaffected by outliers); or

    - The **average** moving range divided by 1.128, which is typically taught in control chart texts.

      - This estimate can be influenced by outlying observations and process shifts, but not to the extent of the "traditional" calculation.

      - If there are no special causes in the process, these two estimates, as well as the "traditional" calculation, will yield approximately the same number.

(Continues)

## EXHIBIT 9A.2 ■ (Continued)

**Trap 5: Choosing arbitrary cutoffs for performance considered "above" average or "below" average**

- Ignoring the "dead band" of common cause variation on either side of an average
  - The dead band is determined directly from the data. As a result, approximately half of a set of numbers will naturally be above (or below) average. The potential for tampering appears again — treating common cause as special cause.
  - Incorrect calculation of the standard deviation can inflate the estimate of the common cause variation and artificially widen the dead band.

**Trap 6: Misreading special cause signals on a control chart**

- Only searching for the special cause at the time period when the control chart gave an out-of-control signal
  - Just because an observation is outside the calculated three standard deviation limits does not guarantee that the special cause occurred then. It is extremely useful to do a runs analysis before construction of any control chart.

**Trap 7: Attempting to improve processes through the use of arbitrary numerical goals**

- Ignoring the natural, inherent capability of the process
  - Whether they are arbitrary or necessary for survival, goals are merely wishes and of no concern to your actual process. Data must be collected to assess a process's natural performance relative to any goal, that is, what it is "perfectly designed" to achieve. It is especially destructive when a goal lies within the common cause range of the natural process output, which results in nonproductive tampering.
  - The most prevalent form of tampering is interpreting common cause over time as special cause, either in a positive or negative sense, for individual deviations of process performance from the goal (Trap 1).
  - The other prevalent form of tampering results from failure to recognize the dead band of common cause around an average in a data summary (Trap 5). This leads to individual performances judged relative to being above or below an arbitrary goal as opposed to being "inside" or "outside" the process, particularly if the goal falls inside the dead band.
    This method has no recognition or assessment of capability, and people inside the system (common cause) can be arbitrarily and incorrectly identified as special causes, once again either in a positive or negative sense, or many times assigned a ranking, which is inappropriate — they are statistically indistinguishable both from the overall average and from each other.

**Trap 8: Using statistical techniques on a time sequence of "rolling" or "moving" averages**

- Another, hidden form of tampering — attributing special cause to a set of data that could contain only common cause.
  - The "rolling" average technique can create the appearance of special cause even when the individual data elements exhibit only common cause.

ever-present factors that affect a process continuously. Special cause variation, as its name implies, arises from factors that are not normally present in the process. From a practical standpoint, we care about the differences because there are different strategies for attacking these different sources of variation.

3. **Though we cannot eliminate variation entirely, we do have tools and methods to help us reduce it to a point where it no longer hinders our work.** The most common tools used to study variation are called *statistical control charts*. Control charts show a time plot of process measurements, along with two control limits that indicate the expected effects of common cause variation on the process. Control limits are calculated from measurements taken on the process.

*Process-Oriented Thinking*

Eliminate the four C's: confusion, conflict, complexity, and chaos.
- Do you ever waste time waiting, when you should not have to?
- Do you ever redo your work because something failed the first time?
- Do the procedures you use waste steps, duplicate efforts, or frustrate you through their unpredictability?
- Is information that you need ever lost?
- Does communication ever fail?

Why?

Improving quality = improving processes.

### Part 2: Everyday Data Skills — Process-Oriented Thinking in a Data Framework

As shown in Chapter 2, by integrating this philosophy into an organization, several sacred cows of data management will be challenged. In addition, inevitable errors will be inherent in a new, initially counterintuitive method of thinking. This is all part of the learning process (Exhibit 9A.1).

Organizations tend to exhibit wide gaps in knowledge regarding the proper use, display, and collection of data. These result in a natural tendency to either react to anecdotal data or "tamper" because of the current data systems in place. Exhibit 9A.2 is a summary of the most common errors in everyday data use, display, and collection as discussed in Chapters 2, 6, 7, and 8. Avoiding these will stop a lot of wasted meeting time.

## REFERENCES

1. Dauten, Dale. 2011. *The Corporate Curmudgeon: Farewell* (blog). http://blog.dauten.com/2011_05_01_archive.html.
2. Middleton, Robert. 2011. "The Thing That Bugs Me Most." *More Clients eZine* (blog) (May 31). http://actionplan.blogs.com/weblog/more_clients_ezine/page/2/.
3. Clemmer, Jim. 1992. *Firing on All Cylinders: The Service/Quality System for High-Powered Corporate Performance,* 167. Homewood, IL: Business One Irwin.
4. Scholtes, Peter. 1996. "Foreword." *The TEAM Handbook*, 2nd ed., v. Madison, WI: Joiner Associates.

5. Clemmer, Jim. n.d. "Why Most Training Fails." www.clemmergroup.com/articles/training-fails/.
6. Snee, Ronald D. 2009. "3.4 per Million: Digging the Holistic Approach: Rethinking Business Improvement to Boost Your Bottom Line." *Quality Progress* (October): 52–54.
7. Berwick, Donald M. 1992. "The Clinical Process and the Quality Process." *Quality Management in Health Care* 1 (1): 1–8.

## RESOURCES

American Society for Quality, Statistics Division. 2000. *Improving Performance through Statistical Thinking*. Milwaukee, WI: ASQ Quality Press.

This is an outstanding introduction to process-oriented thinking and written at a level where it could easily be used as an organizational text for internal seminars at all levels. It contains an excellent example of using statistical thinking to control a brittle diabetic's condition.

Balestracci Jr., Davis. 2008. "An Underrated Test for Run Charts: The Total Number of Runs Above and Below the Median Proves Revealing." *Quality Digest* (October). www.qualitydigest.com/magazine/2008/oct/department/underrated-test-run-charts.html.

Balestracci Jr., Davis. 2011. "From Davis Balestracci — What's Wrong with Our Data? Part 2: The Human Dimension." *Harmony Consulting, LLC Newsletter* (November 14). http://archive.aweber.com/davis_book/JhWMc/h/From_Davis_Balestracci_.htm.

This article demonstrates another way to lead a dialogue about data and offers powerful examples.

Balestracci Jr., Davis. 2012. "From Davis Balestracci — I am shocked…shocked…!" *Harmony Consulting, LLC Newsletter* (April 30). http://archive.aweber.com/davis_book/8VIWE/h/From_Davis_Balestracci_I_am.htm.

This article presents an interesting way to consider educating your organization after achieving critical mass.

Balestracci Jr., Davis. 2013. "Some Days, If We Couldn't Laugh, We'd Cry: Five-Minute Humor Therapy." *Quality Digest* (July 24). www.qualitydigest.com/inside/quality-insider-column/some-days-if-we-couldn-t-laugh-we-d-cry.html.

This article, offering Deming's "beatitudes," is intended to help you keep your sense of humor during transformation.

Carey, Raymond G. 2003. *Improving Healthcare with Control Charts: Basic and Advanced SPC Methods and Case Studies*. Milwaukee, WI: ASQ Quality Press.
Carey, Raymond G., and Robert C. Lloyd. 2001. *Measuring Quality Improvement in Healthcare: A Guide to Statistical Process Control Applications*. Milwaukee, WI: ASQ Quality Press.
Carnell, Mike. 2004. "Six Sigma Mambo." *Quality Progress* (January).
Carnell, Mike. 2008. "3.4 per Million: Forget Silver Bullets and Instant Pudding." *Quality Progress* (January).
Executive Learning. 2002. *Handbook for Improvement: A Reference Guide for Tools and Concepts*, 3rd ed. Brentwood, TN: Healthcare Management Directions.

This is a particularly outstanding resource that contains virtually every quality improvement tool you would consider using and all the examples are from healthcare.

Gregerman, Alan. 2007. "Unlocking Genius in Yourself and Your Organization." *Journal for Quality and Participation* (Summer): 9–13.
Hacquebord, Heero. 1994. "Health Care from the Perspective of a Patient: Theories for Improvement." *Quality Management in Health Care* 2 (2).

Hoerl, Roger, and Ronald Snee. 2002. *Statistical Thinking: Improving Business Performance*. Pacific Grove, CA: Duxbury.

This book provides a more in-depth look at statistical thinking, emphasizing improvement of business processes. It gives a sound improvement process framework, explains basic quality tools, describes some of the standard computer packages (Excel, Minitab, JMP), and offers clear, in-depth explanations of traditional basic statistics.

Joiner, Brian L. 1994. *Fourth Generation Management: The New Business Consciousness*. New York: McGraw-Hill.

Langley, Gerald J., Kevin M. Nolan, Clifford L. Norman, and Lloyd P. Provost. 2004. *The Improvement Guide: A Practical Approach to Enhancing Organizational Performance*, 2nd ed. San Francisco: Jossey-Bass.

Maccoby, Michael, Clifford L. Norman, C. Jane Norman, and Richard Margolies. 2013. *Transforming Health Care Leadership: A Systems Guide to Improve Patient Care, Decrease Costs, and Improve Population Health*. San Francisco: Jossey-Bass.

QI Macros. n.d. "Excelerating Lean Six Sigma." www.QIMacros.com.

QI Macros, a quality improvement statistical package, is the brainchild of Jay Arthur. He has designed a software package that acts as an Excel add-in (it works directly off one's *current* work sheet). I have tested his calculations, and they are correct (many of the less expensive packages, frankly, cannot be trusted). In addition, he provides good customer service and has a lot of information on the Website that puts the package in the context of an organizational quality improvement effort, especially Six Sigma. You can also download it free for 30 days.

Scholtes, Peter R., Brian L. Joiner, and Barbara J. Streibel. 2003. *The TEAM Handbook*, 3rd ed. Madison, WI: Joiner/Oriel.

Wheeler, Donald J. 1993. *Understanding Variation: The Key to Managing Chaos*. Knoxville, TN: SPC Press.

Wheeler, Donald J. 2003. *Making Sense of Data: SPC for the Service Sector*. Knoxville, TN: SPC Press.

Wheeler, Donald J. 2004. *The Six Sigma Practitioner's Guide to Data Analysis*. Knoxville, TN: SPC Press.Wheeler, Donald J., and Sheila R. Poling. 1998. *Building Continual Improvement: A Guide for Business*. Knoxville, TN: SPC Press.

Wheeler has been one of my virtual mentors over the years. His books have a refreshing practicality. Visit Wheeler's Website, SPC Press & Statistical Process Controls, Inc. www.spcpress.com.

## EDUCATING A CULTURE ON IMPROVEMENT

The following thread of eight newsletter articles (to be read sequentially) will shed light on the frustrations of educating a culture on improvement and suggest a possible design of educating a culture around the value of safety.

1. Balestracci Jr., Davis. 2011. "From Davis Balestracci — Back to the Basics through Another Lens." *Harmony Consulting, LLC Newsletter* (May 30). http://archive.aweber.com/davis_book/1X0_A/h/From_Davis_Balestracci_Back.htm.
2. Balestracci Jr., Davis. 2011. "From Davis Balestracci — 20 Years of Proof: The More Things Change, the More They Remain the Same." *Harmony Consulting, LLC Newsletter* (June 6). http://archive.aweber.com/davis_book/Mhag./h/From_Davis_Balestracci_20.htm.
3. Balestracci Jr., Davis. 2011. "From Davis Balestracci — New Results = New Conversations, Part 2." *Harmony Consulting, LLC Newsletter* (June 27). http://archive.aweber.com/davis_book/OtmdU/h/From_Davis_Balestracci_New.htm.

4. Balestracci Jr., Davis. 2011. "From Davis Balestracci — Quality: Everyone Doing His/Her Best?" *Harmony Consulting, LLC Newsletter* (July 25). http://archive.aweber.com/davis_book/ADapE/h/From_Davis_Balestracci_.htm.
5. Balestracci Jr., Davis. 2011. "From Davis Balestracci — Apply Plan-Do-Study-Act to Your Improvement Process?" *Harmony Consulting, LLC Newsletter* (August 8). http://archive.aweber.com/davis_book/IwALo/h/From_Davis_Balestracci_Apply.htm.
6. Balestracci Jr., Davis. 2011. "From Davis Balestracci — Continuing Your Journey to Getting the Respect You Deserve." *Harmony Consulting, LLC Newsletter* (August 22). http://archive.aweber.com/davis_book/LG_zo/h/From_Davis_Balestracci_.htm.
7. Balestracci Jr., Davis. 2011. "From Davis Balestracci — More Crazy Conversations…to Get You Respect." *Harmony Consulting, LLC Newsletter* (September 5). http://archive.aweber.com/davis_book/Dy4X2/h/From_Davis_Balestracci_More.htm.
8. Balestracci Jr., Davis. 2011. "From Davis Balestracci — Big Dots to Little Dots: Making Your Job Much More Interesting and Effective." *Harmony Consulting, LLC Newsletter* (October 17). http://archive.aweber.com/davis_book/ORAZM/h/From_Davis_Balestracci_Big.htm.

CHAPTER 10

# The Ins and Outs of Surveys: Understanding the Customer

**KEY IDEAS**

- Surveys are only one method of obtaining customer feedback and should not be used exclusively.
- Long surveys that collect a lot of vague information with no specific objective or proposed actions are relatively worthless.
- It's not "how we are doing" but understanding true customer needs that is important.
- Open-ended feedback is far more valuable for improvement and designing surveys to measure the effects of the subsequent improvement effort.
- Surveys are most useful for testing conclusions made in face-to-face interviews.
- Customers can only judge what they have received and may not know what they really want; they may even unintentionally lie to you.
- If you must do surveys, there is a robust 12-step process for designing and using them.
- Act on customer feedback!
- Customer satisfaction must evolve to customer involvement and integration into an organizational balanced scorecard.

## MORE THAN ONE METHOD FOR CUSTOMER FEEDBACK

It seems I can't turn around without someone in a store, hotel, or e-commerce merchant wanting to know how I judged their service or what it would take for me to buy their service. Most of the time, things are adequate. The transaction accomplished what I wanted — no more, no less. I don't have a strong opinion one way or the other, and I'm at a loss to tell them how to improve. I'm now at the point where I ignore most of them.

When a survey is planned, many questions are typically brainstormed about "how the customer might feel" (rank from 1 to 5) and "oh, yes, that would be nice to know too" (age, gender, day of the week born, favorite color, shoe size, etc.). They probe the customer experience from every imaginable angle. Although admirable, this approach usually results in a long, unwieldy, amorphous survey that generally gets a return rate of 5 to 30 percent.

The key to successful customer feedback is to ask about the few aspects of the customer experience that matter the most and *do something about them*. By asking about everything under the sun, you're establishing the expectation that you'll take action on everything, which is impossible. You are also telling your customer, "Your time isn't very valuable, so the imposition of this long and boring survey should be no problem for you." Focus on a few vital issues. The dilemma is that most organizations don't know what the few vital issues are.

Imagine you have the data in hand. What are you going to do with them? Remember, data are a basis for action: Vague data with vague objectives yield vague results. Are you committed to use what you learn, and how would you use it?

Generally, one's knowledge after a survey isn't useful and doesn't present any particular surprises (except perhaps, "We were rated 4.56 on this last time, but only 4.42 this time. What happened?"). It is also a waste of time to ask what you already know, especially if you are not going to do anything about it. This is not a useful customer focus. Instead the focus is on the score and meeting some arbitrary numerical goal. It also tends to bring out the "What happened? Who's to blame for this score?" mentality, or sometimes, the decision is to send it out again and see if the results are better; that is, a higher number.

Again, these comments refer primarily to mailed, written surveys or self-selected "Tell us how we're doing!" surveys answered independently, not those asked orally by an interviewer in person or over the phone. The assumptions of survey designers tend to differ from the answerer's understanding of what is being asked. It is hard to tell what those assumptions are and equally difficult to develop an unbiased, unambiguous question. People's responses to mailed surveys tend to reflect their current, transient reactions. One does not know how the customer may have felt in the past and is unable to probe for such important information. Generally the customers' comments that could be captured after answering a survey question would be far more interesting.

"Before-and-after" surveys merely represent two points in time. How does one explain the numerical difference? Do the differences mean anything? Are they due to common causes or special causes? Or is it just another case of insanity, doing what you've always done and expecting different results?

The people who designed the survey sometimes put their own (generally positive) spin on survey results to confirm their entrenched perceptions. If they don't like the results, they may send out another survey or blame the customer because "the customers don't know what they want anyway."

In fact, customers do know what they want. However, *it may not be what they need*. Customers often need education to learn their real needs. Heero Hacquebord lists education as his first principle for improvement of quality in healthcare: "Improving quality includes customer education, because the customer does not always know what he or she needs. The customer does, however, judge what he has received, and can only specify what he wants based on his past experiences, or what he has heard others experience."[1]

What should be done instead? Generally open-ended comments are more useful, especially when kept in the customer's language, and give insight into what the customer is actually thinking. Transforming organizations increasingly conduct face-to-face focus groups with both internal and external customers.

*Customer Focused Quality* (see Resources) by Mowery and colleagues provides some excellent guidelines for focus groups. It also contains a good summary of many methods for understanding customer needs (Exhibit 10.1). Can you think of any better way to

EXHIBIT 10.1 ■ Tools to Aid in Understanding Customer Needs

| Methods | Advantages | Disadvantages |
|---|---|---|
| Internal brainstorming | Multiple ideas from internal sources. Lots of ideas quickly. | Can be misled by the internal paradigms of your organization. |
| Casual comment cards | Collect large amounts of information from many customers in an unobtrusive way. | Can be somewhat difficult to administer. Workers may simply fail to listen or record casual comments if they do not see the effect they are having. |
| Interviews and focus groups | Allow for specific dialogue with customers. Facilitate completion of thoughts and clarification of meaning. | Require a considerable amount of the customer's time. Several interviews may be required to understand the attitude of "many" customers. Facilitators need to be skilled to avoid "group think" and domination by vocal participants. Surveys may be required to verify what is learned. |
| Friends' comments | Excellent source of honest opinions and ideas | Only provide one point of view. Must be supplemented with other information. |
| Observing other businesses with the same customer base | Allows you to pick up on ideas that may have been missed by others in your industry. Good source of innovation by understanding the need that is being addressed. | Not totally reliable. Needs to be supplemented by other methods. |
| Surveys | Collect comments and opinions from large numbers of people. Good for validation of ideas from other methods. | Responses are often superficial and polarized. Somewhat intrusive. No chance for dialogue and explanation. |
| Pilot studies | Provide a method to stop bad ideas before the customer is affected. Also provide a means to observe customer/product interaction | May prevent rapid deployment of new ideas. Require ideas be fundamentally complete before product study is done. |
| Mystery customer | Allow management to experience and evaluate service experiences from a customer's perspective. | Risks being used as a tool of fear. May also be subjective. |

Source: Neal Mowery, Patricia Reavis, and Sheila Poling. © Copyright 1994. *Customer Focused Quality*, 74–75. Knoxville, TN: SPC Press. © 1994. Used by permission of SPC Press. All rights reserved.

find out how your processes should work? Another good resource is Burchill and Brodie's *Voices into Choices* (see Resources).

One must ask questions, listen, and have the wisdom to probe deeper to understand the customers' real needs as opposed to what they may be superficially and literally asking for. Once again, focus on open-ended questions and record comments in the customers' language. If you want to grab your customers' attention, ask them what they like and don't like. It's that simple. Asking simple, open-ended questions of this sort enables customers to dictate the content of their feedback. You will hear what's important to them, and this is exactly the sort of feedback you want. Trends in open-ended feedback will inform you on the issues that customers care most about, something that many organizations don't understand.

Craig Cochran[2] has three favorite open-ended questions that he feels will quickly point the way to improvements that matter to your customers:

1. Do you have any problems with our products or services that you haven't told us about?
2. Is there anything you think we do particularly well?
3. What could we do in the future that would make your experiences with us easier?

Open-ended feedback doesn't help you make fancy charts, but do you really need more fancy charts to cover the walls of the conference room? No, you need improved customer satisfaction and loyalty. Open-ended feedback will reveal exactly what actions lead to long-term success.

Open-ended feedback follows the same rules as most traditional numerical data: It tends to clump into categories. Use an affinity process (see Brassard in Resources) to cluster the feedback into categories and themes and apply Pareto analysis to the results. Your opportunity areas will quickly emerge. Focus resulting surveys and action on these.

## A Cultural Expectation of Management?

In the case of hospitals, Quint Studer in *Hardwiring Excellence* (see Resources) advocates that executives and middle managers (coordinated with the appropriate supervisors) phone *every patient* (or family contact) at home on the day of discharge. This offers a chance not only to "make things right" but at the same time gather important information on how to improve the hospital experience for future patients, find consistent system issues, and possibly avoid a readmission for this patient and future patients.

How could a process like this not improve the patient's and family's experience? The information is also used to develop a scripted phone call on key issues, in other words, a standardized process whose purpose is deep organizational improvement and not just a marketing gimmick to let the customer know your organization cares.

## Act on the Feedback

Whatever you do, *act on your opportunities*. Action is the most critical step of the entire process. It starts with identifying trouble areas. Problems that are revealed through feedback must be addressed immediately. This is the business equivalent of triage: Stop the bleeding and stabilize the patient. Let's hope you won't discover too many issues that require this immediate first aid, but it is better to learn of these proactively while the customer is still your customer and not a former customer.

Surveys are best used to test the conclusions drawn from the data gathered face to face. Input these opportunities into your corrective and preventive action system and track them to completion. Treat every improvement action as a mini-project with assigned tasks, responsibilities, time frames, resources, and reviews.

You need to communicate widely. The final communication about your improvement will be to your customer: "Here's what we've done based on your feedback." These may be the most important words you ever say, and you don't have to use a traditional customer survey to say them.

Benchmark customer feedback tools with other organizations. There's no virtue in being original. Borrow good ideas and approaches as you see them. See what other people are doing and adapt the methods to your own needs.

If some of you struggle with this more proactive approach to getting customer feedback, the following sidebar may help you see the wisdom of knowing how to read between the lines and underscore why I've been insisting that anyone interested in quality improvement must have the wherewithal to keep learning relentlessly: *It's all about changing your belief system to view and understand issues through the "world of the solution."*

## TWELVE BASIC STEPS OF SURVEY DESIGN

As Craig Cochran put so succinctly, "If you like defusing explosives, you'll love creating surveys."[2] Here is an up-front summary of the problems with most surveys:[3]

- The wrong people are surveyed.
- The wrong questions are asked.
- The questions are asked the wrong way.
- The questions are asked at the wrong time.
- Satisfaction and dissatisfaction are assumed to be equally important.
- Those who did not buy or use the product/service are not surveyed.
- Surveys are conducted for the wrong reasons.
- The results are generalized to groups not surveyed.
- Surveys are used as a substitute for better methods.
- The results do not enable focused, direct improvement actions.

So how does one ask the right questions, in the right way, of the right people, and at the right time so one knows exactly what to change?

Quality surveys are built on two types of expertise: Your business process knowledge plus a survey specialist's technical knowledge. Survey planning can be completed quickly and without a lot of formality. Doing your homework will ensure the most useful survey results at the lowest cost. Survey goals and objectives are the key to the entire effort. Writing the questions is an important and visible element in your survey development.

You need to make 12 key decisions in three areas: establishing goals and objectives, constructing the survey instrument, and finalizing survey logistics.[4]

### Establishing Goals and Objectives

#### Step 1: Determine the Survey Purpose

Ask yourself what you will do with your newly acquired information and how it will be used. One of the worst outcomes is collecting information that is never acted on. Formalize your intent by completing the following phrases:

- I want to do a survey because…
- I intend to use the information I am seeking by…

## Why Your Customers Lie to You

In 1985 the Coca Cola Corporation spent gobs on the best marketing research money could buy and asked thousands of people their opinion. Armed with overwhelming statistics and clear answers from a huge number of people, they launched New Coke.

### $4,000,000 Down the Drain

Coca Cola spent $20 per person on 200,000 people in focus groups, testing, market surveys, and the blind taste test. And the results that came back were totally wrong.

The same thing will happen if you ask your customers "What do you want?" If you ask them if they prefer to meet on the phone or in person, or how much they are willing to pay, or what color they want, you'll get the same answer — the wrong one. They will cheerfully give you their best answers to what they want, just like the Coca Cola 200,000 did. And when you offer them what they said they wanted, they will turn their backs on it, leaving you in the dust. If you don't believe me, ask Coca Cola about the storm of public protest they had to contend with and the fact that a year later, New Coke held less than 3 percent of the market.

### Did 200,000 People Lie?

No, 200,000 people didn't lie. Each person gave the best answer he or she could, sipping at different unmarked cups of a cold cola beverage, blindfolded while paid consultants sat around with clipboards, measuring their response.

Asking questions of your customers is one of the absolute best ways to get clear guidance for your business. But don't ask them what they want. Because you and your customers live in different worlds. You've already traveled through the problem your business solves. Maybe you aren't yet enlightened, maybe you still struggle, but you understand the world of the solution, so to speak. Your customers, however, haven't gotten there yet. That's why they're coming to you.

You may ask me if I prefer a wool coat or one of those big, bulky ski jackets. And my preference is completely irrelevant if you're taking me up Mt. Everest. You know what I need, I don't.

So, if your customers have such excellent information and guidance for you, and yet they won't follow their own advice when you offer it back to them, how do you get clear, useful answers from them that you can implement in your business? The answer requires you to be a little more intimate. It also requires you to be stronger in the captaincy of your business.

### Keys to Questioning Your Customers

**Ask about problems, not solutions.**

Your business solves a problem. Your customers are familiar with that problem. So ask them about the problem. They don't know the solution yet. So don't ask them what the solution should look like. Because whatever answers they give you won't apply.

What are they struggling with? Where are they stuck? Where are they frustrated? What don't they like? What are they trying to accomplish? What would they like to be different? These questions are powerful for three reasons: (1) They create an empathetic connection because your customers are able to be heard in the midst of their frustrations. (2) They create more empathy in you as well, because you are reminded of what it was like before you got so good at what you do. And (3) the answers show where your customers have the biggest pain, struggle, or misfortune. If you have something that will help them with that and it works, they'll come get it. So ask and ask

(Continues)

> (Continued)
>
> and ask those questions about the problems. Get as much information as you can. Don't answer, don't fix. Just listen.
>
> **O Captain, My Captain**
> Armed with clear answers about the struggle, your job is to create and offer strong solutions that work. You are the expert in your business. People are coming to you for care, guidance, and help. They want to be able to trust you, to lean into your support and care. So be the captain of your ship and offer your customers what you know will help. Remember to first ask about the problem and then to take captaincy of the solution. Do that and your customers will never lie to you.
>
> Source: Adapted from Mark Silver. 2006. The *Business Heart eZine*. (December 20). Reprinted with permission.

- The information to be gathered will enable me to decide…
- I am prepared to implement change as a result of this survey because…

### Step 2: Identify End Users

Ask yourself who will use the results and how the information will be communicated. Define the survey audience by completing the following phrases:

- The users of the survey results include…
- The group(s) I will provide with information includes…
- They want the information so they can…
- The way(s) they like to receive information includes…

### Step 3: Identify Information Needs and Logistics

It is time to determine what specific information is needed and when you will need it. Identify every element of data that will be collected and its added value. Avoid the tendency to gather information that is merely interesting or might be good to know. To determine the criteria, you can ask yourself, "What will enable me to make decisions and take action?" Then complete the following phrases:

- The information I really need is…
- I need this information because…
- My top-priority information needs are…

Once you have prioritized your information needs, logistics about timing and frequency need to be considered through answering the following questions:

- How soon will I need information from this survey?
- How often does significant change occur in my process, my customers or their lives, or in the environment in which this process operates?
- How often do I need updated information to manage my process or program?
- How often do survey users need updated information?

The time period between surveys should be short enough to give you reliable information, but long enough that your customers will not feel bothered. This emphasizes the need for excellent data requirements, definitions, and database design because comparisons over

time can be tricky. Some questions to answer regarding data-tracking decisions include the following:
- How will we track performance over time?
- How will we provide staff access to survey data while protecting confidential information?
- What if our criteria requirements change over time?

### Step 4: Determine Resource Requirements
Ask yourself if you have the capability to deliver a survey that meets your overall expectations. The following questions will help you make decisions about resources:
- What is the value of the information I am seeking?
- What are the potential consequences on organizational resources of the decisions I will make based on this information?
- What is the cost of not having survey data?
- What staff and other resources are currently available?
- What staff and other outside resources do I need?

### Step 5: Determine Who Will Conduct the Survey
Should you use a neutral third party for credibility and candor? Whatever you decide, continue with the remaining seven steps, the next of which are concerned with constructing the survey instrument itself.

## Constructing the Survey Instrument
### Step 6: Determine Who Has the Needed Information
Whom should you consider surveying? In most cases, you will gather data from one or more subsets of the entire universe of people you can contact. You can make an intelligent choice of whom to survey, ensuring better accuracy and lower costs, by considering the following questions about your audience:
- Who has the information I need?
- Is my customer base composed of two or more discrete groups, or are all my customers fairly similar?
- Who decides whether to use my products or services?
- Do I have current addresses or phone numbers?
- Who is the key group(s) I need information from?
- Shall I randomly ssample from my entire customer base or survey only certain types of customers?

It is important to understand whom your sample represents to draw appropriate conclusions from the data. If you wish to generalize from the sample to the population it represents, the sample must be randomly selected. Random selection tends to ensure the most representative sample (and will probably generate the highest credibility among users), but is not necessary or desirable in every case.

Depending on your overall customer base or the decisions you are facing, you may want to concentrate your survey on a particular segment rather than a random selection of your entire customer base. This is especially true if your customer base is characterized by distinct segments rather than homogeneity. Applying the Pareto principle as a starting point, who are the 20 percent of your customers accounting for 80 percent of your interactions or sales?

### Step 7: Select an Appropriate Survey Type

The survey method you select depends largely on the time available, customer characteristics, the information you wish to obtain, and the costs you are willing to incur. Answering the following questions will help you make decisions about survey type:

- What format will get the needed information at the lowest cost and effort and within the time frame I need?
- How will limitations of survey types impact my ability to make key decisions?

*Written surveys* are the most commonly used because of their lower cost and labor requirements. This type of survey allows the customer more time to respond, but there is no opportunity to clarify intent. Because no interviewer is available to coach the respondent through the questions, it is important for questions to be ordered properly and for clear directions to be given. There are other considerations for written surveys. For example, surveys personally and courteously handed to customers during the service-delivery process have higher response rates. Surveys available for pickup at the service-delivery location are often only completed by customers who have had a very favorable or a very unfavorable experience. This, of course, creates a different type of bias.

In particular, mail surveys can suffer from low response rates. Ways to boost survey returns include:

- Reducing respondent barriers to survey return through such means as short surveys (faster to fill out) and postage-paid, preaddressed mailers (easier to mail).
- Using postcard or telephone reminders to follow up with respondents who have not returned their surveys.
- Providing incentives, such as gifts or chances to win prizes, for returning surveys.
- If an up-front random sample has been chosen, aggressively follow up with phone calls after the initial mailing and subsequent postcard reminder so that at least 80 percent of the chosen sample has ultimately responded.

*Face-to-face interviews* are often conducted to explore issues that are not easily understood and when information cannot be gathered from a written or telephone survey. Face-to-face interviews also allow the interviewer to assess nonverbal responses and ask follow-up questions. These interviews are often used to gain insight into customer needs and requirements as well as to determine which services are most important to them.

*Telephone surveys* consist of a series of questions and answers presented in strict sequence by a trained interviewer. The strength of telephone surveys lies in their interactive nature: Respondents can ask for clarification about the questions, and surveyors can quickly spot any problems with survey administration.

Telephone surveys provide the fastest turnaround and allow you to troubleshoot problems not detected in the pretest. Telephone surveys are best used when all segments of the survey population are known to have telephones and they should be conducted during the time of day when respondents will be available to talk, which may be after 5:00 p.m.

*Focus groups* are small-group conversations moderated by a neutral facilitator. They can provide valuable, in-depth, detailed reactions to new concepts and ideas. Questions tend to be open-ended. The results are largely qualitative and cannot be generalized to the entire population unless extreme care is taken when recruiting respondents. Try to avoid recruiting a group with diverse membership because the members then have little in common and it is much harder to get a sensible contribution from all participants. One use of focus groups is to provide a quick and fairly inexpensive way to identify the issues to be addressed in a subsequent mail-out or telephone survey.

*Key informant interviews* are face to face or by telephone with leaders in a field whose responses can be assumed to apply generally to others in that field. Open-ended or quantitative questions can be used.

### Step 8: Design the Survey Questions

Survey results will be meaningless unless you ask the right questions. Ideally they are based on the seven preceding steps and *anticipated analysis methods*. Consider the following when designing questions:

- How is this question relevant to the purpose of the survey?
- Is the question clearly worded?
- Will the question be easily understood by my customers?

The question must contain enough specifics so the respondent can give a meaningful answer. Compare, for example, the following two questions: "How would you rate our service?" and "How would you rate the timeliness of our computer-repair services?" Answers to the former will be difficult to act on, whereas answers to the latter tell you clearly what, if anything, needs to change.

### Types of Questions

Two types of questions are generally asked on written surveys — open-ended questions and closed-ended questions. Open-ended questions allow the customer to respond to a question in his or her own words. They can be a rich source of information, especially when you may not know all the possible answers that respondents might choose. However, you must consider how you will analyze the results of open-ended questions, for you will need a coding system to quantify open-question responses. An affinity process, putting each individual comment on a sticky note and clustering the morass of notes into themes (see Brassard in Resources), is also extremely useful.

Closed-ended questions offer the customer a choice of specific responses from which to select. Multiple choice, rating scale, and yes/no questions are examples of closed-ended questions.

The questions you ask your customers must be properly worded to achieve good end results. Try to begin all of your questions with how, what, when, where, why, or do. Avoid the following:

- Leading questions: They inject interviewer bias.
- Compound questions: They may generate a partial or nonresponse.
- Judging questions: They can lead to guarded or partial responses.
- Ambiguous or vague questions: They produce meaningless responses.
- Acronyms and jargon: These may be unknown to the respondent.
- Double negatives: They will create misunderstanding and are especially confusing to non-native English-speaking respondents.
- Long surveys: They discourage respondent participation.

### Step 9: Choose the Data Analysis Design and Reporting Format

As a final check on the instrument, build the tables and charts, and fill them with test data. Ask the question, "If these tables and charts are filled in, will I be able to perform my desired analysis and make the decisions I've planned?" Other useful questions to address include the following:

- What type of analysis will I need to perform? How simple or sophisticated should it be?
- Who will analyze the data? How long will it take?
- For automated analysis, what format must the survey results use?

You may need to iterate between steps 8 and 9 to ensure you will have the data needed to meet your survey needs.

## Finalizing Survey Logistics

### Step 10: Clarify the Sample Size and Selection

Sample size is driven by many factors, including the survey type you have chosen, the complexity and relative homogeneity of your target audience, and in some cases the margin of error you and your users are willing to tolerate in this survey. Answering the following questions will clarify your sample size:

- How many completed surveys do I need?
- How many people must be contacted to get the needed number of completed surveys?
- How will we reach them?

*Large samples are not necessary for many surveys.* A sample of 40 to 50 surveys is often quite adequate, and 100 suffice in most cases. At this point in the process you should consult a survey expert to ensure that your approach is well grounded.

You may need to iterate between steps 6 and 10 to ensure you are reaching the right number of desired respondents.

### Step 11: Decide Data-Entry Methods

Once survey data are collected, ensure that the data are accurately recorded so they are ready for analysis. Specific design tools are available to increase the ease and accuracy of data entry. You can consult a survey specialist for ideas. To help you make decisions about data entry, answer the following questions:

- Who will perform the data entry?
- How much time will it take?
- Will we use a spreadsheet program, a database program, or a survey-analysis software program?
- How will we ensure data quality and accuracy?

### Step 12: Pretest the Survey

Before distributing a survey to your customers, *always* pretest the survey. No matter how confident you are in the survey design, pretesting will help you to:

- Determine whether your instructions are understood;
- Identify questions that may be misunderstood or that are poorly worded;
- Determine whether rating scales are understood;

- Determine how long it will take your customers to complete the survey; and
- Determine the customers' overall level of interest in completing the survey.

One method to pretest your survey is through a pilot group process. Pilot group participants should be representative members of your survey's target audience. The pretest should be administered in person, with participants understanding their role.

You will want to look for questions not answered, several responses given for the same question, and comments written in the margins. All are signals that the question may not have been understood and may need revision.

You should conduct follow-up group discussions with your survey team to gain additional insight into your survey product's strengths and weaknesses and to identify suggested improvements.

## MORE ON SAMPLE SIZE

What is being discussed in this chapter is a totally different issue from the type of survey that is used to estimate a literal percentage in an opinion poll. In that case, there are statistical formulae to yield sample sizes in the context of needing to know the actual percentage today of recipients who will respond positively to this question within, say, plus or minus 5 percent with 95 percent confidence.

For the type of survey being described in this chapter, the issue isn't estimation, but information. So when people ask me what sample size they should use, I answer, "Enough," and tell them to use whatever will give them some degree of confidence in the result and an ongoing process to increase their degree of belief in the result.

Once issues are identified, smaller surveys can then be designed on specific issues to track progress on whether the actual measure of customer satisfaction is increasing. And once again, all you need is "enough." I would rather have 50 people surveyed monthly (or even 10–15 weekly) and plot the 12 monthly "dots" to track progress than 600 surveys received in December that are then compared to the 600 surveys received the previous December.

It's much better to randomly choose a sample of 50 every month and aggressively follow up to make sure at least 80 percent of them respond than, as in the case of the annual December survey, send out 2,000 hoping you will get 600 back (a biased sample) because that is the sample size some statistical formula gave you.

The issue with which to be concerned is moving the process average, not estimating it, which is very different from what is typically taught in formal statistics courses. The ongoing repeated small sample size will affect the variation limits seen in the control chart, but that isn't the concern — it's "moving the needle." If a major effort is being made to work on the issue, the progress will be visible regardless of the variation. The following is a good example of a typical well-meaning, but useless survey process.

## STOPLIGHT METRICS REVISITED

It has taken healthcare a while to see the wisdom of getting customer feedback. However, I see far too much emphasis on customer satisfaction scores obtained by a new *expensive* healthcare subindustry: organizations hired to routinely send out patient surveys and summarize them (using only the results from people who *choose* to fill out the surveys), meanwhile establishing benchmarks and judging an organization's performance vis-à-vis these benchmarks.

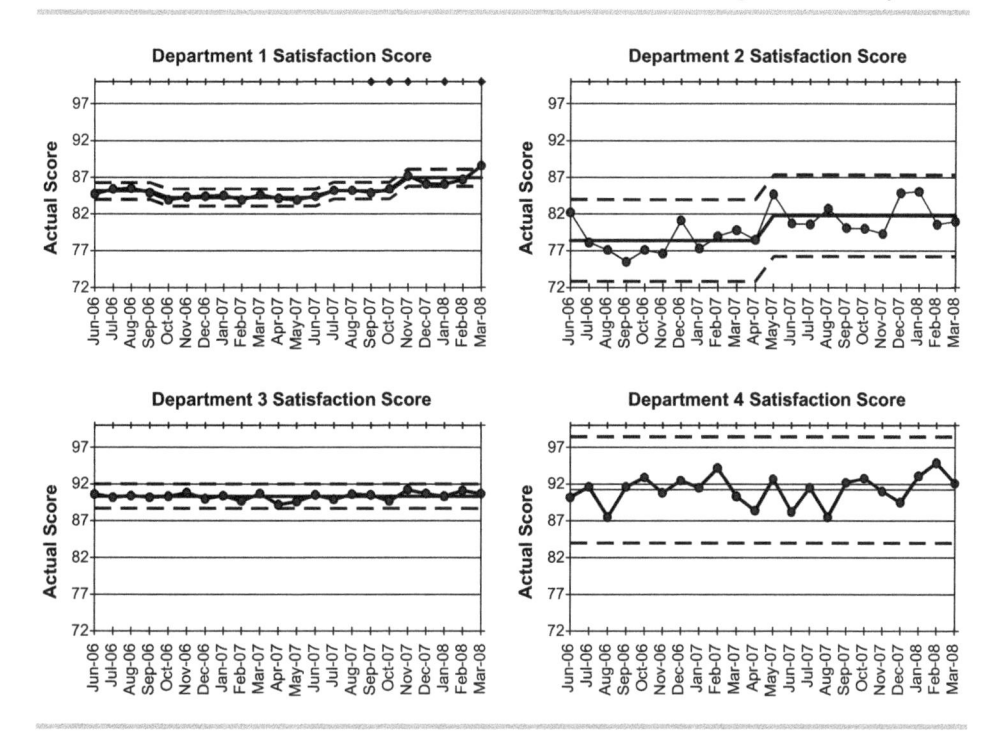

EXHIBIT 10.2 ■ Control Chart of Actual Satisfaction Score — Four-Department Comparison

I've heard of several instances of a disturbing process used for feedback: "Red," "yellow," and "green" arbitrary goals are set in terms of desired percentile performance, and it is measured weekly, at which time each department is visited by the executive team and receives a red, yellow, or green flag to post in their department.

The following is an actual scenario that summarizes customer satisfaction survey performance for four individual departments within a health system. No one had ever plotted the data like this before. The first set of graphs presented in Exhibit 10.2 shows the four control charts (on the same page and same scale) of the actual satisfaction score.

After some rocky initial performance, Department 1 improved over its initial scores, as did Department 2. Departments 3 and 4 are stable. It is also interesting to note the variation in common cause bands: plus or minus 1 for Department 1, plus or minus 5 for Department 2, plus or minus 1.5 for Department 3, and plus or minus 7 for Department 4.

Things get more interesting when the actual percentile performance (based on rankings for similar departments in the surveyor's benchmarking common database) is plotted and compared (Exhibit 10.3). Similar conclusions are made as those from using the actual scores.

Recently, there has been an increasing emphasis on percentile performance, and it is not unusual to have the red, yellow, and green goals all within the common cause. Now look at Department 4's control chart. I put them on the same scale, but I also knew that the range of numbers was restricted to 0 to 100 percent. I have no idea what Department 4's goals were, but this is a true lottery where they were changing nothing and getting a number between 0 and 100 percent.

In case you are intrigued, Exhibit 10.4 is the control chart with the actual limits calculated from the data, which are slightly wider than 0 to 100 (actually 60 ± 93).

**376** CHAPTER 10

**EXHIBIT 10.3** ■ Control Chart of Resulting Percentile Ranking — Four-Department Comparison

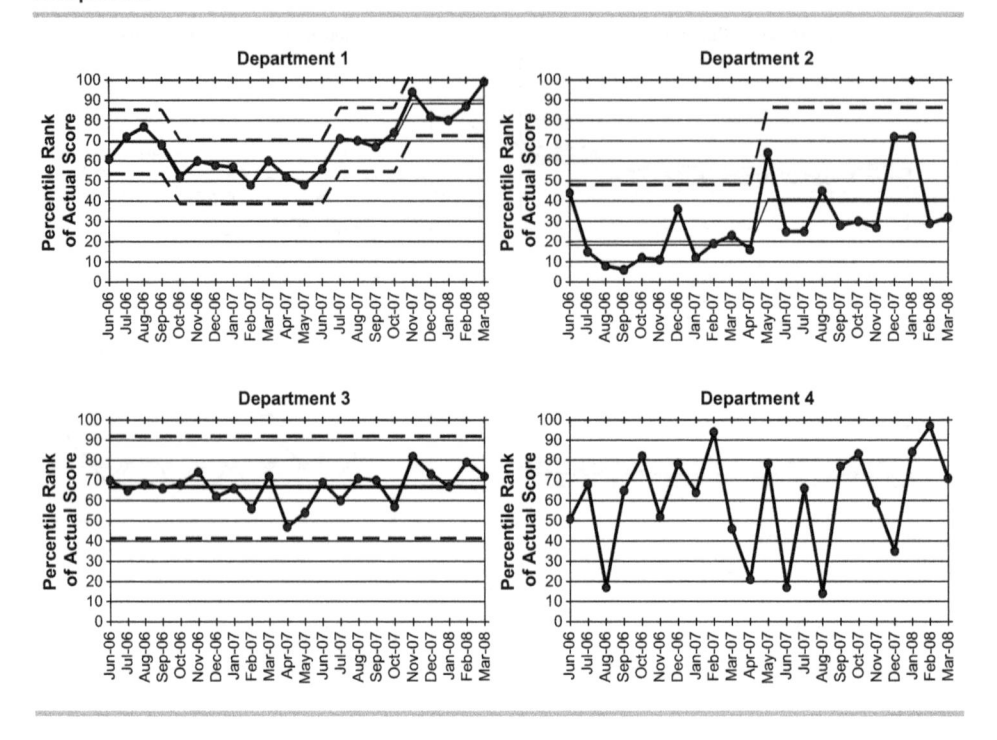

**EXHIBIT 10.4** ■ Can You Believe This?

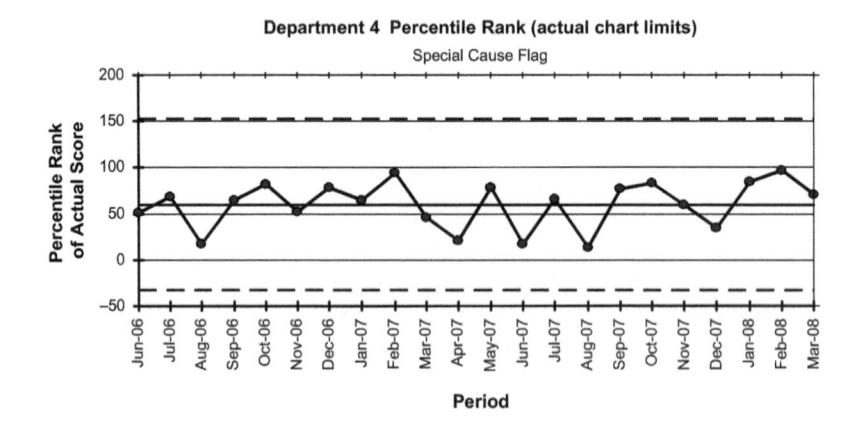

This is a perfect example of a point made repeatedly by W. Edwards Deming that statistics on performance by themselves do not improve performance. There was no formal organizational strategy to improve satisfaction other than the flag feedback process coupled with the exhortation of "Do better" when the result was yellow or red. And this leads to another point that Deming made often: A goal without a method is nonsense! It would be interesting to see what an employee satisfaction survey's results would be in this work culture.

## SUMMARY

*Surveys are an acceptable tool if what customers want is already known.* Sometimes organizations can learn more about their customers in a 90-minute focus group or a 15-minute interview than they will ever find out in a decade of surveys. The right time to survey is after determining what customers want, designing the product or service to meet those expectations, and determining that what the customers got is what they wanted.

Surveys need to be designed to allow you to make intelligent decisions about what needs to be improved. Good survey questions provide four answers:

1. What was expected or wanted;
2. What was experienced;
3. The level of satisfaction with the product or experience; and
4. The degree of relative importance of this variable.

Customer satisfaction is neither objective nor easily or accurately measured. It is also not quickly or easily changed. It takes time for an attitude shift. Because of the high inertia factor inherent in changing human perception, many customer satisfaction survey efforts, as currently practiced, can only be a lagging indicator, not a leading or current one. To put it differently, customer satisfaction surveys are not early warning systems. If you cannot take action on customer perceptions within a few weeks of the perceptions being formed, there's a strong chance that you will lose your window of opportunity or even the customer.

The solution is to focus customer satisfaction efforts on the detailed input that comes from focus groups, customer visits, customer complaints, and so on, addressing issues when they arise, rather than waiting until overall satisfaction measures are affected.

### Beyond Customer Satisfaction to Customer Involvement[5]

Beware of wanting to measure customer satisfaction without making customer input and involvement a fundamental part of your business. Without such a customer orientation, measuring satisfaction is pointless. Even if the numbers are valid, they aren't actionable because they give no clue as to why customers are satisfied or not and what might be done to improve things.

### Step 1: Identify Your Customers

This falls into two parts: finding out who the customers are (as opposed to who they are assumed to be) and deciding who the customers should be. The first part involves examining company databases for customer information, polling sales and field personnel, and actual customer visits. The second part involves discussion among the senior leadership team, perhaps in conjunction with board members or outside analysts and consultants, about where the company sees itself heading. The company may want to strengthen its position in a particular market or move into new markets. Different goals involve different customers.

### Step 2: Talk to Customers

As repeatedly emphasized, you need to talk to customers to identify major issues in satisfaction and dissatisfaction. There is no substitute.

### Step 3: Ascertain Issues

You must find out how widespread the issues are. In-depth methods have a lot of time and expense involved, and as a result they can only be carried out on a fraction of the customer base. This risks mistaking the issues of a minority for those of the customer base as a whole. *Surveys are most effective when used in this role*, because they contain precise, actionable questions rather than vague, unactionable ones.

Even when improvements are made, the proof is in the customers' reactions to them. Steps 2 and 3 need to be repeated, this time paying special attention to whether customers' issues and attitudes have changed. Sometimes it is best to simply collect input and look for a positive change. Often it is useful to ask customers directly if they have noticed any changes, and if so, what they think of them. Again, in-depth interviews followed by broad surveys are the most efficient means of getting the information.

## Satisfaction and the Scorecard

Your organization must institutionalize the measurement of customer satisfaction into its daily fabric. Difficult as it is, this is not a one-time process. A true commitment to continuous improvement means that it will be necessary to keep the flow of customer information coming in. Only when this information flow is firmly established does it make sense to consider a companywide summary measure of customer satisfaction reportable at the board level. For the reasons mentioned previously, such a measure should be a set of metrics capturing different aspects of satisfaction, for example:[5]

- Percentage of highly satisfied customers;
- Percentage of highly dissatisfied customers;
- Cost of dissatisfied customers;
- Levels of expectation;
- Perceived value for the money; and
- Brand loyalty.

Customer satisfaction is a subtle, complex attitude shaped gradually by repeated experiences with a company's products and services. The most direct effect on it comes when a company involves the customer at all levels of operations, and it is that process of involvement that drives customer satisfaction. But remember that quality cannot be surveyed into a product or service. As you consider solutions based in quality improvement theory, take the steps to build quality into products and services from the beginning through integrating customer feedback. Heed the warning from the title of one of my favorite survey articles: "Are Your Surveys Only Suitable for Wrapping Fish?"[3]

## REFERENCES

1. Hacquebord, Heero. 1994. "Health Care from the Perspective of a Patient: Theories for Improvement." *Quality Management in Health Care* 2 (2): 70.
2. Cochran, Craig. 2006. "Don't Survey Your Customers!" *Quality Digest* (September).
3. Miller, Ken. 1998. "Are Your Surveys Only Suitable for Wrapping Fish?" *Quality Progress* (December): 51.
4. Zimmerman, Richard E., Linda Steinmann, and Vince Schueler. 1996. "Designing Customer Surveys That Work." *Quality Digest* (October).
5. Rosenberg, Jarrett. 1996. "Five Myths about Customer Satisfaction." *Quality Progress* (December): 57–60.

## RESOURCES

Brassard, Michael. 1996. *The Memory Jogger Plus+*. Methuen, MA: GOAL/QPC.
Burchill, Gary, and Christina Hepner Brodie. 1997. *Voices into Choices: Acting on the Voice of the Customer*. Madison, WI: Joiner Associates.
Carnell, Mike. 2003. "Frontiers of Quality: Gathering Customer Feedback." *Quality Progress* (January).
Cochran, Craig. 2006. "Don't Survey Your Customers!" *Quality Digest* (September). www.qualitydigest.com/sept06/articles/06_article.shtml.
Miller, Ken. 1998. "Are Your Surveys Only Suitable for Wrapping Fish?" *Quality Progress* (December): 47–51.
Mowery, Neal, Patricia Reavis, and Sheila Poling. 1993. *Customer Focused Quality*. Knoxville, TN: SPC Press.
Rosenberg, Jarrett. 1996. "Five Myths about Customer Satisfaction." *Quality Progress* (December): 57–60.
Studer, Quint. 2003. *Hardwiring Excellence*. Gulf Breeze, FL: Fire Starter Publishing.
Zimmerman, Richard E., Linda Steinmann, and Vince Schueler. 1996. "Designing Customer Surveys That Work." *Quality Digest* (October). www.qualitydigest.com/oct96/surveys.html.

AFTERWORD

# Just Between Us Change Agents

As I discussed in Chapter 3, the inherent frustration of the change agent role exposes you to the constant danger of being infected with the "victimitis virus," as shown by the following behaviors:

- Treading lightly around certain issues or avoiding them altogether;
- Not feeling free to suggest specific solutions;
- Trying many different solutions without any of them working;
- Complaining bitterly but unable to take action;
- Seeing new options as too complicated to implement;
- Always hoping things will change and get better; and
- Feeling like you are between a rock and a hard place.

Victim behavior can be seen as an occupational hazard of being a change agent. Unfortunately, in the organizational culture, everyone but the change agent has the luxury of exhibiting these victim behaviors. In fact, any public exhibitions of these types of behaviors by change agents will act as a deterrent to organizational transformation. Those darn humans will agree with your frustration and then promptly lose respect for your change-agent role. Your own victim behavior has just supplied them with a convenient excuse for not changing.

The caution, however, is against *public* exhibitions of victim behavior. That does not mean you don't have the right to, collegially and behind closed doors, vent inevitable frustrations with colleagues, accept the frustrations for what they are, depersonalize them, and then take a deep breath and get on with dealing with them effectively.

See the truth in your situation. Own your results even when they are undesirable. Use the past to learn, not justify, and do whatever it takes to move forward. Do this all without judgment, facilitating this same process with workgroups to own their circumstances and results. It is tempting to confuse activity (number of teams and projects, number of courses taught, number of people trained) with impact. Remember that you are the learning and growth sub-business of your organization and you need to take charge of making quality improvement the strategy for having the organization attain its results. Your behavior also needs to telegraph clearly to the culture that you are committed to clear organizational $R_2$ results.

Some sobering questions quality professionals may need to ask themselves regarding their work cultures when faced with yet another frustrating situation include:

- What can I control, and what can't I control in this situation?
- Have I been wasting time or energy on things I can't control or influence? Am I blaming the person and not the process?
- What are my perceived barriers to results? Are they necessarily real?
- What am I pretending not to know about my accountability in this situation?
- Where are the areas of joint accountability that may lead to the ball getting dropped? What can I do so that won't happen?
- Have I confronted the things or people that need confronting in a depersonalized manner? Have I allowed whining, including my own, to go unchallenged? Have I held myself accountable for holding myself accountable?
- Have I held myself accountable for appropriately holding other people accountable? Have I offered appropriate peer coaching in the moment related to behaviors seen as neither committed to organizational success nor stated cultural values (personal success)? Have I let the people have the lion's share of the credit for any successes I facilitate?

## A BELIEF SYSTEM FOR CHANGE AGENTS

The job of a quality professional or change agent is inherently frustrating. Quality professionals are generally underappreciated and they often find themselves in no-win situations. The quality professional's job title should probably be changed to "corporate piñata."

During transitions such as what healthcare is currently experiencing, quality professionals need a belief system to help balance their needs and create a much-needed inner peace to handle it all. When you feel the frustration of being a change agent, remind yourself that people don't dislike change for other people, but they dislike being changed themselves and everyone is doing the best they can.

In assessing the current state of your organizational quality role, here is an additional tough question to ask yourself: "How can current in-house education be redesigned and delivered to create an appropriate activating event to obtain the needed changes in people's, the organization's, and if necessary, my own beliefs, to drive the desired consequential behaviors to produce $R_2$ organizational results?"

## 10 COMMANDMENTS

Now that you have made it through the book, I hereby ordain you as a deacon of the church of those darn humans. The following is a list of commandments I created, but remember the most important one is to bless us darn humans:

1. Thou shalt love thy neighbor and realize that we are all just plain folks.
2. Thou shalt have no more than 10 percent jerk time, keep it behind closed doors, and ask thyself what else it will it take.
3. Thou shalt learn from thy jerk time, especially if thy neighbor feeds back to thee appropriately, and thank thy neighbor for any feedback.
4. Thou shalt attack thy neighbor's behavior, not thy neighbor.
5. Thou shalt sincerely commit to thy organization's success and thy neighbor's success.
6. Thou shalt commit to surrendering to the fact that thou can only change thyself.

7. Thou shalt realize that quality may be very interesting to thee, but that thy neighbor's job takes up 100 percent of their time.
8. Thou shalt not personalize thy neighbor's jerk time.
9. Thou shalt love jerks but make them accountable for their behavior.
10. Thou shalt swallow thy ego a dozen times before breakfast and another dozen times before lunch and resist any urge to blame or whine publicly.

## THE PARADOXICAL COMMANDMENTS

I discovered The Paradoxical Commandments (see sidebar) almost 10 years ago. As I've said in understanding resistance, without emotion, there is no investment. It could be so easy in our jobs to take personally the stated reasons people throw at us, become cynical and harden our hearts; but this would also neutralize our passion and we would lose all feeling — the joy as well as the sorrow. Trust me, it's not just about quality improvement.

---

### The Paradoxical Commandments

People are illogical, unreasonable, and self-centered.
*Love them anyway.*

If you do good, people will accuse you of selfish ulterior motives.
*Do good anyway.*

If you are successful, you will win false friends and true enemies.
*Succeed anyway.*

The good you do today will be forgotten tomorrow.
*Do good anyway.*

Honesty and frankness make you vulnerable.
*Be honest and frank anyway.*

The biggest men and women with the biggest ideas can be shot down by the smallest men and women with the smallest minds.
*Think big anyway.*

People favor underdogs but follow only top dogs.
*Fight for a few underdogs anyway.*

What you spend years building may be destroyed overnight.
*Build anyway.*

People really need help but may attack you if you do help them.
*Help people anyway.*

Give the world the best you have and you'll get kicked in the teeth.
*Give the world the best you have anyway.*

© 1968, renewed 2001, by Kent M. Keith.

APPENDIX

# The Physician's World

## KEY IDEAS

- Quality assurance traditionally collects data to identify perceived individual negative variation and to correct outliers.
- Quality improvement collects data to expose process variation, discuss it, and reduce that which is *unintended* and *inappropriate*.
- The statistical framework needed for quality improvement (analytic) is generally not taught as part of medical education.
- Clinical trials are a specialized subset of quality improvement.
- After a significant clinical result is obtained in a formal trial, it is put into an environment where variation is minimally controlled, especially the human variation of applying the result.
- The enumerative statistical framework of clinical trials is inappropriate in an everyday practice environment.

No one is against quality. Yet the word *quality* can bring to mind negative associations from experiences with monitoring programs such as quality assurance (QA) and compliance audits, motivation programs, or managed care standards. When these perceptions of quality are considered in conjunction with *statistics*, another word often associated with negative academic experiences, it is not surprising that the current emphasis on quality improvement (QI) is perceived as a passing fad.

## QUALITY ASSURANCE VS. QUALITY IMPROVEMENT

Quality measurement and improvement have been part of practice activities for years through QA departments, peer review, and so on. However, QA and QI differ in their approaches and the contexts in which they operate.

The key distinction is process-oriented thinking (QI) vs. results-oriented thinking (QA). Typically, QA is a peer-review process that concentrates solely on observed outcomes and uses traditional statistical analysis of these results to identify alleged nonconforming outliers. QA's goal is to maintain a current standard of medical performance by sorting so-called bad performers from good. In this context, improvement takes place by revising individual performances to meet the standards set by external organizations.

QI takes a more fundamental approach: Healthcare is a *process* that leads to an output. QI acknowledges that results vary, but considers variation to be mainly the result of process breakdowns or unwitting lack of knowledge rather than outright failures (incompetence) by individuals. Attributing blame or sorting out poor performers is not the focus. QI looks closely at data from the processes to identify significant undesirable sources of variation and prevent similar occurrences. Improvement comes not only from outside research approved by external organizations. It also comes from finding hidden improvement opportunities (positive variation) in current work processes and the development of robust practices.

Exhibit A.1 uses traditional statistical normal (bell-shaped) curves to illustrate the contrast between QA and QI. The area under the curves represents the range of results. The QA "before" curve shows a distribution of results obtained, both good and bad. A predetermined number, commonly 1 to 5 percent, is identified as the significant outliers. Attention is focused on the outliers, and those seen as responsible are told to correct the outlying behavior.

Making this correction is not so simple, especially where human psychology is involved. It's not as easy as saying, "If they can do it, you can do it. Let's have results instead of alibis." To motivate true change, people will require an answer to their natural question, "What should I specifically do differently from what I'm doing now?"

There also seems to be a universal sequence of reactions by physicians when faced with QA data that suggest a change in practice (the first three are stated reasons as explained in Chapter 3):

1. "The data are wrong."
2. "The data are right, but it's not a problem."
3. "The data are right, it's a problem, but it's not *my* problem."
4. "The data are right, it's a problem, and it's my problem."

As shown in the "after" curve (see Exhibit A.1), the action attempts to chop off the left end of the distribution. At best, this leads to only a small increase in overall average

**EXHIBIT A.1** ▪ Quality Assurance vs. Quality Improvement: Traditional Statistical Normal Curves

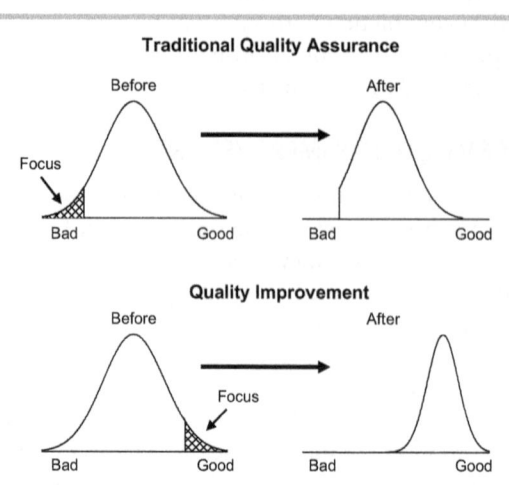

*Note:* Traditional QA focuses on removing the poor performers, while QI focuses on the top performers to improve the work of all employees.

quality. This seemingly arbitrary selection and judgment is usually not based in sound statistical theory but on the poor and inappropriate application of techniques learned in most required statistical courses. Although such analyses are well-intended, many become lotteries as has been demonstrated with examples throughout this book.

This QA mind-set has created a somewhat ingrained climate of defensiveness and lack of cooperation, particularly among physicians. The potential of the high achievers to influence the other processes generally is not recognized and therefore lost.

In QI the focus shifts from the negative end of performance to the other, positive performance end of the curve. QI identifies the 1 to 5 percent of people who consistently achieve superior results, including those who may not realize they are even doing so. This identification is often referred to as *best practices* or *benchmarking*. Thus QI's shift in focus can identify practices from which all can learn and benefit, resulting in not only higher, but also *more consistent* quality.

What about those who truly may be poor performers? These persons are still identifiable with QI. They sort themselves out if and when they do not cooperate in the improvement implementation.

QA certainly has a role in QI. However, its energies are redirected to a positive application rather than the outlier or "bad apple" mentality. QA's purpose changes to one of expanding and providing the underlying measurement system used to monitor process performance. Data from the QA system currently used to rank people or departments can be used either to make immediate adjustments to the process or identify QI opportunities.

The role of statistics also changes between the two contexts. In QI, statistical thinking becomes more important than statistical tools. Instead of being a set of tools for analyzing results, statistical thinking becomes an umbrella to encompass the entire improvement process.

In summary, there are two quality dimensions in healthcare. The first is the quality of the healthcare outcomes themselves (the traditional focus of QA). However, QI adds a second aspect: the study of process quality. Processes must work together as a system to deliver care. QI results are also measured in terms of customer needs and experiences. Examples of customer needs include good quality diagnosis, access, and treatment processes as well as operational and financial services such as medical record transportation, dictation, and patient billing. Exhibit A.2 is a comparison of the two facets.

Significant improvement opportunities arise because quality fails when any one of these processes fails, even in the case of excellent outcomes. For example, a practice's excellent clinical results can be negated by poor processes that cause significant delays, unnecessary visits, or poor communication that causes unnecessary duplication. When examined in this context, traditional healthcare delivery and its management can be seen as two virtually parallel processes whose independence has created much waste and inefficiency.

The core business of medical practice is to deliver healthcare to customers and to meet obligations to insurance payers and the overall community. The entire system must be studied and optimized as a whole instead of separating healthcare delivery and healthcare management. This separation unwittingly optimizes separate processes to meet separate specific goals while the organization and its customers suffer.

A primary benefit of using QI is the potential for discovering waste in a process. Variation creates waste, such as work done more than once with no value added or a process involving more steps or staff than are required to meet customer needs. By focusing

EXHIBIT A.2 ■ Comparison of Peer Review (Quality Assurance) and Quality Improvement

| Characteristic | Peer Review (Quality Assurance) | Quality Improvement |
|---|---|---|
| Object of study | Physicians | Processes |
| Types of flaws studied | Special | Common and special |
| Goal | Control | Breakthrough |
| Performance referent | Standard | Capability/need |
| Source of knowledge | Peers | All |
| Review method | Summative (enumerative) | Analytic |
| Functions involved | Few | Many |
| Amount of activity | Some | Lots |
| Linkage of design, operations, and business plan | Loose | Tight |
| Tampering | Common | Rare |

on the whole spectrum of variation rather than simply the negative end, inefficiencies can be found in processes throughout the system. Waste reduction, of course, equals improved resource allocation, with time, energy, and money used more appropriately.

## DEMING AND JURAN

W. Edwards Deming and Joseph Juran are considered the two primary quality giants of the 20th century. They provided the two predominant quality philosophies or offshoots followed by most organizations that implement the QI model. The late Deming was an American statistician who became an internationally known consultant. He originally established modern sampling methods for the U.S. Census and served as an advisor to the Japanese census in post–World War II Japan.

During that time, he also took part in the education of Japanese scientists and engineers on methods of quality control. Although unsuccessful with similar quality training efforts in post-war America, he found a willing audience in Japan. Japan's subsequent QI successes are well known.

Transformation is fundamental to Deming's approach. He emphasized application to management practices as well as the structure of management and work processes. Their alignment is crucial and must be accomplished via a well-understood, broadly communicated strategy grounded in the synergistic interaction of four elements: (1) appreciation of a system, (2) psychology of intrinsic motivation, (3) understanding of variation, and (4) use of planned data collection to test improvement theories.

Another American, the late Juran, also took part in post-war Japanese industrial education. Juran was an electrical engineer who also obtained a law degree and established the Juran Institute, an internationally known quality consulting corporation. Juran's approach was heavily based in projects, planning, tools, and implementation that minimize disruption to current structures.

In deference to an organization's existing management structure, the Juran approach adds additional structure and a relatively formal approach to identifying, solving, and implementing improvement efforts. It is an empirically derived strategy developed from judicious, keen observation of work cultures.

## CLINICAL TRIALS VS. QUALITY IMPROVEMENT

Many physicians will argue that the process-oriented approach of QI is invalid because it doesn't follow established procedures of rigorous double-blind clinical research. I have heard this, and you have no doubt heard this (see Chapter 3 for the discussion on stated reasons). My response is generally, "You're right, doctor. Nor could it be, nor should it be." Let's look at *research as a process* and this includes clinical trials.

In research, all input variations are *tightly controlled* such that observed differences in the intentionally varied control and treatment groups can be attributed to the methods input of the clinical trial process and no other. In addition, a formal part of the process is writing an excruciatingly detailed protocol to ensure the following:

- There is a clearly designed overall trial objective that frames appropriate operational definitions for data elements.
- Standard statistical research techniques will be used for analysis, resulting in clear collection, analysis, and interpretation data processes.
- For multiple clinical centers (clinical trial process "environment" input), common data forms are developed with the operational definitions clearly spelled out to reduce inappropriate and unintended data bias.
- *These previous three issues are all defined before one patient is randomized.*
- If needed, an occasional data process audit may be conducted to determine whether inappropriate and unintended biases have crept in.
- Appropriate patients are randomized into the trial. The patient-to-patient variation cannot overshadow any proposed benefit of the treatment. In this way the clinical trial process "people" input is tightly controlled.
- The requirements of the "machines" and "materials" inputs are specifically spelled out.

Proactively controlling all of this variation is inherent in the process and expensive; thus clinical trial research is expensive.

Research statistics is actually a specialized subset of process-oriented statistics. Research makes the assumption that it is possible to sample from an underlying infinite population to estimate its underlying truth, which should then be universally applicable. By inherently forcing variation to be controlled, it has the luxury of ignoring the everyday factors lurking to compromise results in busy, uncontrolled practice environments.

Methods unique to research are based on the assumption of an underlying population being estimated. This is the context generally taught in most required introductory statistics courses. The naive assumption is that one can continuously sample from a stable population to estimate parameters. Good research inherently creates such a stable process where this is temporarily possible. But what changes in the transition from a research environment to an everyday environment?

After a significant result is published, researchers lose control over how clinicians use it. This is called the *inference gap*, defined and explained in Chapter 6. To complicate matters further, the result resembles the process of Exhibit 1.1 (see Chapter 1), where there is rampant variation of all kinds waiting to exert their influences above and beyond the clinical considerations.

There will be variation in how people interpret and apply the result as well as lack of rigor in how data are collected to evaluate it. This human variation virtually guarantees that they won't necessarily achieve the same results as reported. This variation could be present in any or all of the six inputs of five processes (the clinical process as well as the data measurement, collection, analysis, and interpretation processes). Any casually collected data will be hopelessly contaminated with these sources of variation.

In understanding any variation gap between the research results and actual results, it becomes necessary *to expose the variation* between individual use and the research use of the protocol and reduce any inappropriate and unintended variation. The presence of this lurking variation and the process of exposing it for all intents and purposes invalidate most standard statistical methods.

## ENUMERATIVE STATISTICS VS. ANALYTIC STATISTICS

There are actually three kinds of statistics, and one way to summarize them in a healthcare environment is as follows:

1. Descriptive: "What can I say about this *individual* patient?"
2. Enumerative: "What can I say about this *specific group* of patients?"
3. Analytic: "What can I say about the *process* that produced both this particular group of patients and its results?"

An *enumerative study* always focuses on the *actual state* of something *at one point in the past*. For example, one can literally summarize the results of all the participants in any clinical trial once it is completed, and because of the way the sample is chosen, consider these patients a random sample of the patients *who were potentially available*. An *analytic study* usually focuses on *predicting the results* of action *in the future*, in circumstances we cannot fully know. *It is this predictive way of thinking that is fundamental to QI.*

However, the process under consideration is different in the clinical trial vis-à-vis the everyday environment. The clinical trial process is concerned only with the effect of the treatment and needs to produce a relatively consistent group of patients. The rigor of the protocol ensures a stable group of patients who can be treated in an enumerative fashion via estimation. We want the process that produced the result in this group of patients to reflect variation only caused by the presence of the treatment. In the context of the future, *at this time*, we want assurance that any group of patients chosen by the same protocol would be similar.

### The Problem in an Everyday Clinical Environment

Once the treatment has been declared to be beneficial and released, it is only part of the subsequent process, which is the daily reality of a practicing physician's everyday process. The diagnosis process *and its interaction with the application process, which includes treatment, is what is producing the result in this group of patients* on whom data is subsequently collected. If there are problems with clinical outcomes, it is the variation in both of these processes that must be exposed, *not* ignored. And it is also the presence of this everyday variation that essentially invalidates the use of statistical techniques that are essential to research.

In summary, clinical trials are concerned with creating a stable population where outside variation is controlled to estimate a result (enumerative). Once a result is obtained, analytic statistics must be used to study the inference gap on this result in relation to the research conditions under which it was obtained. In addition, crucial to the understanding and subsequent application is the exposure and study of the manifestations of uncontrollable outside variations, hardly a stable infinite population because most of it cannot be anticipated.

# About the Author

Davis Balestracci Jr., MS, began his career as an internal industrial statistical consultant, most significantly with 3M, where he received several corporate awards for his innovative teaching and applications of statistical methods. After being exposed to W. Edwards Deming's philosophy in 1983, his interests evolved to a broader application of statistics and cultural psychology to develop leadership capabilities to transform organizations. Since 1992 his primary involvement has been with healthcare.

Davis holds a bachelor of science degree in chemical engineering and a master of science degree in statistics yet describes himself as a "right-brained" statistician. (He is a pipe organist and has also done graduate work in orchestral and choral conducting.)

He is well known for his provocative, challenging, yet humorous and down-to-earth public speaking style. He is a regular speaker at Institute for Healthcare Improvement forums in the United States and Europe. People attending his presentations appreciate his acute awareness of the daily realities of implementing statistical approaches to quality and cultural transformation, including the inherent frustrations of dealing with "those darn humans."

In 1995 at the invitation of Dr. Donald Berwick, Davis participated in a project sponsored by the Harvard Institute for International Development. He was part of a team that taught healthcare improvement methods to 80 participants from Egypt, Israel, Palestine, Morocco, and Jordan.

In 2001 he became an independent consultant, naming his company Harmony Consulting, LLC, to reflect his unique synthesis of left-brain (analytical) and right-brain (psychological) approaches to quality as well as "the passion of Beethoven composing symphonies" with which he approaches his work. (When visiting the consulting firm's Website, www.davisdatasanity.com, select the "brain" in the left margin to view a demonstration of this concept.)

In addition to his domestic work in the United States (36 states), he has consulted and given seminars in Israel, Palestine, Vietnam, Norway, Denmark, New Zealand, and Australia. From 2003–2007, he developed a special relationship with the national health services of England and Wales doing extensive statistical education as a major part of government-sponsored improvement initiatives.

Davis was the chair of the Statistics Division of the American Society for Quality in 2003–2004 and since January 2004 has regularly shared his unique approach writing regularly for *Quality Digest* (www.qualitydigest.com).

# Index

Note: *ex.* indicates exhibit

## A

Above average and below average, 54
    analysis of means (ANOM), 55, 56*ex.*
    bar graph comparison of coin flip performances, 54–55, 54*ex.*
    bar graph comparison of coin flip performances, with quartile lines, 54–55, 55*ex.*
    bar graph comparison of coin flip performances, with standard deviation lines, 54–55, 56*ex.*
    SWAGs (statistical wild a** guesses), 55, 249–251
    WAGs (wild a** guesses), 55, 249
Accident data example, 33–35
    ANOM comparison, 292, 293*ex.*, 294*ex.*
    ANOVA table, 292*ex.*
    Bartlett's test, 288–290, 291*ex.*
    common cause variation, 24*ex.*, 34–35, 214–215
    control charts and analysis, 214–215, 215*ex.*
    data analysis, 187–190, 188*ex.*, 190*ex.*
    and data collection strategies 1–3, 145–147
    Levene's test, 288–290, 291*ex.*
    Pareto diagrams, 312, 312*ex.*
    Pareto matrix, 145–146, 146*ex.*
    run charts and analysis, 33–34, 34*ex.*, 146–147, 146*ex.*, 188–189, 189*ex.*, 191*ex.*, 289*ex.*
    S-charts and analysis, 288–294, 290*ex.*
    special cause rules, 216–219, 216*ex.*
    special cause strategy error, 33, 188–190
    stratification, 35
    trend analysis, 33, 34*ex.*, 190
    two-out-of-three rule, 217, 217*ex.*, 218*ex.*
    year-over-year plot, 189*ex.*
Adverse drug event example, 326–331
    C-chart and analysis, 326–327, 328*ex.*, 329*ex.*, 330*ex.*
    data, 327*ex.*
    data after educational intervention, 329*ex.*
    Pareto matrix, 330
    run chart and analysis, 326, 328*ex.*, 330*ex.*
Analysis of means (ANOM), 245
    accident data example, 292, 293*ex.*, 294*ex.*
    to analyze rates and percentages, 247–248
    analyzing rare events, 261–262
    antibiotic managed care protocol example, 251, 253–256
    applied to patient satisfaction comparisons, 58–61
    coin flip example, 56*ex.*, 57
    comparing 20 group practices, 57*ex.*
    in comparison of percentage performances, 57, 60*ex.*, 61*ex.*
    for continuous data, 265–268
    county healthcare case study, 63, 63*ex.*, 284–286, 285*ex.*, 286–288

C-section scenario, 263–264,
    263*ex.*, 264*ex.*
ER lytic data example, 337–338,
    337*ex.*, 338*ex.*
ER unpredictable admit case study,
    270–281, 272*ex.*, 273*ex.*, 276*ex.*,
    277*ex.*, 278*ex.*
patient satisfaction data, 58–61,
    60*ex.*, 61*ex.*
p-charts, 251, 253–256
regional target model example, 266–267
vs. research, 246–247
u-charts, 248–249, 249*ex.*
versatility of, 281–282
Analysis of variance (ANOVA)
    accident data example, 291–292, 292*ex.*
    cardiac mortality example, 170, 171*ex.*
    county healthcare case study, 283–286,
    284*ex.*
Analytic statistics, 4
    vs. enumerative statistics, 174, 176, 390
    objectives and methods, 176–177
    sources of uncertainty, 176
    *See also* Process-oriented statistics
Antibiotic managed care protocol example,
    249–251, 250*ex.*
    ANOM calculation, 251, 253–256
    correct protocol analysis, 254*ex.*
    incorrect protocol analysis, 251*ex.*
Autry, James, 88, 94
Average moving range, 211–212

**B**

Bacteremia example, 40
    bar graph analysis, 42*ex.*, 230*ex.*
    c-chart and analysis, 232–233, 233*ex.*
    control chart, 232*ex.*
    moving and median moving range, 232*ex.*
    run chart and analysis, 40, 42*ex.*, 231*ex.*
    trend analysis, 230*ex.*
Bar graphs
    above and below average, 54–55, 54*ex.*,
    55*ex.*, 56*ex.*
    bacteremia example, 42*ex.*, 230*ex.*
    computer uptime example, 41*ex.*
    county healthcare case study, 62*ex.*
    C-section scenario, 222*ex.*, 263*ex.*
    guideline compliance scenario, 25, 26*ex.*
    infection rate example, 43*ex.*
    inferior to run charts, 40–42, 41*ex.*, 42*ex.*
    patient satisfaction data, 58*ex.*
    standard deviation, 54–55, 56*ex.*

Bartlett's test, 288–290, 291*ex.*
Belief systems
    10 commandments, 382–383
    for change agents, 382
    and changing adult behavior, 344–345
    changing self-defeating, 78
    "conscious business," 116
    and cultural handcuffs, 89, 121
    cultural mantras for reinforcement,
    125*ex.*, 126
    driven by behaviors, 87–88
    effects on behavior, 74–76, 345
    and feedback, 84–86
    leadership educational moments,
    122–124
    model for behavioral change, 76–78,
    98, 344
    and organizational culture, 76–78
    paradoxical commandments, 383
    and resistance to change, 79–83, 308
    transition red flags, 122
    "unconscious business," 116
    using a cultural audit to effect change,
    89–92, 90*ex.*, 91*ex.*, 92*ex.*
Benchmarking, 17–18, 54
Berwick, Donald, xx, xxii, xxiv–xxv, 3, 4, 130
Binomial distribution, 250
Block, Peter, 70, 110, 114–115
Box-and-whisker plots, 287–288, 287*ex.*
Brown, Mark Graham, xxi, 158
Budget example, 47–50
    scatterplot, 48*ex.*
    variance to budget control chart, 48, 49*ex.*
    variance to budget run charts, 48, 49*ex.*
Budgeting, as a process, 47–50
Bypass survival rate example
    p-chart and analysis, 256–257, 256*ex.*
    run chart, 258*ex.*
    special cause test, 257
    2 × 2 table, 258–260, 258*ex.*, 259*ex.*

**C**

"Can Chance Make You a Killer?," 61
Cardiac arrests example, 38–40
    plotting the dots, 38, 39*ex.*, 40
    run chart and analysis, 38–39, 39*ex.*
    2 × 2 table, 260*ex.*
Cardiac mortality example
    analytic statistics, 170–171, 170*ex.*, 171*ex.*
    comparative histogram, 170*ex.*
    run charts and analysis, 172, 173*ex.*, 174
    special cause variation, 178

useless statistical analysis, 170–171, 170*ex.*
Causal analysis. *See* Root cause analysis
C-charts, 232–233
    adverse drug event example, 326–327, 328*ex.*, 329*ex.*, 330*ex.*
    bacteremia example, 233*ex.*
    ER unpredictable admit case study, 274*ex.*
    *See also* Control charts
Change agents, 78, 82–84, 93, 96, 300, 381–383
    *See also* Leadership
Charts, 164–165
    *See also* C-charts; Control charts; I-charts; P-charts; Run charts; U-charts
Clemmer, Jim, xx, 6, 12, 71
Clinical trials, 389–391
Cochran, Craig, 366
Code 13 example, 88–89
Cognitive therapy, 74, 76–78
Coin flip example, 56*ex.*, 57, 178–179, 178*ex.*, 179*ex.*
Common cause, 9, 21, 355, 359
    calculating limits, 29, 33, 66–67
    calculating standard deviation, 214
    coin flip example, 178–179, 178*ex.*, 179*ex.*
    computer uptime example, 200–201
    hiding special causes, 36, 183, 204, 205*ex.*
    inherent, 182–183
    medical information calls example, 186–187
    recognizing sources of variation, 202–204
    representation of limits, 212
    and sequence of three error, 32
    as a source of process errors, 13
    strategy of the Pareto matrix, 25, 36–38
    in a time perspective, 182
Commute time example, 182
Complaints example, 45–47
    control chart and analysis, 46, 47*ex.*
    eight in a row rule, 45, 46*ex.*
    run charts and analysis, 45, 46*ex.*
    treating common cause as special cause, 46
Complexity, 355
Computer uptime example, 40, 195–196
    bar graph analysis, 41*ex.*
    calculating common cause limits, 200–201
    calculating moving range, 198, 199*ex.*, 200*ex.*
    control chart and analysis, 201–202, 201*ex.*
    data measurement, 196*ex.*, 197*ex.*
    run chart and analysis, 41*ex.*, 196, 197*ex.*
"Continuous Improvement as an Ideal in Health Care," 4
Continuous quality improvement (CQI), xix, 298–299
Control charts, 21, 225–227
    accident data example, 214–215, 215*ex.*
    bacteremia example, 232*ex.*
    and common cause, 202–204, 203*ex.*, 212
    computer uptime example, 201*ex.*
    C-section scenario, 221–222, 223*ex.*, 228–229, 229*ex.*
    departmental procedures example, 202–203, 203*ex.*
    ER lytic data example, 337–338, 337*ex.*, 338*ex.*
    ER unpredictable admit case study, 276*ex.*, 277*ex.*, 280*ex.*, 281*ex.*
    FSH test ordering example, 195*ex.*
    medical information calls example, 184, 186*ex.*
    nosocomial infection example, 235–236, 236*ex.*
    patient survey example, 208–209, 210*ex.*, 211*ex.*
    patient transfer time example, 332, 333*ex.*
    regional target model example, 266–268, 267*ex.*
    and standard deviation, 218–219, 224
    unexpected deaths example, 238*ex.*, 239*ex.*
Conway, James, 6
County healthcare case study, 61–64
    ANOM and three standard deviations, 286–288
    ANOM comparison by county, 63, 63*ex.*
    ANOM for 21-county rank scores, 285*ex.*
    ANOVA for rank data, 284*ex.*
    bar graph of sums, 62*ex.*
    box-and-whisker plot, 287*ex.*
    five-number summary, 287*ex.*
    Friedman test, 283–286
    individual ranking data, 283*ex.*
    rank sum data, 62*ex.*
Crosby, Philip, 12
C-section scenario, 220–221
    bar graphs, 222*ex.*, 263*ex.*

control charts and analysis, 221–222, 223*ex.*, 228–229, 229*ex.*
p-chart ANOM by physician, 263–264, 264*ex.*
performance of 35-month baseline ANOM, 263*ex.*
run charts and analysis, 224, 228–229, 228*ex.*, 265, 265*ex.*
summary statistics, 222*ex.*
2 × 2 table, 265*ex.*
Cultural handcuffs, 89, 121
*Customer Focused Quality*, 364
Customers
keys to questioning, 368
tools for understanding needs, 365*ex.*
why they lie, 368–369
*See also* Feedback; Surveys

**D**

Dana-Farber Cancer Institute, chemotherapy overdose, 6–8
Data, 21
aggressiveness, 148, 149*ex.*
analysis process, 152
avoiding inappropriate use of anecdotal, 138*ex.*, 157
collection process, 151–152
conflicting mental models about, 155, 155*ex.*
everyday strategies for using, 164–165
four processes, 149–151, 150*ex.*
guideline compliance analysis, 25, 26, 26*ex.*
guideline compliance scenario, 25–26, 27*ex.*
guideline compliance sorting, 28–30, 29*ex.*, 30*ex.*
interpretation process, 152–153
inventory considerations, 162*ex.*
limits, 239–240
measurement process, 151, 154–155, 158, 159*ex.*–161*ex.*
necessary for understanding processes, 22–23
presentations, 23, 24*ex.*, 180
proper use of, xxi, 157–158
questions for evaluating, 171, 239–240
and statistical traps, 22
tampering, 23, 24, 175
Data collection, 141–142, 311
as a data process, 151–152
eight questions for effective, 153–154

evaluating overall measurement system, 158, 159*ex.*–161*ex.*
as a process problem, 13, 132
process-specific, 139
in a service culture, 183–184
Strategy 1: Exhaust existing in-house data, 142–143, 149*ex.*
Strategy 2: Study the current process, 143–144, 149*ex.*
Strategy 3: Cut new windows, 144–145, 149*ex.*
Strategy 4: Designed experimentation, 147–148, 149*ex.*
summary of, 165*ex.*
use of flowcharts, 137
Dauten, Dale, 93, 94
Deming, W. Edwards, xix, xxii, xxiv, 5, 12
and organizational transformation, 388
red bead experiment, 32
*The Deming Dimension*, xix
Demotivators, 107–108, 108*ex.*, 110, 116
Departmental procedures example
common cause strategies, 203
control chart and analysis, 202–203, 203*ex.*
run chart, 204*ex.*
stratified histogram, 204, 205*ex.*
Dew, John, xxiii
DMAIC (define, measure, analyze, improve, control), 17
Dot plots. *See* Histograms
Drug error example, 9
Dueck, Rodney, xxv, 85, 87

**E**

Education. *See* Training
Eight in a row rule, 27, 28*ex.*, 45, 46*ex.*, 192, 192*ex.*, 217–218
80/20 rule. *See* Pareto principle (80/20 rule)
85/15 rule, 5, 343, 354
Ellis, Albert, 74, 76–78
Empirical Rule, 294–295
Employees
and demotivators, 107–108, 108*ex.*, 110, 116
"Employee Manifesto," 114*ex.*–115*ex.*
reasons for resistance, 321–322
resistance to standardization, 308
seven elements for empowerment, 117
"SuperMotivation Survey," 112–113
teaching process language to, 137, 138*ex.*, 139

*See also* Leadership; Management; Organizational culture; Organizational transformation
Enumerative statistics, 4, 174, 176, 390
Envelope thickness example, 154–155, 154*ex.*, 181
ER lytic data example, 334–338
    ANOM comparison, 337–338, 337*ex.*, 338*ex.*
    control charts and analysis, 337–338, 337*ex.*, 338*ex.*
    data, 334*ex.*
    histogram and analysis, 335, 335*ex.*
    run charts and analysis, 335, 335*ex.*, 336*ex.*
    scatterplot, 336*ex.*
ER unpredictable admit case study
    admit data, 269*ex.*, 271*ex.*, 279*ex.*
    ANOM analysis, 270–281, 272*ex.*, 273*ex.*, 276*ex.*, 277*ex.*, 278*ex.*
    C-chart, 274*ex.*
    control charts, 276*ex.*, 277*ex.*, 280*ex.*, 281*ex.*
    histogram by day of week, 268–270, 270*ex.*
    histogram by time of evening, 268–270, 271*ex.*
    I-chart, 274*ex.*
    run charts and analysis, 272–273, 274*ex.*, 275*ex.*
*Escape Fire*, xxii

## F

"Faulty Systems, Not Faulty People," 7–8
Feedback, xxiii, 72–74, 116
    360-degree process, 84–86
    customer surveys, 363–364, 366
    integrating more proactive, 122, 123*ex.*
    *See also* Surveys
*Firing on All Cylinders*, 6, 12
Fishbone diagrams. *See* Ishikawa diagrams
Fishers exact test, 261–262
Five C's, 3–4
Flowcharts, 134–135, 311
    as aids in understanding variation, 137
    deployment, 135–136, 136*ex.*
    detailed, 135
    and too much detail, 137
    top-down, 135
    universal process flowchart, 3, 3*ex.*, 71
Four C's, 1, 17, 359
Four-out-of-five rule, 217
*Fourth Generation Management*, 12, 352
Friedman test, 62, 283–286
FSH test ordering example, 192–193
    control chart and analysis, 193, 195*ex.*
    holding the gains, 193–195
    run charts and analysis, 193, 194*ex.*

## G

Glasser, William, 74
Goals, arbitrary numerical, 202, 242
Guideline compliance scenario
    bar graph analysis, 25, 26*ex.*
    basic scenario, 25–26
    compliance data, 28, 29*ex.*
    determining median, 28, 30*ex.*
    project history, 26, 27*ex.*
    run chart and analysis, 29, 30*ex.*
    trend analysis, 26, 26*ex.*

## H

Hacquebord, Heero, xxiv, 157, 364
*Hardwiring Excellence*, 103, 116, 366
Healthcare
    changes needed in, xxii
    examples of waste in, 14
Histograms, 311, 316–317
    departmental procedures example, 204, 205*ex.*
    ER lytic data example, 335, 335*ex.*
    ER unpredictable admit case study, 268–270, 270*ex.*, 271*ex.*
    examples of stratified, 319*ex.*
    regional target model example, 266, 267*ex.*, 268*ex.*
Hospital wait time example, 43–45
    calculating common cause limits, 66–67
    control chart, 68*ex.*
    plotting the dots, 44, 44*ex.*
    run chart and analysis, 44, 44*ex.*
    traffic light report, 31*ex.*
    treating common cause as special cause, 43–44

## I

I-charts, 184, 201, 232–233
    ER unpredictable admit case study, 274*ex.*
    importance of moving range, 198
    instructions for analysis, 213*ex.*
    patient survey example, 211, 211*ex.*
    vs. p-charts, 257
    performance review example, 206*ex.*
    *See also* Control charts
Incidents, 232
Infection rate example, 40

bar graph analysis, 43*ex.*
run chart and analysis, 40, 43*ex.*
Inference gap, 176, 390
Institute for Healthcare Improvement (IHI)
100K Lives Campaign, xxi
and quality improvement, 2
Ishikawa diagrams, 311, 314
"ask 'why?' five times" analysis, 315*ex.*
cause-and-effect diagram, 315*ex.*

**J**
Joiner, Brian, xxi, 12
on special cause reactions, 298
Juran, Joseph, 4, 5, 12, 79, 140*ex.*, 302
and organizational transformation, 388–389
on project journeys, 299–300
Rules of the Road, 321–324

**K**
Kerridge, David, 3, 17
Kotter, John, 102

**L**
Lab test turnaround time example, 144–145
Lao-Tzu, 17
Leadership
10 percent jerk time factor, 93–94
and accountability, 94–96, 106*ex.*, 120–121
changing me to change them, 119*ex.*
and creating an empowered culture, 96, 101–102
creating awareness for, 349
creating educational moments, 122–124
creating leadership and organizational accountability toward clear results, 119*ex.*
cultural mantras, 125*ex.*, 126
dangerous beliefs of, 86
eight errors to avoid, 102–103
facilitation/dialogue process, 82*ex.*
four levels of dysfunction, 87
integrating more proactive feedback, 122, 123*ex.*
key questions for QI, 117–118
major steps to transformation, 16*ex.*, 349–351
vs. management, 103
manifesto for leaders, 105*ex.*
mantras for effecting change, 70
mood map, 106*ex.*
need for clear results, 83–84

"The 100 Percent Responsibility Exercise," 119–120, 120*ex.*
"paperboy wisdom" mantra, 93–94
resistance to change, consequences of, 81
resistance to change, understanding, 79–83
role in QI, 19
seven elements for empowerment, 117
steps for taking charge of change, 124, 126
team role, 118–119
what can be done, 97*ex.*, 98–99
"What Should I Keep Doing, Stop Doing, and Start Doing?" analysis, 118–119, 120*ex.*
*Leading Change*, 102
Lean, xix, 13–14, 17, 72
Lean Six Sigma, xix
Leape, Lucian, 6–8
Least significant difference, 284–285
Lehman, Betsy, 6–8
Levene's test, 288–290, 291*ex.*
Limits, 239–240
*Love and Profit*, 88

**M**
Management
"Are You Trying to Make Your Organization or Team into Something You're Not?" checklist, 109
"Change Checkpoints and Improvement Milestones," 111
"Employee Manifesto," 114*ex.*–115*ex.*
four primary practices, 103
four secondary practices, 103
implementing QI, 15, 16*ex.*
vs. leadership, 103
levels of commitment to QI, 104–105
obtaining customer feedback, 366
"Outstanding Teams Checklist," 110
principles for successful QI, 15
skills required for improvement and transformation, 65*ex.*, 66
Studer's nine principles, 103–104, 104*ex.*
"SuperMotivation Survey," 112–113
*Managerial Breakthrough*, 79
May, Matthew E., 301
Mayfield, Stephen, 71
Median, 188–189, 190*ex.*
Median moving range, 66, 198, 200*ex.*
vs. average moving range, 211–212
bacteremia example, 232*ex.*

medication error data example, 219–220, 221ex.
    patient survey example, 210ex.
    patient transfer time example, 332
Medical information calls example, 184, 186–187
    common cause variation, 186–187
    control chart and analysis, 184, 186ex.
    data measurement, 184
    data summary, 185ex.
    stratification data, 185ex.
Medication error data example, 35–36, 219–220
    common cause strategy, 35–36
    control chart, correct, 221ex.
    control chart, incorrect, 219, 220ex.
    moving ranges, 220ex.
    run chart and analysis, 35ex., 219
    special causes hidden in common cause variation, 36
Middleton, Robert, 342
Miller, John, 95
Moving range, 66, 67ex., 198
    bacteremia example, 232ex.
    calculating, 199ex.
    medication error data example, 219, 220ex.
    patient survey example, 210ex.
    patient transfer time example, 332

## N

Neave, Henry, xix
Never events, 11
Nolan, Tom, 236
Normal distribution, 294–295
Nosocomial infection example
    control chart and analysis, 235–236, 236ex.
    occurrence chart, 234ex.
    run chart and analysis, 235, 235ex.

## O

Operational definitions, 151, 155–157
Organizational change. *See* Organizational transformation
Organizational culture
    and accountability, 94–96, 106ex.
    and belief systems, 76–78
    "conscious business" belief systems, 116
    creating an empowered, 96, 101–102
    cultural audit, 89–92, 90ex., 91ex., 92ex.
    and cultural handcuffs, 89, 121
    and Ellis's model for results, 76–78
    employee resistance to standardization, 308
    four levels of dysfunction, 87
    integration of improvement into, xx–xxi
    Juran's Rules of the Road for change, 321–324
    need for clear results, 83–84
    and need for feedback, 72–74
    no secrets in, 88
    and project traps, 309
    and the pyramid model of quality, 86–87
    and resistance to change, 79–83, 320–321
    seven elements for empowerment, 117
    and standardization, 325
    and toxic effects of 360-degree feedback, 84–86
    and trust, 92–93, 93ex.
    "unconscious business" belief systems, 116
    *See also* Leadership
Organizational transformation
    code 13 example, 88–89
    Deming's four elements of, 388
    facilitation/dialogue process, 82ex.
    Juran's Rules of the Road, 321–324
    laws of, 17
    major steps to, 16ex., 349–351
    need for clear results, 83–84
    phases of change process, 98, 344
    vs. quality improvement, 347ex.
    roadblocks to, 121
    social consequences of change, 79
    steps for leaders, 124, 126
    transition red flags, 121–122
    via remedial journey, 300, 319–320, 321ex.
    *See also* Leadership
Organizations
    effects of belief systems on behavior, 74–76
    evaluating overall measurement system, 158, 159ex.–161ex.
    four needs of, 86
    and goal of continuous QI, 345–347
    introducing change, 69–70
    summary of skills to be routine, 348ex.
    symptoms of "corporate craziness," 71, 71ex.
Ott, Ellis, 247

## P

"Paperboy wisdom" mantra, 93–94
The Paradoxical Commandments, 383
PARC, 162–163
Pareto principle (80/20 rule), 1, 5, 139,
    140*ex.*, 311, 354
    accident data example, 312, 312*ex.*
    analysis contrasting frequency vs.
        cost, 314*ex.*
    diagram of patient complaints from
        comment cards, 313*ex.*
    diagram of reasons for delays in
        discharge, 313*ex.*
    importance of identifying, 306
    as language of statistical thinking, 24–25
    matrix, 36–38, 37*ex.*
Patient satisfaction data
    ANOM comparison charts and analysis,
        58–61, 60*ex.*, 61*ex.*
    stacked bar graph for survey result, 58*ex.*
    System 19 chart, 59*ex.*
Patient survey example, 207–209, 211
    control chart and analysis, 208–209,
        210*ex.*, 211*ex.*
    data results and statistics, 208*ex.*
    I-chart, 211, 211*ex.*
    moving and median moving range,
        210*ex.*
    run chart and analysis, 208, 209*ex.*
Patient transfer time example, 331–334
    control chart and analysis, 332, 333*ex.*
    data, 331*ex.*
    moving and median moving range, 332
    run chart and analysis, 331–332, 332*ex.*
P-charts, 251, 253–256
    bypass survival rate example, 256–257,
        256*ex.*
    C-section scenario, 263–264, 264*ex.*
    vs. I-charts, 257
    *See also* Analysis of means (ANOM)
Percentages, common traps, 207
Performance review example, 205, 207
    data tables, 205, 206*ex.*
    I-chart, 206*ex.*
    run chart, 206*ex.*
Physicians
    core knowledge for, 352
    and QA mindset, 385–388
    and QI training, 351
Plan-do-check-act (PDCA), 306, 307*ex.*, 308
Plan-do-study-act (PDSA), x, xv, 139,
    177, 306
    rapid-cycle, 310–311, 311*ex.*
Plotting the dots, 28–29, 174–176,
    240–241, 282
    *See also* Common cause; Scatterplots;
        Special cause
Process analysis
    and breakdowns and delays, 133
    and complexity, 133–134
    flowcharts, 134–137, 136*ex.*
    and inefficiencies, 133
    and mistakes and defects, 133
    and problem solving, 132–133
    and variation, 133
Process behavior chart, 184
    *See also* Control charts
Processes, 1
    all work as, xxii, 5–6, 8–10, 129
    and arbitrary numerical goals, 202, 242
    behavioral, 74
    breakdowns in, 4, 6, 71
    budgeting, 47–50
    data analysis, 152
    data collection, 151–152
    data interpretation, 152–153
    data measurement, 151, 154–155, 158,
        159*ex.*–161*ex.*
    demotivators, 107–108, 108*ex.*, 110, 116
    and not people, 6–8, 298
    problem sources, 12–13, 14, 132, 354
    questions to ask about, 137, 138*ex.*, 139
    research and clinical trials, 389–391
    seven deadly sins of improvement, 299
    six sources of input, 9, 32, 149
    and standardization, 302–303, 306,
        307*ex.*, 325
    stratification via Pareto matrix, 36–38
    and suppliers, 298, 352, 354
    and time, 179–180, 181–182
    universal process flowchart, 3, 3*ex.*, 71
    use of data, 149, 150*ex.*
Process-oriented statistics, 4, 177–178
Process-oriented thinking, 1, 4–5, 6, 12,
    19, 359
    in the context of defining QI, 158
    and deep-level fixes, 242–243
    false barrier between clinical and
        administrative issues, 351–352
    five-stage plan for improvement, 303*ex.*
    Joiner seven-step method for
        improvement, 304*ex.*–305*ex.*,
        320*ex.*, 321*ex.*
    statistical perspective inherent to, 164

Projects
    diagnostic journey, 299–300, 300*ex.*
    evaluation criteria, 301
    five-stage plan for improvement, 303*ex.*
    Joiner seven-step method for improvement, 304*ex.*–305*ex.*, 320*ex.*, 321*ex.*
    and organizational transformation, 324
    and QI efforts, 353
    remedial journey, 299–300, 300*ex.*, 319–320, 321*ex.*
    seven deadly sins of process improvement, 299
    traps, 309
Pyramid model of quality
    base, 73*ex.*, 74–76
    "engine," 72, 73*ex.*
    "fuel," 72–74, 73*ex.*
    and organizational culture, 86–87

## Q

QI. *See* Quality improvement
"Qualicrats," xx
Quality, 385
    of execution, 354
    problems caused by differing operational definitions, 155–157
    skills needed for, 19–20
    of target values and features, 354
Quality assurance, 2–3, 245–246, 385–388, 386*ex.*, 388*ex.*
Quality improvement
    blaming processes, not people, 6–8, 298
    clinical trials vs., 389–390
    common mistakes in, xix
    and complexity, 355
    as a continuous goal, 345–347
    and 85/15 rule, 5, 10, 343, 354
    frustration caused by eight leadership errors, 102–103
    implementing, 15, 16*ex.*
    importance of customer needs, 107
    importance of statistical skills, 23–25
    incorporating statistical thinking, 65*ex.*, 107
    key concepts needed to create a universal improvement language, 353–359
    key questions, 117–118
    leadership roles, 19
    levels of executive commitment, 104–105
    manufacturing processes applied to service, 130
    motivating people, xxiii–xxiv
    and organizational transformation, 2–3, 17
    and Pareto principle, 5, 24–25, 139, 140*ex.*, 354
    principles for successful change, 15
    principles to create culture for improvement, 6
    and process, 1, 353
    process problems, 4, 12–13, 14, 354
    and process-oriented thinking, 4–5, 6, 353, 359
    pyramid model, 72–76, 73*ex.*
    vs. quality assurance, 2–3, 245–246, 385–388, 386*ex.*, 388*ex.*
    reaching critical mass, 350–351
    requirements, xxiv, 117–118
    scientific approach, 355
    and statistical analysis, 158, 162–163
    steps for taking charge of change, 124, 126
    theory, 297–298
    three key concepts, 2
    tools for, 311–319
    vs. transformation, 347*ex.*
*Quality Improvement: Practical Applications for Medical Group Practice*, 202, 298

## R

Ralston, Faith, 71, 71*ex.*, 119
Ranking, 33, 54, 245
    county healthcare case study, 61–64
Rare events, 234–235
    analyzing, 261–262
    nosocomial infection example, 235–236
    unexpected deaths example, 236–238
Red bead experiment, 32
Reengineering, xix
Regional target model example, 266–268
    ANOM analysis, 266–267
    control charts, 266–268, 267*ex.*
    data chart, 266*ex.*
    histograms, 266, 267*ex.*, 268*ex.*
Rolling averages, 50–53, 53*ex.*
Root cause analysis, 11, 232
    Dew's seven root causes, xxii–xxiii
    identified via diagnostic journey, 299–300
    use of flowcharts, 136
Run charts, 21, 26–27, 65, 226–227
    accident data example, 33–34, 34*ex.*, 146–147, 146*ex.*, 188–189, 189*ex.*, 191*ex.*, 289*ex.*

adverse drug event example, 326,
    328*ex.*, 330*ex.*
bacteremia example, 40, 42*ex.*, 231*ex.*
budget example, 48, 49*ex.*
cardiac arrests example, 38–39, 39*ex.*
cardiac mortality example, 172,
    173*ex.*, 174
coin flip example, 178, 178*ex.*, 179*ex.*
complaints example, 45, 46*ex.*
computer uptime example, 40, 41*ex.*,
    196, 197*ex.*
counting the length of runs, 190–192,
    191*ex.*
C-section scenario, 224, 228–229, 228*ex.*
departmental procedures example, 204*ex.*
ER lytic data example, 335, 335*ex.*, 336*ex.*
ER unpredictable admit case study,
    272–273, 274*ex.*, 275*ex.*
FSH test ordering example, 193, 194*ex.*
guideline compliance scenario, 30*ex.*, 39
hospital wait time example, 44, 44*ex.*
infection rate example, 40, 43*ex.*
invalidated by rolling averages, 50–53,
    53*ex.*
medication error data example, 35*ex.*
nosocomial infection example,
    235, 235*ex.*
number of procedures coded by day of
    the week, 204*ex.*
patient survey example, 208, 209*ex.*
patient transfer time example, 331–332,
    332*ex.*
performance review example, 206*ex.*
superior to bar graphs, 40–42,
    41*ex.*, 42*ex.*
"Run to Space," xxiv–xxv

## S

Scatterplots, 311, 315–316
    budget example, 48*ex.*
    charges vs. length of stay, 316*ex.*
    potential deceptiveness of linear
        regression, 316, 317*ex.*
    showing relationship but possibly
        needing quantification, 318*ex.*
S-charts, 288–294, 290*ex.*
Scholtes, Peter, 297, 346
Scientific approach, 355
Sentinel events. *See* Rare events
Sequence of six rule, 32
Sequence of three error, 32

Services
    measuring processes in, 130–131
    process inputs, 131–132
    process outputs, 131, 131*ex.*
Seven in a row test, 256*ex.*, 257
Shewhart, Walter, 212
Six Sigma, xix, xx, 12, 13, 17, 72, 203
Snee, Ron, xix
    common mistakes in training, 348
Special cause, 9–11, 21, 355, 359
    accident data example, 216–219, 216*ex.*
    coin flip example, 178–179
    eight in a row rule, 27, 28*ex.*, 192, 192*ex.*
    graphs of trend possibilities, 31*ex.*
    hidden in common cause, 36, 183,
        204, 205*ex.*
    indicated by run length, 191–192
    Nolan's rule, 236
    point inside upper limit, 216*ex.*
    point outside upper limit, 216*ex.*
    seven in a row test, 256*ex.*, 257
    in a time perspective, 182
    trend rule, 27, 27*ex.*, 28
    two-out-of-three rule, 217*ex.*
Spitzer, Dean, 108
Standard deviation, 217–219
    as balancing error risk, 212
    bar graph comparison of coin flip
        performances, with standard
        deviation lines, 54–55, 56*ex.*
    Bartlett's test, 288–290, 291*ex.*
    calculating common cause, 214
    Empirical Rule, 294–295
    Levene's test, 288–290, 291*ex.*
    myths, 224
    S-charts, 288–294, 290*ex.*
    and significance, 214
    two-out-of-three rule, 217, 217*ex.*, 218*ex.*
    why three, 252–253, 286–288
Standardization
    and organizational culture, 325
    as a process, 310, 325
    process for understanding at a local level,
        307*ex.*
    of processes, 302–303, 306
    training issues, 306, 308
Statistical analysis, 357*ex.*–358*ex.*
    eight common traps, 357*ex.*
    PARC, 162–163
    proper application to QI, 158, 162–163
Statistical thinking, 17

as a basis for statistical theory, 243
importance of in QI, 65*ex.*, 107
need for, 22
and organizational transformation,
    349–350
and Pareto principle, 24–25
skills needed for, 23, 163
*See also* Common cause; Special cause
Statistics
    and benchmarking, 18
    Friedman test analysis, 62, 283–286
    objectives and methods for analysis,
        176–177
    and process problems, 14
    proper application to QI, 158, 162–163
    purpose of, 152–153
    realities of, 22
    risks of not understanding, 23
    role of in QI, 387
    tampering, 23, 24, 175, 202
Step change, 32
Stratified histograms. *See* Histograms
Studentized range, 285
Studer, Quint, 103–104, 116, 126, 366
*SuperMotivation*, 108
Suppliers, internal and external, 298,
    352, 354
Surveys, 363–364, 366
    acting on feedback, 366–367
    close-ended questions, 372
    control chart of percentile ranking,
        375, 376*ex.*
    control chart of satisfaction scores,
        375, 375*ex.*
    and customer involvement, 377–378
    and customer satisfaction, 378
    design steps, 367–374
    face-to-face interviews, 371
    focus groups, 371–372
    four key answers, 377
    key informant interviews, 372
    open-ended questions, 366, 372
    pilot group process, 374
    sample size, 374
    Step 1: Determine the survey
        purpose, 367
    Step 2: Identify end users, 369
    Step 3: Identify information needs and
        logistics, 369–370
    Step 4: Determine resource
        requirements, 370
    Step 5: Determine who will conduct the
        survey, 370
    Step 6: Determine who has the needed
        information, 370–371
    Step 7: Select an appropriate survey type,
        371–372
    Step 8: Design the survey questions, 372
    Step 9: Choose the data analysis design
        and reporting format, 373
    Step 10: Clarify the sample size and
        selection, 373
    Step 11: Decide data-entry methods, 373
    Step 12: Pretest the survey, 373–374
    telephone, 371
    tools to aid in understanding customer
        needs, 364, 365*ex.*, 366
    types of questions, 372
    written, 371, 372
SWAGs (statistical wild a** guesses), 55,
    249–251
Systems
    all work as, xxii
    as group of related processes, 131, 353
    teams as a part of, 297–298

**T**

Tampering, 23, 24, 175, 202
*The TEAM Handbook*, 12, 17, 137, 298, 302,
    346
Teams, 355
    as part of larger systems, 297–298
    realities of, 309
    role of in QI strategy, 345–347
10 percent jerk time factor, 93–94
Time
    common vs. special cause, 182
    effect of on process, 179–180
    envelope thickness example, 181
    importance of studying, 181
    variation in, 181–182
Total quality management (TQM), xix
Toyota Production System, xix, 14
Traffic lights, 29, 31*ex.*
    case against, 43–45
Training, 341–342
    changing adult behavior, 344–345
    chief medical officers, 351
    common mistakes in, 348
    and 85/15 rule, 343
    physicians, 351
    problem with training the trainer,
        343–344

self-sufficiency an unrealistic goal of, 342–343
summary of skills to be routine in all organizations, 348*ex.*
transition phase, 345
Trend
    bacteremia example, 229–230, 230*ex.*
    four-out-of-five rule, 217
    graphs of special cause terms, 31*ex.*
    meaning, 32–33
    rule, 27, 27*ex.*, 28
    statistically defining, 27*ex.*
    two-out-of-three rule, 217, 217*ex.*, 218*ex.*
    *See also* Two point trends
Two point trends, 38–40, 39*ex.*, 180
Two sigma, 214
2 × 2 table, 258, 258*ex.*
    bypass survival rate example, 258–260, 259*ex.*
    cardiac arrests example, 260*ex.*
    C-section scenario, 265*ex.*
Two-out-of-three rule, 217, 217*ex.*, 218*ex.*

## U
U-charts, 248–249, 249*ex.*
Uncertainty, 176
*Understanding Variation*, 257
Unexpected deaths example, 236–237
    control charts, 238*ex.*, 239*ex.*
    data analysis, 237
    run charts, 238*ex.*
    tabulation of unit deaths, 237*ex.*
Universal process flowchart, 3, 3*ex.*, 71

## V
Vague, problems with as a strategy, xxi–xxii
Variation, 21
    appropriate reaction to, 241–242
    common cause, 9–11, 175, 202–204
    effect of time on, 179–180, 181–182
    envelope thickness example, 154–155, 154*ex.*
    fundamentals of, 356*ex.*
    importance of context, 33
    key ideas, 355, 359
    level 1 fix (incident), 9–10
    level 2 fix (process), 9
    level 3 fix (system), 9, 11
    nonquantifiable human, 12–13
    perceived, 23
    as a process problem, 150
    reducing, 1
    special cause, 9, 10, 175
    *See also* Common cause; Special cause
*Voices into Choices*, 366

## W
WAGs (wild a\*\* guesses), 55, 249
Walinsky, Adam, 341
Wheeler, Donald, 184, 257
"Why the *Vasa* Sank," xx

## X
X-MR chart, 184
    *See also* Control charts